# Blood, Guts and Gore

# Blood, Guts and Gore

## Assistant Surgeon John Gordon Smith in the Waterloo Campaign

Edited by Gareth Glover

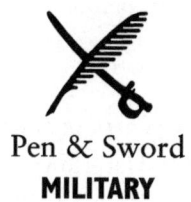

Pen & Sword
**MILITARY**

First published in Great Britain in 2022 by
Pen & Sword History
An imprint of
Pen & Sword Books Ltd
Yorkshire – Philadelphia

Copyright © Gareth Glover 2022

ISBN 978 1 39909 721 5

The right of Gareth Glover to be identified as Author of this work has been asserted by him in accordance with the Copyright, Designs and Patents Act 1988.

A CIP catalogue record for this book is
available from the British Library.

All rights reserved. No part of this book may be reproduced or transmitted in any form or by any means, electronic or mechanical including photocopying, recording or by any information storage and retrieval system, without permission from the Publisher in writing.

Typeset by Mac Style
Printed and bound in the UK by CPI Group (UK) Ltd,
Croydon, CR0 4YY.

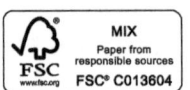

Pen & Sword Books Limited incorporates the imprints of Atlas, Archaeology, Aviation, Discovery, Family History, Fiction, History, Maritime, Military, Military Classics, Politics, Select, Transport, True Crime, Air World, Frontline Publishing, Leo Cooper, Remember When, Seaforth Publishing, The Praetorian Press, Wharncliffe Local History, Wharncliffe Transport, Wharncliffe True Crime and White Owl.

For a complete list of Pen & Sword titles please contact

**PEN & SWORD BOOKS LIMITED**
47 Church Street, Barnsley, South Yorkshire, S70 2AS, England
E-mail: enquiries@pen-and-sword.co.uk
Website: www.pen-and-sword.co.uk

Or

**PEN AND SWORD BOOKS**
1950 Lawrence Rd, Havertown, PA 19083, USA
E-mail: Uspen-and-sword@casematepublishers.com
Website: www.penandswordbooks.com

# Contents

*List of Plates*   vi
*Preface*   vii
*Acknowledgements*   ix
*Comments on the Present Version of John Smith's Work*   x

**Chapter 1**   Ordered to Belgium   1

**Chapter 2**   Marching to Join the Army   26

**Chapter 3**   Preparations for War   46

**Chapter 4**   War Clouds Gather   54

**Chapter 5**   Retreat   61

**Chapter 6**   The Day of Waterloo   67

**Chapter 7**   19 June   77

**Chapter 8**   Mont St Jean Farm   93

**Chapter 9**   March to Paris   108

**Chapter 10**   Paris in Peace   132

**Chapter 11**   Normandy   145

**Chapter 12**   Neufchatel-en-Bray   177

*Bibliography*   252
*Index*   253

# List of Plates

1. A Review at Hounslow Heath by Denis Dighton.
2. The Crown & Thistle, Abingdon-on-Thames.
3. The Cavalry Barracks at Canterbury.
4. Dutch schuyts.
5. A Surgeon and an Inspector of Hospitals.
6. Study of Sir Frederick Ponsonby by Thomas Heaphy.
7. Frederick Ponsonby's Waterloo Sword.
8. The 12th Light Dragoons by Denis Dighton.
9. Captain William Hay, 12th Light Dragoons, circa 1820.
10. A view of Quatre Bras on 19 June 1815 by Thomas Stoney, with corpses still littering the ground.
11. Farm of Quatre Bras just before it was shamefully destroyed.
12. Courbevoie Barracks.
13. The Waterloo Memorial to the 12th Light Dragoons. One of the first memorials to include the names of all ranks killed.
14. Surgeon's Regulation Case circa 1812.
15. Chateau Marais, Argenteuil.
16. Chateau Puteaux before its final destruction after a fire in 1881.
17. Chateau de Bacqueville.

# Preface

John Gordon Smith (1792–1833), professor of medical jurisprudence, was born in 1792 and educated at Edinburgh, graduating from the university in 1810 with the highest honours in medicine. He entered the army as a Hospital Mate on 25 April 1811, becoming the Assistant Surgeon of the 11th Light Dragoons on 11 March 1813 and then transferring as Assistant Surgeon to the 12th Light Dragoons on 28 October 1813, with which regiment he served at the Battle of Waterloo, when he received the thanks of Colonel Ponsonby for his services to the wounded. He then continued caring for the wounded at Mont St Jean farmhouse for some days, before catching up with the regiment on the road to Paris. He retired from the army on half-pay on 25 December 1818 and settled in London.

Here he found it difficult to establish himself in practice, as he held a Scottish degree only and was therefore not entitled to practise in England. He accepted the appointment of physician to the Duke of Sutherland and resided with him for four years, occupying his leisure in composing a work on forensic medicine. At the same time, he acted as surgeon to the Royal Westminster Ophthalmic Hospital. He also lectured on medical jurisprudence at the Royal Institution of Great Britain in 1825 and again in 1826 and also at the Mechanics' Institute. In 1829 he was elected the first professor of medical jurisprudence at the London University (now University College) in Gower Street. None of the licensing bodies in London required any evidence of instruction in forensic medicine and there was consequently no class. Smith lectured for two years and then resigned his office. Smith fought hard, but again unsuccessfully, to place Scottish and English degrees and licences in medicine upon an equal footing. For a time he edited the *London Medical Repository*. He unfortunately died in a debtor's prison, after 15 months' confinement, on 16 September 1833.

He published, besides various contributions to the *Edinburgh Medical and Surgical Journal*, *De Asthmati* (Edinburgh, 1810); *The Principles of Forensic Medicine* (London, 1821); *An Analysis of Medical Evidence* (London, 1825); *The Claims of Forensic Medicine* (1829); and *Hints for the Examination of Medical Witnesses* (1829). He then wrote his two-volume *The English Army at Waterloo and in France*, published in London in 1830, the text of which forms the basis of the present publication.

WorldCat.org, registers the existence of just twenty-two copies of this work worldwide, all of which are held in prestigious libraries, many connected to renowned universities. Copies in private hands are exceptionally rare and are virtually never seen for sale, therefore it is high time that a revised single-volume edition is published, allowing the general public to enjoy this work.

John Gordon Smith did not write of battles, for he saw little of the fighting, but his work is full of the pathos of the suffering of the wounded and dying in the aftermath of the carnage. Beyond the fascinating description of the medical care he and his colleagues were able to provide for those in need, he also offers an excellent 'behind the curtains' expose on life as an officer in King George's army in the campaign of 1815 and the three subsequent years they remained in France as the 'Army of Occupation'. In the original work, Smith hides the identities of all of those he talks about, only offering initials, which on investigation have been proven to be false, making identification extremely difficult. In almost all cases, however, following intensive investigation, the identities of most have been fully discovered. Unfortunately, as many of the records of the 12th Light Dragoons are not extant, little can be done to identify the other ranks whose names he had obscured, nor one major incident regarding an elopement and marriage which has proven particularly stubborn and it has been impossible to identify the main characters involved.

Beyond these minor issues, this book provides an invaluable description of life as a junior medic in a cavalry regiment in the 1815 campaign, covering many aspects of army life rarely, if ever, covered in most military memoirs. It is both a pleasure and a privilege to be able to bring John Smith's work to a wider audience.

# Acknowledgements

Any complicated work such as this requires the help and advice of many people to bring it to fruition and a number of people and organisations deserve my grateful thanks.

Firstly, I must thank my niece Shauna Williams, who resides in Ireland and kindly agreed to travel to the National Library of Ireland in Dublin to photograph the original work for me to transcribe; and to the staff at the library, who aided her greatly in facilitating this. I must also give my grateful thanks to Mary my wonderful wife, who kindly agreed to patiently type out the original text for me to work on.

I must also thank my editor Rupert Harding, who believed in this project when few saw its potential and resolutely saw it through to fruition.

I often rely on the good services of Ron McGuigan, who patiently searches to find answers to the most complex questions. I have never had the pleasure of meeting Ron, but I regard him as a good friend, who is always willing to help. On the very few occasions that even Ron is left unable to come up with an answer, I can be certain that the information simply does not exist. I must also thank my good friend Robert Burnham who is always happy to bat theories and ideas back and forth without openly calling me an idiot.

Finally, I must also thank Andrew Bamford, who has written two excellent books relating to the 12th Light Dragoons and who kindly and generously gave me copies of his notes made on the regiment during the 1815–18 period.

Gareth Glover, Cardiff 2021

# Comments on the Present Version of John Smith's Work

This version contains by far the greater proportion of the original two volumes, but not all. The original two volumes approximate to 160,000 words, which was deemed too long by the present publishers. The task of reducing the size of the work was greatly aided by the fact that the final 25,000 words or so of volume two consists of a novelette of a Georgian love story, which has no bearing on the memoirs of John Smith and has been removed in total. Elsewhere, Smith occasionally wanders off into long descriptions of places which are of no real use today, or he makes long footnotes which are more relevant to a Georgian reader than to modern eyes. These have been reduced greatly in size, although a smattering of this material has been retained to maintain continuity. The original chapters have not been retained, but a new simpler and more relevant chapter system has been introduced. The overall effect is to reduce the overall size to one that is far more manageable but has not lost its original flavour in any way.

Smith hides the names of all of the characters in his story, both presumably to maintain the anonymity of those he describes, but also undoubtedly to avoid the threat of litigation. Smith reduces the names of both people and places to initials; the identity of the places has been easily reconstructed via official letters and the memoirs of those who served in the regiment, but in the case of people it is patently obvious on checking the initials given, that the people mentioned are rarely given the correct initials, making identification much more difficult. To aid the reader I have consistently added the correct name, or correct spelling of towns in [ ] to help the flow of the book, hopefully making it a far less frustrating and confusing read. I have also avoided the temptation to add further information into the main text but have done this purely via the medium of footnotes, which I find far more satisfactory and much less disruptive to the reading experience than endnotes.

# Chapter 1

# Ordered to Belgium

I have been induced, at this distant period, to record transactions, which, however interesting at the time of their occurrence, or rotted long afterwards in the memory, have now, for a considerable time, been fading. My written journal has been lost; and pursuits, of a nature scarcely compatible with vivid recollections, have contributed, perhaps too successfully, to eradicate impressions, which I first received about fourteen, and was removed from nearly twelve years ago. Nevertheless, as I have the *misfortune* to be the keeper of a memory that rarely forgets anything, I will not affect to be unable, even at this distance of time, to reduce to *paragraphs* some of those reminiscences which have casually interested the social circle, and have, even to the surprise of the narrator, created a sensation, in which he himself barely participated.

The private history of important transactions, as well as of conspicuous personages, is always amusing and sometimes instructive. The economy of military men, when actively engaged, on occasions of deep interest, will always be productive of matter, attractive to those who sit at home and who learn but confused accounts of what may be going on. Things perfectly familiar to us, I have found incomprehensible to *others*; and I confess to have been amused with the *naivete* of queries put to soldiers by intelligent men, who never saw any military *apparel* beyond a review at Hounslow.[1] There is occasionally an awfulness, but more frequently an apparent insignificance, attached to the proceedings of a large army on active service, which are, both of them, highly interesting. I will not say, that when a Yorkshire man is placed in a hussar saddle, reduced to the clothes on his back and the provender slung over his shoulder, with the prospect of *cutting six*[2] at a native of Orleans [France], in ten minutes, that

---

1. Hounslow Heath was regularly used for Military Reviews attended by the Royal family with easy access from Windsor.
2. There were six approved different sword cuts in the exercise of cavalrymen.

2  Blood, Guts and Gore

he is exactly the *character* he would be upon the Doncaster racecourse;³ but I am sure he is the same *person*. For my own part, on some of the occasions I am about to describe, I should have thought any hovel in England enviable quarters.

The reader will not however, thank me for prolonging these preliminary observations. Passing over, therefore, for the present, several years, (during which I had been engaged, with as much advantage to myself as to the public service, in a *medical* capacity in the peninsula⁴), I shall introduce my narrative, as commencing with the early part of the eventful year, 1815. Many will recollect how the metropolis was at that period, the scene of popular tumult, on the occasion of certain measures projected by government, with regard to the regulation of the corn market. The present Lord Goderich,⁵ (then President of the Board of Trade) attracted a considerable share of odium; and his proceedings were not only censured by the nobility of London but animadverted upon by those who were at too great a distance for their execrations to reach his ear, or their stones to break his windows. On a dead wall, adjoining the capital of Berkshire,⁶ I was amused with an inscription *a la Hunt*, which pointed out the propriety of '*Robinson's ribs forming a gridiron to broil Castlereagh's heart on.*'

To this town and neighbourhood, my regiment (a cavalry one⁷) was, in consequence of these riots, ordered, by forced marches, to repair; and we remained there, in hourly expectation of proceeding to London.⁸ The Oxford Blues⁹ had left their usual and enviable quarters, for the duty (of

---

3. Doncaster racecourse is one of the oldest horse racing establishments in England, having races as early as the sixteenth century. It is famous for two major races, the Doncaster Cup and the St Leger Stakes.
4. He served in the Peninsula from 1811 to 1814, mostly at General Hospital locations.
5. The Honourable Frederick John Robinson was Vice President of the Board of Trade in 1815 and joint Paymaster of the Forces. His Corn Importation Bill successfully passed through Parliament in February 1815, a protectionist measure which imposed minimum prices on imported wheat and other grains, preventing them undercutting the price of home-produced grain. Robinson was granted a peerage in 1827, becoming Viscount Goderich. On the death of Canning in that August, King George IV asked him to form a government, but he was a failure, his premiership lasting only 144 days.
6. The county town of Berkshire was Abingdon-on-Thames until 1867.
7. He belonged to the 12th (or the Prince of Wales') Regiment of Light Dragoons.
8. On 25 March, the regiment was in the vicinity of Reading, four troops in Reading, two (Wallace and Webb's Troops) at Maidenhead and two (Sandys and Andrew's Troops) at Henley. The regiment numbered 502 rank & file and 441 horses.
9. The Royal Regiment of Horse Guards.

all others most unpleasant to English soldiers) of laying the strong hand upon their fellow citizens. John Bull had at the period in question, a very erroneous opinion of the character and feelings of his defenders. It was too much the custom even then for ignorant persons to abuse and for the intelligent to dislike them.

While anticipating the highly repugnant order to approach the turbulent metropolis, the newspapers one morning announced that Bonaparte had escaped from Elba! For a single day, we (*militaries*) were in common with the rest of our countrymen, abandoned to every degree of wonder and astonishment at this unexpected event. I recollect that the squadron-mess, to which I at that time belonged, met as usual in the principal inn of the town,[10] and talked this exploit over with as much indifference as might have been due to the escape of Sir F[rancis] Burdett from the Tower, or of Lord Cochrane from the King's Bench.[11] Next morning, however, things assumed a different aspect *quoad nos* [with regard to us]. Something like a warning for foreign service reached us and we learnt that the colonel,[12] 'A warrior (as will in due time be seen) for the working day', had arrived at headquarters. To me, who at that time knew this honourable and gallant character more by report than personal observation, such an event appeared to be in the ordinary course of affairs. I was, however, somewhat mistaken: for afterwards I knew my chief too well, to suppose that he would care about making himself visible when nothing was *to be done*. He arrived, however, and some of our outpost associates went to pay their duty to him.

On Saturday, 19 March (I think[13]) 1815, our detachment proceeded, not to quell a London mob (as the unexpected *retour de L'Empereur* [return of the Emperor] had done more for that purpose than the appearance of

---

10. The principal inn was the Crown and Thistle at Abingdon-on-Thames.
11. Sir Francis Burdett, a reformer, was found guilty of libelling the House of Commons in 1810 and troops were required to arrest him and take him to the Tower of London. When released in 1815 there was a great fear of a large demonstration which could potentially turn riotous, but Burdett chose to avoid the crowds and took a boat up the Thames and the crisis was averted. Lord Cochrane was a friend and supporter of Burdett, but Burdett kept him at arm's length after Cochrane had proposed some form of military action in his defence in 1810. Cochrane was in King's Bench, the prison for debtors, having been found guilty in 1814 of a major fraud on the Stock Exchange.
12. Lieutenant Colonel the Honourable Frederick Ponsonby 12th Light Dragoons, was actually a colonel in the army.
13. The Saturday was 18 March 1815. He seems to be one day out consistently in his dates.

the whole British army would perhaps have accomplished), but to embark for Belgium. Our march, which in its rapidity, seemed to betoken the spirit of the emergency, furnishes few incidents worthy of record. But as I do not pretend to quote adventures, my recollections being confined to the everyday and hourly occurrences of the interior of military life perhaps I may find readers if I indulge in a few descriptions of a comparatively humble nature.

Our first halt was at the miserable but well-known town of Hounslow,[14] where our temporary commanding officer[15] exhibited so little tact as to higgle [sic] about sixpence per head in the dinner charge the effects of which were rather severely visited upon the party. He was laughed at by the subalterns who witnessed the bargain but consoled himself with the idea that they were but 'boys', who little knew the care he was taking of them.

Before we assembled at the headquarters inn, Lieutenant [Goldsmid][16] and I took a stroll in Osterley Park,[17] and round the skirts of the town, in the course of which he led me to a spot whence several roads branched off, and there demonstrated the manner in which he had brought a London tailor to terms upon a former occasion. As well as I can recall the story, it was to the following purport:

On the arrival of the regiment, the year before, from the continent, one of the first places in which they became objects of notice to the London tradesmen was this same town of Hounslow. There, many of the officers appointed tailors, bootmakers, saddlers and others of that *genus*, to come to them, in order to clear off old scores and to commence new.[18] Among the good customers was a Captain C[oles],[19] but my present companion, the lieutenant, happened to have gone through the peninsular campaigns, without the cordial consent of some of the above-mentioned tribe. In the very same inn, where, on the present occasion, we had bargained for

---

14. Hounslow village was the first halt on the great coaching road from London to Bath. It was also the site of a large cavalry barracks, constructed during the Napoleonic Wars. It is highly likely that the regiment quartered there.
15. Major James Bridger commanded the regiment during its march to the coast.
16. Lieutenant Albert Goldsmid 12th Light Dragoons.
17. They walked in the grounds of the beautiful Georgian pile of Osterley House designed by Robert Adam, now a gem in the National Trust portfolio.
18. To pay off outstanding debts and to order new uniforms.
19. Captain William Cowper Coles 12th Light Dragoons.

a cheap dinner, the greedy tradesmen met their customers, and among them was a celebrated West-End tailor, who had no great regard for my friend the lieutenant, having (as he, the said tailor alleged) been rather cavalierly treated by him on former occasions. Our officer (whom, for brevity's sake, I shall call G[oldsmid]) happened to enter Captain C[ole]'s apartment and was by the latter informed that such and such a tailor had been there, and would return within a certain time, so that if G[oldsmid] wanted anything, he could take the opportunity to give his orders.

The effect of this information was an immediate exit through a window (the room being on the ground floor) which gave issue to the stable-yard, the saddling of his horse and a message for Dick E[Fulton[20]], a brother officer, to repair forthwith to Hounslow Heath where he would learn something of great importance. Out sallied my friend to a spot, where, with no little exultation, he informed me there was a clear start into four different counties and where he would have the tailor at his mercy, inasmuch as he could not have taken out a writ in *more than two*. Dick did not fail in the appointment. The lieutenant offered terms, Dick explained to the tailor how matters were, how G[oldsmid] was already *a cheval* on the heath and prepared for flight in any direction whatever. A promissory note was gladly accepted, the writ cancelled and the lieutenant marched into the west of England[21] with all the honours of peace, as well as of war.

Now to our dinner. I forget what we had to eat; but whatever it was, I am not inclined to think that we got much harm by it. The bargain about the sixpence secured us against any hazardous luxuries of the *cuisine*, and not only so, but ensured us the very worst bottle of wine mine host could find in his cellar. This we had sense enough to discover on tasting the first glass and we decidedly objected to proceeding one drop farther. The lieutenant ordered a change; we only changed from bad to worse. A second change was insisted upon and we had absolutely got in the landlord, blown him up and agreed to give eight shillings a bottle (for port!) before we should be fairly sacrificed to the honour of

---

20. Dick being a shorthand version of Richard, Lieutenant Richard Fulton was the only officer named Richard in the regiment and he was of equal rank to Goldsmid.
21. The regiment had been stationed at Dorchester before being ordered towards London. William Hay described Dorchester: 'it was the most horrid, dull, stupid inland town I had ever known.'

the odd sixpence. For my own part, finding the wine unswallowable, I retreated at an early hour, but others of the party remained, in the sure and certain hope of bettering their condition, by raising the price of their indulgence. Next morning some were left seriously ill in bed and the exhibition made by others told very expressively, what may be done by the saving of sixpences.

Our route lay across Kew Bridge; and just at the east end of Brentford, we met a gentleman driving a curricle,[22] to which was harnessed a pair of rather spirited horses.[23] The animals were not a little agitated at the sight and clatter of the cavalry, and there would have been *a charge*, without doubt, had not the driver reined up to let us pass. Our commandant, who was remarkably near sighted, was on the point of giving the gentleman some very unceremonious advice, when we had the good fortune to recognise his late Royal Highness the Duke of Kent.[24] The only subaltern who had been able to march with us, was immediately ordered to the rear, to ascertain that the troops were in a proper state of regularity, before the Royal Duke should have an opportunity of seeing them. In doing so, the wine that had been forced down his throat the evening before, began to take effect, just as the Royal Field Marshal had an opportunity of witnessing it. Whether he saw the accident or not, we never heard. The young gentleman is now a field officer, and a great ornament to his majesty's service.

On we went for Bromley, which was to be our resting place for the night; but, somewhere about Clapham Common, we lost our way and what was rather singular, could find no one capable of directing us.[25] At length we trotted past Deptford, in which neighbourhood was residing a young lady, to whom at the time, I *believed myself* to be very much attached and for whom I absolutely had at the moment a poetical epistle in my valise. When I set out in the morning, I did not know which way we were to go and it was not till we arrived near the place

---

22. A curricle was a light two-wheeled chaise large enough for a driver and only one other.
23. Note by Smith – About eight in the morning, HRH was going from town.
24. Edward Augustus Duke of Kent, was the fourth son of King George III. He was made a Field Marshal in 1805.
25. Note by Smith – Though none of those we met could tell us the way to Bromley, the stage coachman and passengers exhorted us to bring *Boney* over as soon as we could catch him. There was *something* in the advice, of which no one at the time could tell the meaning.

that the notion of an interview occurred to me. I now, however, stated to the commanding officer (the saver of sixpences) that, as I was passing very near the residence of a particular friend, I wished to take leave. G[oldsmid] desired me to take what I liked, provided I took myself to Bromley by dinnertime. So I cantered off to beat up Miss [?]'s[26] quarters. 'Gone to church!' was the answer, (it was Sunday morning). I put up my charger and in the conspicuous uniform (a thing the damsel held to be an abomination) of the dragoons, paraded up and down till I had an opportunity of astonishing her with my appearance, 'Is it *possible*? What brought *you* here?' were the enquiries. 'A tolerably good horse', was the reply. 'Where are you going?', 'I really do not know, but I believe *abroad*. I have brought a letter for you, which I thought I might as well take the opportunity of delivering in person, as it may be some time before another occurs.' So we kept walking about and talking for an hour, at the end of which I was obliged to take my leave and I am very sure my fair friend was glad of my departure. She had been brought up with an unlucky idea; too prevalent at the time, that no man could be good for much who wore the *King's livery*.

At Bromley nothing remarkable occurred. I forget what sort of a dinner we had, but I remember that our little party was exceedingly merry. We were waited upon, not by a gentleman dressed like a professor in the University of London, but by 'neat-handed Phillises',[27] with whose general aspect and deportment we were much pleased. Coming off a duty march, we were not much inclined to dress for the ceremony; yet, as some alteration of garb is always attended to when practicable, we agreed not to change, but to turn our jackets inside out. When we met after this little metamorphosis, our appearance was so irresistibly droll, both in the eyes of ourselves and the handmaids, that we could hardly eat our meal on account of the incessant laughter proceeding from both parties. Calling the guests to order, reprimanding the servants (in the way in which both were attempted) only added to the hilarity. After dinner, the senior officer came from another inn, where he was billeted, to take his wine with us. Not being at all in the secret of our innovations upon the article of dress, his astonishment was so genuine and its expression

---

26. It is impossible to be certain of this lady's identity.
27. A term used by John Milton, indicating young ladies with small delicate hands.

so unaffectedly ludicrous, that one of the damsels absolutely lost her senses and went into fits of really convulsive laughter! In which we the more effectively joined as we had anticipated the surprise and our sides were stronger and fitter for the task than those of the poor females. Of course, we did not exhibit out of doors in this costume; nor had we any desire to leave a scene so merry as the interior of the house. The whole establishment planted themselves wherever they could, to get a peep at the gay fellows going to fight Bonaparte and wherever we moved there was a head to be seen, or a giggle to be heard. We went to our rooms amid roars of laughter at night; and when we came down next morning, with things on as they should be, the recollection of the preceding day was still too much for decorum. We left the town of Bromley, perhaps the merriest party that ever entered it; and though within three months, the head of one of these cheerful individuals was laid low among the heroes of Waterloo, I am now (at the distance of fourteen years) almost unable to record the incident, in itself perhaps trifling enough, with any sort of gravity.

Our next halting-place was Rochester; where we arrived on the day appointed for the launch of a line-of-battleship from Chatham; if I remember rightly, she was 'the *Howe*.'[28] It was a sort of coincidence that the first of the troops, ordered to meet the disturber of the peace of Christendom, should have come to the place where a specimen of Britain's other force was to be exhibited, in a situation of efficiency, for the first time. I shall quote in the sequel; but I am the less disposed to omit this one, as our halt in Rochester produced nothing worthy of notice. We were billeted in different inns and on the following morning, I had the bad luck to pry into a little bit of scandal, in the most innocent and unintentional manner conceivable.

One of my brother officers had sneaked off from the mess at an unreasonably early hour the evening before, upon some frivolous pretext of duty or fatigue, which we had been rather the less inclined to question, as he was a married man, whose wife was somewhere on the line of march. At all events, we did the best we could without him and sought our own repose at the usual time. Before we moved off next day, I strolled to the inn where this gentleman was quartered, dressed precisely as *he*

---

28. The 120-gun HMS *Howe* was launched at Chatham on 28 March 1815.

was, though in person we were not much alike. I was standing in the gateway, with my face to the street, when a gentle tap was given to my shoulder and a soft voice uttered, 'I say!' This brought me round and oh! imagine if possible, with what expression of countenance the exclamation was made, 'Good gracious! I beg your pardon Sir, it isn't you.' [I replied] 'Yes, but it is though, *myself*, and *nobody else*.' I now complimented her (a not a very handsome, but rather a neat-looking chambermaid) gave her a wink of re-assurance and said that I would send the gentleman to her. I found him just about to mount his horse and told him that the chambermaid had given me a message for him. 'The devil she has! What is it?' [I replied] 'You shall hear as we ride on; but I think you ought to take leave.' 'Well, if you will ride with me, I will explain it all!' [to which he replied] 'My dear fellow, there is no occasion whatever; it is all explained already. You have the greatest knack,' he replied, 'at finding out every body's business of anyone I ever met with.' 'Well, but I don't think Mrs H[eydon][29] will call this your business when she comes to hear of it; and you know where are no secrets in regiments.' We did ride together, all the way to Sittingbourne; in the course of which, I was duly informed of the particulars and promised not to tell the wife. All that I can say of Sittingbourne is that we entered it on a Tuesday, found all sorts and descriptions of artillery pouring into it, and left it on Wednesday morning.

This was my first visit to the count of Kent, the kitchen garden, (as Surrey may be called the pleasure ground) of England.

From Sittingbourne we proceeded to Canterbury, a city which I approached with all the feelings and anticipations of a young man romantically inclined and habituated to look upon the relics of antiquity with something like poetic interest. Our party marched in upon the Wednesday; but the whole regiment (as it had proceeded in separate detachments) did not assemble there till Friday. Of the beauties of the ecclesiastical metropolis, however, I am not going to say a word: there are printed guides for visitors and I must confess that, under the circumstances in which I was placed, I either acquired very imperfect notions of the city and its curiosities, or other matters have since driven them from my

---

29. There were two officers in the regiment with a surname beginning with H, Lieutenant William Heydon, who had been a lieutenant for ten years already and would not gain a captaincy for another ten years yet and Lieutenant William Hay. Hay was certainly not married, leaving Heydon as the likely candidate.

recollection. I did not pass the three days alluded to in much of a poetical manner; so that it will be better for all parties if I proceed to discuss matters *a la militaire.*

On Friday, about noon, the last detachment marched in; and the whole regiment was assembled in a field near the barracks,[30] for an operation of a very important and interesting nature; in order to do justice to any allusion to which, it is necessary that I introduce a digression.

Our corps was the first, *of any description*, which, (on the news of Bonaparte's re-appearance in France) had been ordered for foreign service. It had returned from the Peninsula but a few months previously and was found, as soon as an inspection was made,[31] to be ready for active duty in any part of the world and we were the second corps that *actually got* to the continent, one other regiment having been upon the coast and ready to embark, when the mandate was received. When we reached Canterbury, we found a third cavalry regiment under similar orders; but we left them there, and several weeks elapsed before we had the pleasure of seeing them on the other side; and I recollect hearing that they had required all this period to accomplish what the [12th Light] Dragoons did in one afternoon. And what was this? *Re-Trooping* the regiment; a ceremonial which, for the benefit of country gentlemen, *yeomanry* and others, I shall endeavour to explain.

On foreign [home] service, a regiment of cavalry consists of ten troops, composed of about seventy mounted men and ten or fifteen dismounted, to supply casualties, furnish servants, &c &c. The whole are seldom if indeed ever sent abroad: two at least and sometimes even four, remaining at home, to form the depot, or source of supply both of men and horses, which the wear and tear of service may demand.[32] During the time of peace, the troops are reduced, both in number and strength, (there being no regiment of dragoons at present in England consisting of more than six troops and these not exceeding forty horses each). When our regiment was placed upon the peace establishment in 1814, it had been reduced to eight troops, which formed the strength of it at the time now referred to; but from these eight,[33] six were to be selected, composed of

---

30. The cavalry barracks built in 1794 were situated at Barton Mills just north of the city.
31. The regiment was inspected at Canterbury, by Major General Sir Dennis Pack.
32. On embarkation, the regiment left 16 sergeants, 5 trumpeters, 113 men and 46 horses behind to form the depot.
33. Note by Smith – The two other troops (making ten) were reformed, and the officers in the old *break*, were re-instated.

the most effective soldiers; and those six were to consist of seventy horses and eighty-five men each. In order to make this new arrangement, every man was *untrooped*,[34] personally inspected by the medical officers and replaced in some one particular troop, there to have his 'local habitation and his name', during the active period before him. A similar ordeal was instituted with respect to the horses and what may create surprise, there was a selection of women! The regiment had a proportion of wives, which amounted to a great inconvenience and four only per troop were permitted to accompany their husbands and to become, in consequence, entitled to rations and quarters. Some female followers are indispensably necessary, for purposes of washing and other services which cannot be conveniently obtained in foreign countries, more particularly when the army is in motion.

Now all this work, under the eye of one of the best officers to whom King George ever confided the command of his soldiers, was accomplished by six o'clock on Friday evening. At seven on the morning of the following day, the six newly arranged troops, forming three fine effective squadrons, proceeded to Ramsgate, where the whole concern, animate and inanimate; right, centre and left; horse, foot and *dragoons*,[35] were put on board the transports, in which they sailed, with a fair wind, to Ostend at an early hour on the morning of Sunday, April 1 [2nd].

I must return to Canterbury, in order to account for my embarkation at Ramsgate; a little paradox, which I hope the reader will not only forgive, but feel somewhat amused with the explanation of it.

As far as the *medical* duties of the trooping business were concerned, they had been performed by the surgeon[36] and myself, the other (senior)

---

34. Note by Smith – Untrooping may be compared to shuffling a pack of cards for a new deal. Every man is thrown into the confused mass, whence he is afterwards taken into regulated hands.
35. Note by Smith – There is a distinction between *horse*, or cavalry, and *dragoons*, which may as well be pointed out, though existing rather in words and deeds. Dragoons are troops capable of acting either *on foot or horseback*, whereas *horse* act only when mounted. Excepting the Household Brigade of Life Guards and Oxford Blues, all the mounted soldiers of the British army are styled dragoons, dragoon guards, heavy and light dragoons. These last are all dressed in blue, the former in red; and though *hussars* and *lancers* are now to be found in our army, they are officially known at the War Office only as *dragoons*, according to their number, 7th, 8th, 9th &c.
36. Surgeon Benjamin Robinson had joined the 12th Light Dragoons in October 1803 and served with them in the Peninsula from June 1811 until April 1814.

assistant,[37] of whom I shall have at least enough to say in the sequel, having taken himself off to London, when we moved from Berks[hire] and having never been seen or heard of since. What he found to do in London, no one could possibly imagine, as he had neither friends nor business there of any known description. We were not sorry for his absence, on the occasion in question, for Larry Murphy [Patrick Egan] had ways of performing, or of spoiling duty, altogether on his own and utterly at variance with those of every other person, civil or military. The only cause for vexation to myself was that, when the order arrived to proceed on foreign service, he had claimed the right of accompanying the regiment, as the opportunity was one which would secure his promotion, whereas by staying with the depot, (as either he or I was to do) he ran the risk of being passed over. As he was some two [one] years my senior, any attempt to overturn this arrangement would have been unreasonable, as well as fruitless. My worthy and kind friend, the surgeon, comforted me with the assurance that, from what he knew of Murphy [Egan], as well as from the opinion generally entertained about his value, there was every chance of his being left behind and that I had better make my arrangements for going. We were aware that Larry [Patrick] had not a horse, having sold his *charger* (a half-starved pony) the day before we left our quarters in the west of England. This might appear to be a very common-place event; but my brother chip [surgeon] forgot, when he put the animal up to auction on *Saturday*, that we had received the order to proceed towards London, by long and forced marches, on the *Monday*. The pony was no sooner knocked down, however, than he recollected this and exclaimed, even in the marketplace, 'Och, what will I do for a horse?' The beast fetched seven pounds nineteen shillings[38] and the purchaser, understanding the state of the case, *kindly* offered to let the recent owner have it again for about double the money; but Larry [Patrick] was perfectly frantic at so barefaced an imposition and swore he would rather walk all the way than be *chated* in such a manner. I believe he did ride a spare trooper and, as he wore no uniform and was never out of bed in time to proceed with the squadron, he had to raise an argument at every *too-bar*

---

37. Assistant Surgeon Patrick Egan was listed on detached service and was not present at Waterloo. Egan had originally been appointed Assistant Surgeon to the 23rd Light Dragoons in April 1809, serving with them at Talavera, before transferring to the 12th Light Dragoons in October 1812 and served in the Peninsula with them from January 1813 until April 1814.
38. About £400 in modern terms.

[toll booth] about passing without payment. Sometimes he was obliged to wait till a straggling soldier, or the baggage came up, in order to obtain a voucher that he was an officer of the regiment gone forward; at other places he was let through as an officer's servant, which the tollkeepers occasionally took the liberty of saying he resembled much more than an officer. At one gate, he recognised in the keeper an old soldier who had experienced his tender mercies in the peninsula.[39] The man totally unprepared for another visit from his doctor, wanted to be paid; 'What! You ungrateful scoundrel, do you pretend you don't know me? Have you forgot how I saved your life at Talavera?' 'Oh, Sir!' was the reply, 'go through and welcome, I did not look at you, or I should have recollected your extraordinary countenance at once: nobody can ever forget it, who has once seen it.'

Up to six o'clock on the Friday evening I remained in a disagreeable state of suspense as to the manner in which I was to be disposed of. My family as yet knew nothing of my movements. At this time, having 'borne the burden and heat of the day', I accosted the major as follows: 'Major, I am in a very unpleasant situation. Murphy [Egan] has not yet made his appearance and I understand he claims the right of accompanying the regiment. I have not had much personal acquaintance with the colonel and I do not like to thrust myself on his notice at this busy moment. Will you have the kindness to ascertain whether I am to go or stay, for my baggage is yet unselected and I have some arrangements of considerable importance to my comfort to make.' The good and gallant man replied: 'Why, is it possible you don't know? You are to go, whether Murphy [Egan] comes in time or not, Colonel [Ponsonby] has had his eye upon you all day and has decided the matter in the proper way, so make your arrangements for marching with us tomorrow.'

The words were scarcely out of his mouth, when all that was useless and provoking appeared in the shape of Larry Murphy [Patrick Egan] himself! He came, just in time, (off the top of a London coach, covered with dust and dressed in a *shabby genteel* sort of barber's clerk uniform of sky-blue) to catch Colonel [Ponsonby] as he was mounting his horse, to leave the busy scene of our somewhat tiresome operations. I said to him, 'Murphy [Egan], you are too late, you are to be left behind with the depot. It is all settled and I must go with the regiment.' 'Jesus,' said the selfish

---

39. The old soldier must have been an ex-23rd Light Dragoons man.

creature, 'this will be the *ruin* of me.' 'Well,' I replied, 'you should have been here to look after your own interest, however, there is the colonel; you had better speak to him; don't take my word for it.' He approached our chief, who had the good nature to listen to his lame story and being one of those generous characters who never could pronounce the word 'No' he got out of the dilemma, by saying he had left the decision of the question to the surgeon, referring Mr Murphy [Egan] to him accordingly.

Larry [Patrick] then returned to me and said, 'I don't care about going,' (indeed, I saw he *could not* go, for he was totally unequipped and dismounted into the bargain) 'but as I know S [Robinson]' (the surgeon) 'would put a spoke in my wheel if he could, I want to see him, as Colonel Ponsonby has referred me to him and hear what he has to say. Where are his quarters?' I directed him accurately and was leaving the barrack-yard (where this scene had taken place) to mind my own business, when he came back, saying he could never find his way to [Robinson]'s without my assistance and desiring that I should go with him. Almost fainting with fatigue (rather of mind however, than of body) and much in want of my dinner, I undertook to show him the way; but to my dying hour, I shall not forget the colloquy which the visit occasioned.

We found [Robinson] at high dinner, up one pair of stairs, at the top of which he made his appearance, with a knife in one hand, a fork in the other and his mouth crammed with beefsteaks, or something else, intended to go further into his interior than the *Murphy* [Egan] which held me by the arm.

'Well, Sir!' exclaimed [Robinson], 'you are come at last.'

'To be sure I am.'

'And why did you not make your appearance before? J[ohn] and I have had to perform the heavy duty of inspecting every man in the regiment, while you have been amusing yourself in London. Pray, Sir, what do you want with me?'

'Why, I want to know whether J[ohn] or I shall go with the regiment, because the colonel say it is left to you.'

'Why then, if it is left to me, I have to say that I consider you have forfeited all right to go and in my opinion, you are not able to go.'

'Not able!! Not able!! what do you *mane*? I'm as able as ever I was in my life and I will go!'

'Very well, Mr Murphy [Egan], as you are so determined about it, I have little more to say, only I must put one or two questions to you. Have you got a horse? have you a kit? are you effective?'[40]

'Sure, I always had a horse.'

'Yes, till you sold him, but have you one *now*?'

'Sure, I can get one in five minutes and I always had a kit.'

'Well Sir, as I know that you have no horse, no regimentals, no equipment of any kind and now know nothing of the actual state of the regiment, which J[ohn] and I have taken *your* share of duty in ascertaining, you must remain here and J[ohn] will go with us?'

'Very well! Mighty fine! All I wanted was to know that you preferred J[ohn] to me. Good morning to you and the divil go *wid* you!'

'Nay,' said [Robinson], 'I do *not* prefer J[ohn] to you, one officer if effective is as good as another; but you are notoriously not effective. J[ohn] I know, has a perfect equipment for foreign service; he has purchased a second horse this afternoon and the commanding office has selected him for the duty before us. You will attend tomorrow at eight o'clock, to take over the charge of the depot hospital and J[ohn] will march with the troops.'

---

40. Note by Smith: The valise of the horseman is strapped behind his saddle; the infantry soldier carries his knapsack upon his own back. Each contains nearly the same articles; such as shirts, stockings, spare shoes, forage cap, &c; but for horses there are a few more requisites; viz currycombs, hand brushes &c. Long after I joined the [12th], a wisp of straw was the only thing employed in grooming; but it was afterwards judged proper to introduce the manufactured articles specified. The horse of a light dragoon is expected to be master of twenty-two stone, jockey weight.

| Estimate | Stone (Jockey weight of 14 lb) | lbs |
|---|---|---|
| 1st A light rider | 12 | 168 |
| 2nd Clothing &c personally worn | 1 (at least) | 14 |
| 3rd 3 days' rations for himself and horse | 5 (and upwards) | 70 |
| 4th Arms, accoutrements, 60 rounds of ammunition, Spare clothing, necessaries, with allowance for personal weight, over 12 stone &c. | 4 | 56 |
| | 22 | 308 |

It is to be observed, that this is a low estimate for what actually occurs on service, upon many occasions of emergency. The corn is carried in a sack, balanced behind the saddle; the hay or straw is packed into nets and slung across the saddle *bow*. Upon field days in France the men were ordered to appear always in *light* marching order; which meant without rations and forage (as in England) but they used to stuff their valises with *hay*, till the trick was found out, and necessaries were *necessarily* packed up on future occasions.

I cannot exhibit the actors upon this occasion in the reality of their performance. For my own part, I could hardly contain my gravity at the mock heroic of [Robinson], as contrasted with the petulance of Murphy. We were not even asked upstairs, (for which I could well account); but Murphy [Egan] turned from the inhospitable door with a thousand Irish exclamations, as to the indignity of his treatment.

'My dear fellow,' said he, as we walked down the street, 'I *knew* I could not go, I *can't* go, I don't *want* to go, you *ought* to go. I am glad you *are* going; but [Robinson] is no friend of mine and all I wanted was a row about it. As you are to be off tomorrow, I hope you will write me an account of proceedings.' Whether I gave Larry [Patrick] any promise to this effect, I have now forgotten; but I know that I was very glad to get rid of him.

I saw nothing of him on the ensuing morning; but instead of being at his post by eight o'clock, I learnt afterwards, that three messages, the last not the most courteous, had been delivered to him by as many non-commissioned officers, before he could make up his mind to leave his couch for the purpose of attending at the hospital. In the course of the day S [Robinson] joined us at Ramsgate; and having seen our nags safely paraded in the hold of *the largest and finest transport* we could select from the fleet, as head-quarter ship, Joe B [James Castley] (the Veterinary surgeon),[41] S [Robinson], and myself spent the day together on shore, all of us, with the addition of the Paymaster[42] and Adjutant,[43] repairing on board the ship to sleep, as we were to sail at a very early hour next morning.

Neither the colonel nor the major embarked with us, though (as will be shewn in the sequel) they were ready to receive us on our arrival at the other side. The presence of neither would have laid us under any unpleasant restraint; but we fared all the better for their absence, in the article of accommodation, which in the event, became of more importance than could have been calculated upon at setting out. Had we been bound for any distant place, or likely to be long at sea, two medical officers would not have been allowed to proceed in the same ship; but we anticipated a short run across and the vessel was appropriated to the regimental staff

---

41. James Castley was originally appointed as Veterinary Surgeon to the 15th Light Dragoons in June 1807, but transferred to the 12th Light Dragoons in August 1809. He had seen extensive service in the Peninsula.
42. Paymaster William Loftus Otway 12th Light Dragoons, also called throughout 'Growler'.
43. The Adjutant was Lieutenant John Griffiths.

generally, commissioned and non-commissioned. We arrived at rather a late hour, on board the transport, on Saturday night, March 31 [1 April]; and scarcely had we descended the companion ladder, when great offence was taken at the master. The fact was, that the rude fellow, having been pretty well insulted in his time, had thought proper to get drunk in the most independent and then *to turn in*, in the most indifferent manner, leaving word, that he would be dammed if he would keep watch, *to please all the officers of the army*. This *calm* determination was the more formidable, as the steward had absconded and not one among us knew where to get bed or blanket, or even where to place them if we had them, nobody having acted quartermaster, in making a previous *reconnaissance* of the ship. Something however, was essential and remonstrances were forwarded to the captain, first of a gentle, but at last of rather a peremptory nature, which procured us the bedding; and we then arranged ourselves in berths, starboard and larboard,[44] the surgeon claiming (as senior) the state-room, left empty by the absence of the commanding officer. For my own part, I would not have exchanged my open berth in the cabin for all his luxury and dignity and we of the πολλοί,[45] enjoyed a midnight laugh there, at his expense.

Although I have said that the Paymaster was of the embarking party, he did not make his appearance till after we had all gone to roost. *Growler* [Otway] (as he was nick-named) entered the cabin about twelve o'clock, none the better seaman for the wine he had taken on board. He was, upon most occasions, an *intolerably* haughty fellow and had the art of expressing himself as if he had been Brian Borou [Boru],[46] instead of a Regimental Paymaster. Upon the occasion in question, he was *enormously* high; and filled with ideas of his own dignity and delicacy, was perfectly frantic at finding, in the berth allotted to him, the full flood of an urn sacred to Bohea,[47] confined however, in a stagnant state, within its brittle banks.

'Steward!' No answer. 'I say, you dammed steward!' Silence still.

'What's the matter, Growler [Otway]?' says B[Castley].

'Why by Jingo, they've put a slop basin full into my bed, on purpose to insult me. Steward!' Still midnight silence.

---

44. Larboard was used for the port or left side of the ship until the 1860s.
45. Greek – The masses.
46. An Irish king 1002 to 1014.
47. A tea urn.

'I have never heard of such insolence', said the occupier of the stateroom [Robinson]; 'let us have the master in directly; as senior officer, I will take the affair upon myself.'

After considerable delay, during which Growler [Otway] sat, with the piece of tea furniture in his hand, upon a camp stool, the master did make his appearance for the first time, not in *full dress*, but drunk, wroth and eloquently impertinent.

'What do you want?'

'The dammed lazy steward to empty this slop.'

'I've got no steward; he ran away yesterday.'

'Then, Sir, as you do not keep a steward, take it directly and empty it yourself.'

'Empty it myself! I'll see you all dammed first. Where are your servants?'

'What? Do you suppose our servants have nothing else to do but clear the leavings out of your ship?'

'Well, if you don't chuse to employ your servants, you can clear them away yourself, it's no business of mine.'

S [Robinson], who had heard the whole colloquy (without interfering), now raised an authoritative voice and exclaimed, 'You, *Sir*! How dare you insult officers of the King's cavalry? You are bound to receive us into a clean ship; but this is no better than a *dung* barge.'

'Why' replied the pot-valiant captain, 'I don't think she is much better when she carries such cargoes as you!'

Here the general laugh became so ungovernable, that silence ensued among the *linguagerent* [*sic* – belligerent?] parties.

We were alive betimes on the following morning; for the event of sailing at a very early hour was one we hardly could be expected to oversleep.[48] Before we went on deck, we called a council of war upon the occurrences of the previous night and unanimously agreed, that 'the captain of the barge' was an impertinent scoundrel, with whom no measures of civility could possibly be observed during the remainder of our abode under his *deck*. With this prejudice we mounted the aforesaid deck, the theatre of our intended scorn, where we discovered our foe busily employed in

---

48. Note by Smith – And we anticipated the disagreeable duty of having to keep an eye upon the master; a duty of which, for my own part, I had some experience.

making the necessary arrangements for our departure, with which he appeared to mingle no ordinary solicitude for the accommodation of the dragoons and (what at the moment rather vexed than pleased us, such was our dislike of him) great anxiety about the welfare of our *horses*. It was touching cavalry men in the tenderest point. If he wished to make the *amende* [apology], a volume of supplicatory letters would not have had the effect of his simple order to '*see if the gentlemen's horses were properly stowed; and to mind that the water and windsails were quite handy!*'[49] This altered the case materially, as to matter of opinion; but the difficulty was yet to be got over concerning who should speak first.

To the honour of the service, I have to record, that the first overture of this nature emanated from *ourselves*. I was sent to the captain and in sufficiently civil, though probably not very condescending terms, asked if we could get the appliances and means of breakfast? Instead of having my eyes most ferociously dammed, I was mildly and respectfully, but certainly in a sailor-like manner, answered, 'Yes to be sure, what would you like to have?' Here the extent of my commission was run and I was obliged to return aft for further instructions. The result was, 'The officers' compliments and if it is convenient, they would be glad of the loan of cups, saucers &c, as they would rather not open their canteens till they get on shore.' 'You can have anything of the sort you like; only, as the steward has run from the ship, I shall be obliged to you if you will order your own servants to attend you.' In the meanwhile, I ought to remark that we had left Ramsgate harbour about six, with a gentle, but fair breeze; and that breakfast was got ready soon after seven, with a voluntary assurance, on the part of Captain *Dung* [the Master], that if he could in any way contribute to our comfort, we had only to let him know.

The breakfast requires no description, unless I add that, instead of having newspapers to read, or politics to discuss at it, we made Captain *Dung* the common theme. We began to suspect that he had been more drunk than insolent overnight and that probably he had taken as much provocation as liquor. We thought that the surgeon [Robinson] had gone rather far in calling a man out of bed to be reprimanded, who owed him no allegiance and that Growler [Otway] himself did not look perfectly

---

49. Note by Smith – At this moment I do not believe the man knew that one of us had left the cabin; in fact, we came upon deck when he was quite unprepared for our appearance.

dignified, sitting with the tea *depot* in his hand. This was the opinion of three out of five; so we resolved, especially as he had it more in his power to annoy *us* than we had it in ours to annoy *him*, to agree to an amnesty; as it was evident that the man was not only sorry for what had occurred, but disposed to make the best amends in his power.

The greater part of the regiment had been very wisely placed onboard small vessels, drawing little water; whereas ours was a magnificent brig, of nearly three hundred tons burthen and draught accordingly. We carried about fifty horses and soldiers in proportion: their numbers however, had nothing to do either with our accommodation or arrangements. In truth, the occasion resembled more the affair of a ferrying across than of a sea voyage; for we had not been long out of sight of the English coast before that of the Netherlands presented itself. I believe we first caught a sight of *Dunkirk*, our destination being *Ostend*. The day was particularly fine, the water smooth and our progress, though not rapid, satisfactory and steady. I do not remember anyone being sick; and we dined upon *picnic*, each having furnished himself with something, which was added to a general muster in the victualling department. The pleasures of the table were considerably interfered with by our approach towards the destined port. All of course, soon began to be anxiety and preparation for leaving a scene in which no long time had been spent; and as much bustle as old soldiers are capable of, or the superintendence of experienced officers will permit, was the order of the afternoon.

But we had reckoned without our captain in the first instance and were now about to be convinced of our error. On we went, in our fine, gallant vessel, commiserating the situation of our friends in the small craft, which had enough to do to keep up with us, till about 4 pm; when, within three or four hundred yards of the pier of Ostend harbour, the *headquarters* of the dragoons, instead of being established in the Hotel of the Emperor [Hotel de l'Empereur], were deposited upon a sand bank. This came of our pride in chusing the largest and deepest lying ship, when we ought to have selected the smallest. This was the end of our 'high notions' as to accommodation. Upon the whole, there was a very pleasant prospect; a lee shore, night coming on, horses to be lost or injured, baggage thrown into the water, confusion and in the event of a blowing night, the probable loss of some of our own lives. It was not quite high water and the greatest of our hopes amounted to getting the ship afloat again and moving off to sea: working her into Ostend was out of the question. Poor *Dung* began to find fault with those who had despatched so large a vessel on such an expedition: 'They ought,' he said, 'to have known better than to *suppose* she could get into Ostend. For his own part, he would not come there again (provided he ever got back) for all the Agents of Transports in England.' The higher the tide rose, we seemed only the better able to set at defiance every attempt at *buoyancy*; and while all our energies were concentrated upon this object, a vessel, apparently about the dimensions of our own, (entangled most probably in a narrow channel which gave no choice of course to steer) came bearing down upon our broadside, with a huge anchor over her bow. This was *truly* formidable. For my own part, although at first provoked at the apparently wanton perseverance in a course that must inevitably run the ships foul, my anxiety was altered to consideration for the animals below, as it appeared to be a *demonstration* that the other one's anchor would go through the side of our ship, like that of a green-house and do damage among the poor *horses*. At all events, I am ashamed to say that at this moment, I derived considerable consolation from knowing that my own cattle [horses] were on the side opposite to the one from which the attack was to come. In the meantime, our consort approached so near, that the danger of being in the way of her gib boom became a consideration; when all immediate fears were removed by seeing her suddenly arrested by the same obstacle which had presented itself in our own way. She grounded close to us.

The tide began to ebb and all chance of floating till morning became hopeless. A boat was got out, and some of the officers went to the town to give notice of our situation and obtain assistance, the means more especially of removing the horses. While the preceding efforts were making in vain, the *little* vessels ran past us and gained the harbour without difficulty, we of headquarters being half ashamed to shew ourselves, in the awkward situation into which our pomposity had gotten us. Our two stuck-fasts were in no long time left in possession of the whole visible German Ocean [North Sea] and our companions at length returned with intelligence that assistance would forthwith be forwarded. The only aid we did receive however, was a small boat, in which was an officer of the Transport Department, who kindly inquired (without coming nearer than was absolutely necessary) how we did. He returned to his dinner and we began to reconcile ourselves to that for which there appeared to be no remedy.

Night closed upon us, but without any alarming appearances as to the article of weather; our situation, therefore, though certainly dangerous, was by no means terrific. We concluded that the wisest thing we could do, was to take up our quarters in the fine large cabin and entertain one another as well as we could, under the circumstances. The conduct of Captain *Dung* (for I have now forgotten, if ever indeed, I knew his proper name) was such as to have gained our entire confidence and we considered it useless to cherish alarm, where such a feeling could only have increased the unpleasantness of our situation. The real difficulty of the moment arose from our not having been provided with more *prog* [food] than was necessary for one day's consumption, calculating as we had every reason to do, (and as the event, with regard to our friends in the other ships, fully bore us out in) that we should have, ere this, been able to avail ourselves of the plentiful resources of fat Belgium. Here however, we suffered no sort of inconvenience; for *Dung*, in the most considerate manner, informed us, that he had a joint or two of fresh meat and the remains of a stock of excellent claret, to all which we were welcome and for which he afterwards would accept of no consideration beyond the price of these articles had cost him. It is but justice to record, that one of our party having left his snuffbox on board in the hurry of disembarking, it was not only taken care of, but forwarded to him by *Dung's* attentive exertions, when it must have been out of his way even to have ascertained where we were. The truth is that, though a coarse seaman in his aspect and manners, he was a gentleman in his feelings.

Day broke and found us still immoveable, if not firm as the Eddystone, or the Bell Rock.[50] The tide, however, was again flowing and we were not without hope that we should be able to escape from the bank and take refuge in deeper water, farther out at sea, for not a sign of assistance had approached us during the night. Whether it was owing to a more dexterous application of our powers, or a more favourable concurrence of circumstances I forget, but we had not been very long engaged in the struggle till the vessel swung off, was put under sail and steered to [a] safer anchorage, where she had (while the weather continued moderate) at least the privilege of *floating*. How our bedfellow got up in the morning I do not

---

50. The third Eddystone Lighthouse off Rame Head in Cornwall was constructed in 1759 and Bell Rock Lighthouse off the Firth of Tay was completed in 1811.

distinctly remember; but I recollect that she did get away undamaged and that the wrecks which took place upon that coast, a few days afterwards, included neither of *us* in the unfortunate number.

Our safety being thus so far provided for, notwithstanding an assurance from Captain *Dung*, that if the weather looked threatening before the means of disembarking came (trying the port with such a ship being preposterous), he would be obliged to take us back to England. We began to think we had the best of it, when compared with the regiment at large. It soon commenced raining most implacably and we knew that our friends on shore were exposed to a march in the open air, spoiling all their accoutrements and equipments, while we were enjoying first a good breakfast, then a pleasant lounge, afterwards no bad dinner and some excellent claret with unparalleled droll stories. We had no songs: we did not want them. Growler [Otway] was an original, of whom I had not seen much up to this period, but as he was in perfect good humour, he amused us considerably. The doctor, as they called him, did all he could to keep up the mirth. Of [James Castley], I have only to say here, that for a perfectly well dried piece of genuine and original wit, I never met with his equal. Of myself it becomes me to say nothing; but my part of the performance was spoken of for years afterwards: the Adjutant possessed great powers of *laughter*; so that each man played his part and the rainy day was all but forgotten. It may be asked, what the troopers had for consolation, while we were so well off? I answer, excellent ship's rations, consisting of beef, bread and rum and little or nothing to do but to enjoy one another's company. Thus passed *Monday*, without the slightest attempt to interfere with us from any point of the compass; and had we gone in search of the North Pole, it is my opinion that no one would have discovered it till we came back again.

Feeling ourselves in comparative safety on Monday night, we turned in with more confidence than we had been able to muster the night before and slept, in all probability, a little sounder. With the following morning our hopes as to extrication were revived. The master of the vessel refused *point blank* to venture near the harbour again: he had received sufficient warning and it was more than the safety of all on board was worth to make the experiment a second time; so, if no aid came from the shore, he must take us back, to be embarked onboard vessels whose draught of water did not exceed the depth over the sandbanks. To have withstood this determination by any opposite one, on our part, would have been madness. However, in the course of the day, advice was received that a *schuyt*[51] would be despatched to our relief, capable of removing the whole of us at once and towards evening she made her appearance, much to our satisfaction, notwithstanding the resignation we had manifested under the untoward nature of our circumstances.

When the 'craft' in question came alongside, she appeared by no means too large to be accommodated between the masts of the headquarter 'barge'; yet into these comparatively narrow limits were we all, *horse and foot*, transferred with a precipitation that was apparently as unaccountable as uncalled for. The afternoon was fine and the sea smooth; but such was Captain *Dung's* uneasiness about his position, in the vicinity of the submarine [underwater] Netherlands, that, which one portion of the ship's crew was hoisting *us* out, another was heaving short the anchor and dropping the sails to be ready for a start; and no sooner were we all bundled into the schuyt, than away they went, as if expecting us to board them, sword in hand. We now found ourselves crowded enough above and our half hundred cattle [horses] still more so below, where there was this advantage arising out of their paved situation, that not one had room to fall, or to lift his foot against his neighbour.

Little incidents like these, are not of themselves worth recollecting, still less perhaps of recording; but they show the realities of life in some of those situations which we strive to avoid, but when placed in, feel no hardship from. Thus, the party which could not find a ship large enough to contain them, but a short time previously, was now perfectly well satisfied with a space not much larger than that ship's cabin. True, an hour or two was the probable extent of our prospect here; but necessity and not selection, was the cause of our resignation.

Whoever has been, not only at sea, but compelled to live in contracted space anywhere, must have observed how the accommodation, which was at first deemed insufficient and intolerable, expanded daily. For my own part, I had on many prior and have upon some subsequent occasions, been crammed, among numerous fellow travellers, into positions which *civil* calculations would have materially enlarged, but which *military* eyes, judgment and admeasurements considered with less apparent, but more

---

51. A barge-like flat-bottomed boat used extensively on canals and in coastal trade.

real accuracy. '*Man wants but little here below*' and in the schuyt we did not 'want that little long.'

As was the case with other regiments and according to a well-known rule, when corps are about to proceed on active service, only a certain and that a small number of soldiers' wives was permitted to accompany each troop. I believe *'sergeants' ladies'* were extra-numerical; and as all the Staff sergeants were embarked in our ship, I recollect that the *beau sexe* mustered comparatively strong upon the deck of the schuyt. It was a large, flat-bottomed and unwieldy barge, of the Dutch fashion, carrying huge sails, one of which was called by a name that sounded like no very polite word in the English language and which, when pronounced with an order 'to hoist', tickled the imaginations and excited the titters of the 'passengers'. It was thought so curious a coincidence, that the order given by the skipper was sometimes quoted, upon after occasions, with a very ludicrous effect.

Even *transported* as we now were, the cross-grained harbour of Ostend would not permit our approach to its interior and we had to leave our craft outside, while we ourselves got ashore in a small leaky boat and found the colonel waiting for his horses. By his kind directions, we gained a hotel and were soon furnished with a *Netherlandische* repast.

Before commencing a new chapter, I beg to remark that I was surprised at finding all the old, smooth, counterfeit halfpence, which had many years before, been annihilated in England, in full and free circulation at Ostend and afterwards in other parts of *La Belgique*: buttons without eyes and all manner of sorts of substitutes for the genuine small coin, or tinker's money of any civilised state. So much and so iniquitously (no doubt) was the exchange against our country, that we were obliged to put up with sixteen francs for a pound note; while ten more afterwards barely amounted to par.

In the course of the evening, intelligence came that the schuyt had entered the harbour; we all repaired to the beach, where, about ten o'clock, we accomplished the task of getting our baggage and horses onshore, a few of the latter notwithstanding the shallowness of water which had been so satisfactorily demonstrated, having had a swim for it: and thus terminated our April fool's day.[52]

---

52. They disembarked on the evening of Monday 3 April.

# Chapter 2

# Marching to Join the Army

On the morning of the 4 [April] we set out, quite a party of pleasure, full of good humour and upon the best terms with one another. Our first halting-place was to be *Bruges*, (distant about twelve English miles from Ostend) to which magnificent and celebrated, though decayed and comparatively deserted city, we proceeded along the edge of the canal. This was not the road usually taken by travellers on horseback and why we preferred it (unless from the greater chance of variety) I cannot say. The monotony of travelling in the Netherlands has been too generally experienced to admit of description in this place; but I used to consider ten or twelve miles there, more wearisome by far, if not more fatiguing, than twice or even three times the distance would be in variegated England. We pass[ed] a drawbridge, but on turning round behold a wide fosse and behind it massive frowning walls;[1] we address ourselves to the journey and at the end of a long straight and level avenue, (the perspective of which is maintained in all its geometrical accuracy) we observe a *spire*. That is the object we are to overtake; it is the mark of town the next, ten miles off, three hours journey but only at the other end of this same avenue, into which we have just entered. 'Come along, let us walk gently, we shall be there in a few minutes.' Many *minutes* elapse, many trees are passed, (for the road is bounded by a row of lofty ones on either side, as well as by a ditch, which separates the whole from and affords the most suitable means of enclosing the adjoining fields) and while we imagine that we have made no progress towards the spire ahead, we turn round and oh! Still more provoking, there appears to be no increase of distance between us and the walls behind. It is next to impossible now to divert our attention from the ponderous undertaking. Surely we have not been misinformed as to the distance! We have been on the road a full half hour and must have gone over two miles, so that there

---
1. The defences of Ostend which were being repaired.

ought to be no more than eight between us and the steeple, yet it looks as small and the air about it is as hazy as at first; and as for the end of the road, the trees are drawn as close together as ever. We now remember to have been taught something about the apparent approximation of parallel lines, when at school and we have since seen the principle beautifully applied in pictures; but all this amounts to no more than theoretical conception, or imitative illustration; now however, we are placed in the very reality and although we ought, perhaps, to admire the source of philosophic inference and the origin of scientific principle, yet we find we have enough to do to save our patience from drowning in the very fountain, as it were of knowledge.

'Onward we marched with measured step' and in course of time actually did reach Bruges. Here, in the ancient *entrepot* of the commercial world, here where the riches of Asia were accumulated till the unlucky discovery of a new way to India round the Cape of Good Hope was made by a *Portuguese* adventurer, here where all the luxuries to which the most luxurious of the ancient inhabitants of the maritime towns of the Mediterranean and of the capital cities of the most celebrated nations were to be had in profusion, we got a good *dinner*! And that is pretty nearly the amount of what I have to say about the cradle of oil painting.[2] We dined I think, at the Hotel de l'Empereur, but for my own part I did not 'take a bed there' having been furnished with a billet upon a respectable clothier, with the aspect of whose domestic establishment I had been particularly pleased when in the earlier part of the day, I went to make good my quarters.

At an early hour (for us English) I retired to my *Bourgmestre's* [Burgomeister] and found that the family (having shut shop and closed commercial transactions for the day) were still out of bed and waiting in their common apartment for the arrival of *the officer*. There might have been various reasons for this, the disclosure of some of which, it is possible the officer would not have considered too complimentary. It would not be difficult to conceive what a substantial English citizen would imagine to be *his* duty towards a French or Russian officer thrust upon his privacy in a corresponding manner. However, as the good people of the *Pay-Bas*

---

2. Note by Smith – Art is said to have been invented by a native of the city above alluded to, who is known in the annals of painting by the name of *John of Bruges*.

had been tolerably habituated to similar intrusions, I verily believe, that a mixture of hospitable feeling and of curiosity formed the cause of their departure from those habits of order and early hours to which they were accustomed. These ran every chance of being overturned, at least for a long time subsequent to the date of our visit; for although I was in all probability, the first officer of the English army who presented the order for accommodation, I shall be readily believed when I declare that it is impossible for me to have been the last.

Supper, the principal meal of families in these regions, had been long over; and I found the *Herr* and his *frau*, with one or more confidential domestics and I think a neighbour or two, seated round a cosy, comfortable and even elegant stove, which diffused a genial warmth throughout the apartment, though the source of this influence was hidden from the eye. We have a foolish saying and a preposterously *pretended* feeling (respecting the *reality* of which I cannot believe) in England, that the *sight* of a fire is indispensably necessary to that association of ideas, denominated comfort, the grand untranslatable English word, I do not think so. I like to see a fire when it is burning clearly and briskly, but nine times out of ten, what can be more gloomy than the aspect of an English grate? My landlord produced the *schnaps*: *will* I, *nill* I, I must partake, the small thimble sized glasses presented nothing so very formidable but that after even a fair quantity of wine, I might venture. This interchange of cordiality was better than a thousand formal introductions, we drank and we drank again and as we could both jabber away in French, so as to understand each other, we kept up a colloquy till a reasonably late hour. One by one, the *frauen* disappeared and at length I was ushered to my *chambre a coucher* [bedroom], by the honest cloth man *in propria persona* [himself].

In the morning I found coffee, liqueurs and all the appurtenances and appliances of a good breakfast prepared for me: and took at least a polite, if not a kind leave of the first Flemish family I had seen. My impressions of the national character were highly favourable, *quoad* [as regards] their disposition. Not doubting that similar receptions were before us (for I learnt from the rest of our party, that they had all experienced corresponding attentions) we set forward well pleased with everything around and in suitable expectation of whatever was in reserve.

*Ecloo* [Eeklo], a large open town or *bourg*, was our next destination; and we arrived somewhere about the middle of the day. There was little or nothing in the aspect of this place to engage our attention, but it afforded much more amusement than we could possibly have anticipated. The master of the auberge where two of us dined, was an artist: we were let it be remembered, now in a country that has a *national* character of devotedness to painting, as the Italians have for music and the French for dancing. We were in the land of the Teniers, of Ostade, Dow, Berghem, Hobbima, the Mieris,[3] and a host of others, the fame of whose works will outlive the canvas, the pane, and the copper to which they were committed by those chosen candidates for immortality. Mine host of the Emperor's Head, or the Black Eagle,[4] (I do not pretend to remember the sign) was an amateur *painter*, though by profession *Aubergiste* [inn keeper], he *said* he had contributed several productions of his pencil to the last exhibition at Bruxelles; and was very eager, while the *roti* was in course of preparation, to do the honours of his little gallery. As the exhibition cost nothing and hunger was an obstacle to criticism, we shall excuse ourselves from introducing anything connected with connoisseurship.

After dinner, we made a patrol through the town; in the course of which we heard the most perfect and delightful trumpet sounds that ever struck on mortal ear. Whence could they issue? From nothing less than instruments of gold, played upon by artists from heaven. Troops in the village we had already ascertained that there were none; we understood that *Louis le desire* [Louis XVIII] was *en garnison* [in garrison] at Ghent,[5] with a heterogeneous jumble of followers and that among the faithful there were some few dozen gentry, styled a *Garde du Corps*, (which I had the honour to fall in with on a subsequent occasion, as will be described hereafter) but *la Garde Royale*, nay, the King of England's Life Guards themselves, whom we knew to be still on the other side of the Goodwin [Sands], could not have trumpeted up to this. Had *L'Empereur d'Elbe*[6] caught all Europe napping? Was it possible that *Napoleon* himself was bringing the captive *Louis* a prisoner in great state, down to the coast, there to superintend his re-embarkation for the ancient town of Dover? Even

---

3. David Teniers the Elder and Younger, Adriaen van Ostade, Gerard Dow, Nichlas Berghem, Meindert Hobbema and Frans van Meiris the Elder and Younger, were painters in the Dutch Golden Age in the seventeenth century.
4. Note by Smith – These signs, it is almost unnecessary to observe, refer their origin to the period when the country formed part of the Austrian dominions.
5. The exiled King Louis XVIII was living at the Hotel d'Hane Steenhuyse in Ghent.
6. Napoleon had been consigned to rule Elba after his defeat in 1814.

upon this surmise, the trumpeting seemed to be beyond the occasion; it was in short, too good for Kings or Emperors either. We could not have surpassed it even in the persons and upon the instruments of our own *regimental* performers and that is quoting a *ne plus ultra* [most extreme example]. Turning the corner of the street, whence these extraordinary notes appeared to issue, we beheld *a rabble*! *a mob*! A collection of vilest blackguards (in appearance) our memories could recall: and in the midst thereof, *twain* [two] ugly, dirty, ragged rascals, with each a common brass trumpet under his nose, sending forth the most exquisite sounds, with perfect indifference and facility! These were followed by two or three correspondents, habilimented much in the style of our London chimney-sweepers on May day or (to describe them, perhaps, with rather more justice and accuracy) like the decoy folks that are to be seen eating fire, *a la Chabert*,[7] or cutting capers at the entrance of a theatrical booth in an English country fair, tarnished lace and dim spangles upon old velvet jackets, with other parts of dress, perfectly uniform and in unison. What then, did all this parade consist of, or amount to? Why readers to a party of conjurors, in more choice language, *jongleurs*, or jugglers. They were to perform that evening for the amusement of the honest bourgeois of Ecloo [Eeklo] and were publishing their advertisement in the manner here described.

A council was now called; and as there appeared no better method of knocking the evening over, we beckoned to the commanding officer and inquired how we should be accommodated in the event of our bestowing *patronage*. The *poor devil* (for after all, he was no better) gratefully and joyfully promised us, not only the best seats, but the best tricks and the best trumpeting, to which we certainly attached a full degree of importance.

When the time arrived, we proceeded to the *spectacle* and found already congregated one of the most motely assemblages that the M[an] of S[orrows][8] ever saw displayed by David Teniers, in one of his hilarious and uproarious masterpieces. Long beards, dirty faces, night-caps, old shapeless hats, mobcaps upon the *frauen*, unmentionables of every indescribable figure, without form, in most instances and in everyone, devoid of fashion. Tinkers and tailors, snobs and tripe sellers,

---

7. Almost certainly refers to General Theodore Chabert, who had a very colourful career.
8. This is the only title of a picture by David Teniers the Younger which fits. It portrays Jesus with his guards before he is taken for execution.

manufacturers of sausages and eaters of the same, fiddlers upon half-pay, chimney-sweepers, *cum plurimis aliis* [with many others], were assembled in an upper room of a very ordinary looking house, situated in a back lane.

The moment we English officers (the *aristocracy* of the occasion) made our appearance, up struck the trumpeters, 'God save great George *our* King;' all the performers pressed forward to conduct us to the '*dress circle*,' otherwise a form in the front and we there seated ourselves, quite patient about the commencement of the juggling, listening to and wondering at the trumpets. One of the accomplishments of the juggler (for he was *primum mobile* [most important mover] on the occasion) consisted in beating the big drum, in a style corresponding to the execution of the trumpeters; and upon this unlikely instrument he 'discoursed most excellent music.' To give any account of his other performances, might justly be considered trifling: suffice it to say, that he perfectly understood his business and amused all the spectators (ourselves most particularly) in a highly satisfactory manner. He seemed to be quite at home, both in the French and Flemish languages, explaining everything for our benefit in the former. On some occasions, it might have been difficult to suppose the tricks practicable without the aid of confederates; but a few of the most amusing were performed, by means of money and other things furnished by our own party.[9]

The next day saw our arrival at *Gand* or Ghent, as the natives spell it, but do not pronounce it:

'*All was bustle, squeeze, row, jabbering and jam.*' For my own part I lost so much time and encountered so much fatigue in seeking my quarters, that I was little inclined to look for the lions of the place,[10] besides, I had no guide, either written or oral; and the city appeared so vast and so full of objects of curiosity, that it would have been impossible to decide where to make a beginning. Here we had expected to find the regiment; and here they had enjoyed an advantage, in which we did not participate, that of having spent two or three days in Ghent, with little or nothing to do but look about them. As we marched in however, we found them marching

---

9. Note by Smith – Ten years afterwards I stumbled upon the same fellow at a Café in the *Palais Royal*, where he was nightly engaged in the exercise of his art, for the amusement of the company. I entered into conversation with him and found that he recollected the great event at Ecloo [Eeklo]; and out of compliment to me, as one of the distinguished visitors on that remarkable occasion, performed an extra trick or two.

10. Lions – the great attractions of the city.

out, to take up quarters farther off and leave room for new-comers. One night, therefore, was all that fell to our share, in the birthplace and favourite city of the Emperor Charles V.[11]

On the following morning we advanced farther into the 'bowels of the land'. Our destination was a small open town beyond Oudenarde [Oudenaarde], called Renaix [Ronse], celebrated chiefly for having been the headquarters of the Duke of York in 1794, after the army retreated from Dunkirk. At Oudenarde [Oudenaarde] I caught a fair sight of 'the lazy Scheldt,' and found my old regiment, the [11th Light Dragoons] quartered there. This was the first corps of the British army which had arrived in the country, though our own was the first that had been ordered on this service; our friends however, got over before us, for when the order reached them, they were at or near the place of embarkation; whereas as the reader is now aware, we had several days' march to perform before we arrived at the place in which we were even *to commence* our preparations. I found at Oudenarde [Oudenaarde] several of the officers I was acquainted with and saw, from the style of *their* accommodation, that was to be expected by ourselves in this article. There were comparatively few of them in the town; and indeed towns, however agreeable or enviable, furnish but indifferent quarters for cavalry, the obvious reason of which is the scarcity of stable room, there being (with the exception of inns) no more than is absolutely necessary for the purpose of the inhabitants themselves, of which it is not usual to deprive them, where the troops are intended for a friendly purpose, unless in cases of emergency: consequently farmyards and therefore villages containing collections of these, are the most suitable places for mounted troops, where it is true, the horses are generally better off than their riders. In the space of nearly four years I do not recollect being above a day or two at a time in a town (unless the little *bourgs* in which our small headquarter establishment was commonly associated deserve that name), the great body of the regiment lying about the country and generally in what were considered execrable quarters, but more about this in due time and proper place.

Renaiz or Renaux [Ronse], being but a short distance beyond Oudenarde [Oudenaarde], the journey was soon concluded; I must not

---

11. Note by Smith – A well-known boast of the monarch was, that he could put Paris in his glove (Gand). Paris at the time, contained within its walls, is said not to be so large as Ghent, though the ensemble of the modern French metropolis is, of course, vastly greater.

call it a march, for this day I happened to be alone, probably, because in so widespread and crowded a town as Ghent, our little party met with a dispersion which rendered it inconvenient, if not impossible, to assign a *point de rendezvous*. I have omitted to observe, that at the *porte cochere* [carriage porch] of a large but no way elegant looking mansion, were two burgher-men in plain attire, standing each with a kind of fowling piece over his shoulder, while a considerable stir was made by a motley group of people passing in and out. I learnt that this was the abode of the *grand monarque*, the king of France himself;[12] whose dinner table was then in the very course of decoration in a room on the ground floor, which operation, I might have a view of, if I chose to look through the window. I confess that his most Christian Majesty's table was a shew I had more frequently read about than beheld, and my curiosity did tempt me to take a *peep*; but that was all,[13] I could perceive no material superiority in point of splendour to what I had often seen at our regimental mess table; but I had no time to make relevant comparisons: for I believe I was beginning to think about my own dinner and the memorandum was rather a powerful one.

'To what vile uses we may come at last,' is an apostrophe, concerning which in my modesty, I have now to cite myself as an example of the applicability. Having been furnished with a billet at Renaix [Ronse], I discovered a good looking and spacious house, with a large courtyard in front, shut in by folding gates; and this was to be the abode of a subaltern in the Duke of Wellington's army, which when English troops last were in the town, had lodged no less a personage than HRH the commander himself! The same family did not indeed, now occupy it; but the building and its accommodation remained nearly in the same state. An old plain sort of man (of whom I saw little) and his still older *frau*, from whom I experienced no lack of attention, in her notable but not very elegant way, composed the family; so as one would say (who did not regard

---

12. Note by Smith – 'Look to de right,' said a French peep-show-man, (whose box was perched upon the balustrade of London Bridge) 'and I vill chow you de grad monarch of France on a horsey back, vid all de nobellity around him; and look to de lef, and I vill chow you King Jorje valking on for, vid all de mob hollarin' after him.' A sailor standing by, gave the box a shove and added, 'look you over de bridge, and I vill chow you your box in de vater.'

13. It was traditional for the French monarchy to be viewed by the public whilst eating their dinner.

the elegancies of language) there was no *fun* to be had at home and we should have perished of town dullness but for one, not very important circumstance which occurred regularly every week, to our ineffable amusement. This was furnished by the most inimitable performer in his line I ever yet beheld. I should say he far surpassed our conjuror; for this fellow conjured in earnest, whereas the other was only in jest. And what is it supposed he was? A player? No: A ballad-singer? No; it was all prose: A Wandering minstrel? No. I will tell at once, a *mountebank*! a *quacksalver*!¹⁴ A man of this sort, without a merry-andrew,¹⁵ or anything to set him off but his own appearance and his peculiar assurance. Let me try first to convey some idea of the former and afterwards, whether I can recollect a specimen of the latter.

Upon the summit of a human figure not five feet high, was placed a huge cocked hat, from beneath the posterior flap of which, descended an English yard of hair, twisted over with something that had once been black, but whether of silk or worsted fabric I never had it in my power to verify. Under the anterior flap of the aforesaid hat was to be seen (and from some distance too) a pair of little twinkling grey eyes; below them again, there was certainly a nose; but whether snub or cocked, or of any other fashion it was difficult to decide, as it was buried in a thicket of foxy-fur which occupied the remaining part of what through complaisance we might have concluded to have been a human countenance, had we not been satisfied on that point by a certain fluency of speech, that indicated a tongue endowed with no common agility. The upper and principal garment was a short tailed red coat; and round the wearer's shoulders, 'as 'twere in scorn of gems,' gold chains, blue ribands &c &c, were suspended several rows of human teeth, all of which he had (as he declared) honestly come by, having wrenched every one of them from the jaws of their original owner, *vi et armis* [violent trespass].

The tooth drawing department however, as far as my observation went, did not seem to be so attractive as certain milder remedies which he offered to an admiring audience: among these was a tooth powder, composed of pounded brickbats and an ointment for the itch, sore eyes and a great variety of other complaints. The powder was not only capable

---

14. A charlatan and a pedlar of false cures.
15. Comic antics.

of keeping the teeth clean, but of curing the toothache; and as for *the tallow* (for I believe it was merely a transmogrification of candle-ends) the story of its virtues he never could find time enough to tell. With these and some other materials of a corresponding nature, he used to take his stand every market day upon a table, in the midst of a gaping and credulous crowd.

'Here you have my celebrated and inimitable dentrifice [toothpaste], formed of the most costly and choice ingredients. It will produce any effect that can possibly be wished for, excepting that of making new teeth grow in the place of old ones. God forbid that I should attempt to impose upon you so far as to pretend that it can work impossibilities! But everything that all other dentrifices put together can do, I pledge *my honour and credit* that this is competent to effect by itself,' &c &c. Then the greasy cylinders being displayed, the mode of using them for disorders of the eyes, for *la gale* [scabies] &c was exhibited by the vendor. How the fellow's assurance could hold out so firmly as to bring him, week after week, among the people whom he so grossly imposed upon, was perhaps not the least wonderful thing among his performances. But so it was, every Wednesday he was at his post and there were some of our officers who attended his demonstrations as regularly as many good people go to church.

One gentleman in the regiment who was very fond of fun and had a considerable turn for mimicry, never failed *Moustache*; and got so much into his favour, that whenever he saw him coming, he used to roar out, '*Place! Place! Pour Monsieur Le General!*' One day in particular I thought myself very fortunate in having nothing to do but attend the lecture; sales were brisk, the *onguent* [ointment] slipped away and the dentrifice was early exhausted. Pointing across the square he informed the audience that his *hotel* was close by, where he believed he still had a small supply of this invaluable preparation, with which he would shortly return and oblige them as far as he could. 'In the meantime,' said he to the captain, 'will you, *mon cher*, have the *amitie* to stay by my property till I come back? I shall be infinitely obliged and happy to do as much for you.' The good-natured captain cheerfully undertook the task, which he scrupulously executed.

It was rather provoking to find the suspicious curiosity with which we were followed about in this place. An officer in particular, could not appear out of doors without a train of followers, who seemed to be at a loss what to make of him; the impressions they had upon their minds, as to the military character of British troops, were to be sure of no great consequence, but they were both unpleasant and unfounded; nor were we at this time, among the partisans of a hostile service. The people were themselves by no means of military habits or pretentions, but exceedingly quiet and apparently kindly disposed. A short period however, served to shew them their error and in the meantime everything went on with harmony and mutual good understanding.

At the end of a week or ten days it began to rain and the state of the country became such that it was difficult, or at all events, disagreeable to communicate with the detached parts of the regiment. One squadron occupied a commune about a league distant, to which I was about this time sent. Dull as had been the town of Renaix [Ronse], it was perfect gaiety compared with my new quarters, in which I found five officers, who absolutely did not know how to pass the day and hailed my arrival as a great event. When the weather permitted (and such permission was not generally to be had after my exile among them) there was the blind wall of a large farmhouse, against which we were fain to knock a handball and deceive ourselves into a belief that we were in a racket court; but alas! the displeasure of the firmament soon deprived us of this resource; and while the bye-roads had become so boggy that repairing to Renaix [Ronse] was a thing not to be thought of and all intercourse with our friends there was cut off, (except by means of a messenger) we were driven to our billets, places where we should at any time, have thought it a grievance to be shut up at night, much more by day. There was nothing for it but invention; and we were reduced to the humiliating necessity of getting the boys of the place to purchase us some marbles, the only weapons of dissipation the little chandlers' shop afforded. These amused us on a barn floor for a day or two. Cards, billiards, books, all were inaccessible and everything around us was lowering, dull and dismal. Still however, we managed to get up what we called 'a mess'; and a queer mess it was.

In a little *cabaret*, there lived an ancient couple, *quasi* landlord and lady, the latter very much humped in the back, but imperturable in the temper. I believe *meine frau* was too proud ever to be angry. Like the rest of the *lordly* genus to which she belonged, she was tolerably well furnished with an opinion on her own behalf and would not be put out of her way. These good people agreed to furnish as good dinners as Belgium could produce, for a sum very moderate in *our* estimation; but which no doubt, in their eyes appeared magnificent. The whole time of the poor little frau was taken up in the serious and formidable business of the *cuisine*, stewing, roasting and boiling till that reasonably late hour at which English gentlemen could, without a breach of etiquette, give relief to the cravings of appetite. Oh! what joy it was to approach near six o'clock! The hour came and with it the soup and bouilli and a great variety of other preparations: but one day was still more like another than the trees along the high road that have been spoken of. *Toujours perdrix*![16] or rather something less acceptable. No remonstrances were available; they were listened to by madame at night, but no alteration appeared on the morrow. At length we thought we had devised a scheme which would infallibly produce some change in our commons, if only for a single occasion. The scheme was this.

The Duke of Wellington having occasion to pass through Oudenarde [Oudenaarde], wished to see the troops which were in the neighbourhood and our regiment with some others, was assembled for the purpose. The night before we informed our hostess that she must positively exert her utmost culinary skill on the ensuing day, as we expected His Excellency to dine with us, ordinary things would not do; and we did not mind some extra expense. She promised fair and kept her word. Many mysterious hints were dropped as to the agreeable surprise prepared for us. We should see in due time, the Duke would be astonished and the *chef de cuisine* immortalised. We had to go home, however, *without* the Duke, a circumstance that admitted of very easy explanation and which did not in fact, seem to be regarded as of any great importance. The good wife's head was full of her own exploit, and we were rather curious to know what was in the wind. Six o'clock came and we assembled for the grand occasion. We began as usual: but this would not do, of course; so there was reservation of corners for the *grand coup*. It was brought in with all due ceremony and solemnity in the form of a huge, unwieldy, shapeless *gateau*, upon which the regimental device had been copied from a soldier's button, pricked with a skewer by the hand of the dame. This was a complete hoax in return; bad as our fare had been, it was now all

---

16. Literally 'Always partridge' meaning always the same

the worse for the abstinence we had observed. We tried the experiment of variety on another occasion, by telling her we expected the Prince of Orange. No better success, the remains of the duke's *gateau* constituted the only deviation.

A laughable little incident occurred on the occasion of the Duke's arrival, in the tribulation of a shoemaker from Renaix [Ronse] who recounted to us, with deep chagrin and considerable pathos, the misfortunes which had attended his laborious endeavours to get a sight of the great English general. In the first place he had made a holiday and dressed himself in his Sunday clothes in honour of the occasion and had left home at a very early hour, in order to be at the place where he had been informed that His Grace had staid [*sic*] all night, ere the Duke could possibly leave it in the morning. Thither he trudged hastily and arrived just in time to learn the mortifying intelligence that the Duke was gone to inspect some fortified place a few miles off. His courage was yet fresh and he followed. Gone again! Which way? To Oudenarde [Oudenaarde], oh, all is now right, that is where the troops are to assemble and it is near home. Arrived at Oudenarde [Oudenaarde] just too late to catch a view there, but the soldiers were within a few yards of the town and the general was on his way to them. 'Sure of him at last, need not hurry now, don't care about the troops, can see them any day at home and a review is a capital occasion; the general having to stand still all the time.' But poor Crispin was not aware that we were merely to be looked at, as we were drawn up by the roadside, while the general passed along the line. So that when he arrived, he had the misery to find the soldiers filing off to their quarters and to hear that the magnet of his attraction had betaken himself again to his travelling carriage, in which he was making the best of his way to dine with Louis XVIII at Ghent.[17]

It was no cause of regret to be ordered away from these dull and even dismal quarters. The demand for accommodation in the area, that is the country between us and the coast, had now become considerable, in consequence of the continued arrival of troops from England; and we

---

17. After the inspection Wellington was pleased to express his 'approbation of their appearance; that he was happy at having again under his orders, a corps which had always been distinguished for its gallantry and discipline and he did not doubt, should occasion offer, but it would continue to deserve his good opinion; and he hoped every man would feel a pride in endeavouring to maintain the reputation of the regiment.'

were moved onwards. In the course of our progress we passed one night in Ninove, a pleasant open town, situated on the Dender, in which the headquarters of the cavalry, under the command of Lord Uxbridge were afterwards established. Our ultimate destination however, was a rich agricultural district, about twelve miles from Bruxelles, in which there was excellent accommodation for the horses. We ourselves were (with the exception of one squadron) very much distributed and widely separated;[18] but this was hardly felt to be an inconvenience when the weather admitted of our moving about. There were no decorations of human origin within reach, but the face of nature was most richly ornamented with those appendages which a fruitful and well cultivated soil will ever produce, in return for the cares of industry. Majestic trees, here and there a thick grove and in some instances a deep forest, features essential to the very existence of the community, inasmuch as they furnished that source of comfort and even of maintenance which we in England have almost forgotten, since the *bowels* of the earth took the place of its surface, in the supply of fuel, luxuriant crops and abodes stored with plenty of all that man or beast could possibly require, were among the objects which it was pleasant to contemplate. The climate was agreeable and at this season uniformly genial. Nightingales were every evening to be heard in all directions, not one here and there but full *choruses* of these melancholy and pleasing little minstrels.

Perhaps I may be allowed to attempt a sketch of the family in which I took up my own abode and among whom I remained with great contentment till the sound of war reached their peaceful domicile and rendered my departure inevitable.

The farm was extensive; the house and offices were large and substantial.[19] The notion of *a gentleman* farmer would have been perfectly incomprehensible to the worthy inhabitants. Mine host was a man of about fifty years of age, his *frau* somewhat younger, who had probably been good looking some years back, for still she was *tolerable* and that is saying much for one of the Belgian fair. There were two grown lads, who assisted their sire in improving his store; and two daughters; the elder somewhat

---

18. The regiment was placed in numerous villages centred around Vollezele, where it arrived before 25 May. Lieutenant William Hay records that they were assembled twice a week for field exercise.
19. This farm was at Tollembeek, two miles from Vollezele.

attractive for a paysanne, the younger not yet either one thing or another, a child running about as wild as a calf and indulged considerably in her little fancies. The elder sister (whose name was Dinah or Diana) had charge of the dairy and the poultry; churned or perhaps rather salted the butter after churning, saw the eggs properly laid, directed the marketing department and made a belle of herself of an evening; [in] short, Dinah was *naturally* fond of dress and particularly of articles that flared and glared. I presented her upon one occasion, with a silk handkerchief, which had been intended for a billet upon my own pocket. Dinah however, put it round her handsome neck and paraded it at church on the following Sunday. She was really handsome, endowed with great good humour and sweetness of temper of a most obliging disposition, but always with an eye open to the 'main chance'. Although *cream* was as plentiful about the premises as ditchy water, I never could obtain as much as I wanted for my breakfast, till I got sufficiently into Miss Dinah's good opinions, to be trusted with it and as for *fresh butter*, it was long indeed ere I could convince her, all disposed as she was to be hospitable (that is for a con-si-de-ra-tion) that it was possible to keep a little bit for *me* out of the salt. Quantities were made every morning, but as fast as *they came*, they were prepared for exportation by being laden with rock salt, in great lumps or crystals.

I once had a few of my brother officers to dine and to eke out the festival, I made an overture to miss for a couple of fowls. They were granted without hesitation and were the very fattest that could be found at the barn door. On requesting afterwards, to know what I had to pay for them, I was charged the enormous sum of two francs![20]

The household (including labourers and one very handsome young female servant) lived all together, and fared the same as to diet, though not in point of lodging. They all observed the Spanish custom of taking a *siesta* after dinner, the members of the family within doors and the employees without; I used to see the boors lying about the farmyard during the heat of the day; and having suspended my too capacious tent to the branch of an apple tree in the orchard, I often took advantage of its seclusion to repair thither, for the purpose of writing.

Two circumstances raised me very high in the estimation of these worthy people. It was clover harvest and the younger son having fallen asleep upon

---

20. Note by Smith – The franc was then current for 11d in Belgium [about £5 today].

a heap of newly cut grass, was brought home in a state of insensibility, to the great distress of a very affectionate, though by no means fuss-making family. Not being applied to for professional assistance and concluding that their medical attendant would be sent for, I considered it improper to interfere and left them to take their own course. This appeared to be a very simple one, consisting in looking at the sick man and occasionally giving him a very useless shake by the shoulders, calling upon him at the same time by name. But poor Peter would not *'come when they did call for him.'* He remained in a state of stupor all the rest of the day and in the course of the night, instead of sending for the doctor, a messenger was dispatched for the priest. I confess that I felt considerable anxiety about the poor fellow, who I now saw stood a foul chance of losing his life, through the misguided economy, stupidity or superstition of his parents; and as soon as the priest had taken leave, I entered the sick chamber and inquired what they were doing for him. As a reason for not calling in a professional man, they declared that it could be of no service, on account of his dangerous state. To this sort of logic, I could not possibly agree and having expressed my confidence that there was more than a chance of saving him, if they would even now, let me try my skill, notwithstanding the ceremony of extreme unction, after which, in some places a heretic might have incurred the vengeance of the church for interfering; the father overruled the mother and authorised me to act as I thought proper. My remedies were successful; Peter recovered his faculties; the thing was considered all but, if not quite a miracle; and I suppose the priest wished the whole of us in purgatory. Although they were a very quiet set and said little, I learnt not only from my servant, (who was regularly inducted into the family circle), but from a variety of signs and testimonials, that I had risen 100 per cent in their estimation. Even the handsome Dinah threw off a considerable portion of her maidenly reserve and national indifference and I verily believe, that I *might* have been successful, had I proposed to qualify her for receiving the pension of a British officer's widow. But not to mention other drawbacks, Dinah in common with the young women of the country, was apt to display an accomplishment, which would have been fatal to domestic peace and comfort, according to *English* notions. Now reader, I will give you as many guesses as you please, but (unless you are that very servant to whom allusion has just been made) you will not stumble on the truth. Did she drink? Nothing I will stake my credit, stronger than skimmed milk. Did she scold? I never heard her raise her voice above its proper level nor did I ever catch her speaking at all, unless it was necessary. Was she unruly? Undutiful to her parents? O dear no: she was their invaluable deputy and much and justly regarded as a kind superintendent of all. Did she encourage young gentlemen? Fie for shame! And *myself* in the house? O, no, no, nothing of that sort. There never came a suitor near the place (whatever may have been the cause) during six weeks or thereabouts, that I was in it: Dinah seemed to be too busy with household cares and occupations to have given much of her time to tender claims. I apprehend that the course of these affairs is rather more sluggish [than] it may be, but also more smooth in the Low Countries; while we poor victims of passion and feeling, are accustomed to go mad and commit ten thousand extravagances. I presume our friends under notice would make a prudent bargain and trust to providence for a sufficient store of *ex post facto* love, to churn and sell butter, to gather fresh eggs and see the fields properly manured. What then, was the grand objection in this case? Was it to yourself, doctor, personally? I think not: for upon the only occasion I ever seized to '*ravish a kiss*,' Smollett somewhere says,[21] I met with no opposition. Besides, I was then only twenty-five, my birthday came round while I was under her father's roof; and though never what may be called handsome, I had youth, health and appearance on my side. Nor had they conceived so very awful an idea of my rank and consequence as would have flabbergasted them. I never studied to be what is called *high*; it would not be natural in me; I am fond of *fun* and seek for it still in all quarters. But I believe I may as well reveal. Mademoiselle (whose cognomen I have been striving, in vain to call to recollection) had been misguided in her *musical education*. She did not play upon the *harp*, nor the *musical glasses*, nor did she *sing*. Still, she had a fancy in the melodious line, *she whistled*! Fact! At all hours and on all occasions, Dinah was whistling, always the same tune and never more than the first part of it.

As a proof of the simplicity of these people and at the same time as an exemplification of the power of curiosity over the female mind, I may allude to a little incident which occurred during my stay. I have already spoken of the tent: that was a great magnet. Everyone who came to the farm was taken to the orchard to see it. As in consequence of its being

---

21. *Tobias Smollett.*

suspended, the pole was not required for its support, there was room for a large table and this was so very great a novelty that sometimes the servants used to steal in to take their dinner upon it. But there was another part of my equipment which astonished them to a much higher degree, this was the *canteen*. Within the compass of a small chest, intended for conveyance on a pack-saddle, was almost everything required for the culinary and menial accommodation of three persons. Such an effort of ingenuity had never been dreamt of in Belgium. Dinah, her mother, her sister, the maid, the father, the brothers, were all confounded, as (article after article) the contents were displayed before them; nor did it end here, for the news spread through the village and many modest hints were given, how much it would oblige if it were possible for a friend who had just dropped in, to be indulged with a glance. I was compelled to delegate my servant to be show-man and I apprehend that John was not displeased with the troublesome office.

Judging from what I saw among these people, they are better off than any other of the same class, whom I have had an opportunity of observing. What might have been the case in Portugal and Spain, before those countries were scourged and devastated by the war which raged so long in them, probably few among us know; we saw misery enough, poverty, with its full train of evils, hunger, nakedness and wandering met us at every step; but I am inclined to think that both the wants and the supplies of the Portuguese in particular, were at all times few. Their country favoured no doubt, in the article of climate, had received little cultivation, though their cities had been enriched by their commercial enterprises. Portugal may be said to produce no corn, no wheat certainly: olives, maize, and pumpkins I have seen growing together in one field; but the whole had the aspect of a sluggard's garden and nature unassisted, seemed to be left to execute her own unchanging agricultural projects as she pleased. From the olive comes the oil for the lamp and for the salad; the maize or Indian corn, when ground and made into bread, I never could eat: horse-beans or dried peas, would furnish an article equally palatable and in my judgement, equally nutritious; for horses it answers very well, particularly when boiled soft. Lean animals I have seen grow fat upon this provender; but because beans act as a powerful stimulus upon them, who would think of such as a substitute for wheat, oats, or even barley? In their beverage these poor people are accustomed to a thin griping wine at the best; and often have I seen the market-folk (who by the way at the time in question, mustered chiefly of the female sex, the men being engaged in the service of their country) squat down to a watermelon, a gourd or a pumpkin; or if a little more luxury was within the reach of their means, it consisted of a lump of yellow bread made from Indian corn, a solitary salted sardinha [sardine].

How the peasantry live in England need not be particularly alluded to, bacon, good wheaten bread, puddings and beer; these form a staff which it is not easy to break. In Scotland, the people are, perhaps not quite so actively laborious. But what does this result from? A less stimulating diet? Or does the *moral* cause operate? Do they eat less (in quality, if not quantity) because they work less? I leave the question to *commissioners of supply* and shall add a few words on the habits of *les Belges*, in collateral circumstances.

My farmer (I wish I could remember his name, for I am confident that it carried the prefix, *le* or *de*) was a sensible man in his station. The lands he cultivated were rich and productive; a considerable part of them lay along the little river Dender and they were all turned to good account. How the relationship between landlord and tenant stood I do not know; but to the best of my recollection, there had been an hereditary contract. He spoke French better than the rest of his family, for they were all *Flams*, and even Dinah could not maintain a conversation in this common currency of European lingo. As for little *Nellikin* the younger sister, she hardly knew six words of the currency and proposed to teach me *Flams spraeken* [to speak Flemish], in which I did take a few lessons from her till I found out that *fingers* were *fingers* in Brabant as well as in England,[22] and so with

---

22. Note by Smith – I can hardly resist the temptation to introduce an anecdote, the subject of which took place several years before, in a general hospital, of which I had the superintendence, in the Peninsula. I had a Scotch orderly, a Glasgow man, who was amazingly fond of snuff and alcohol (that modification of it called whiskey being pro tem out of his reach). However, my coadjutor required great watching, for he was the main prop of the hospital during my inevitable absences. On a certain morning I found that several men of the German Legion had been admitted; and that one in particular was dangerously ill, to the best of my recollection of typhus fever. Anxious to know the precise state of my patient and unable to converse with him to my own satisfaction, I proclaimed for an interpreter. A non-commissioned officer made his appearance and said he could do the required duty. Mustard, my Glasgow man, followed me to the bedside with a tray of medicines and surgical appliances and lent a most attentive ear to the colloquy. My questions were such, that, in translating them for the understanding of the patient, there appeared to be little or no change. *Mustard* at length grew quite

regard to other things. Madame, *meine frau*, could talk a little, so far as on a Sunday, when there was most regularly, if not religiously, a pot of stewed veal on the fire, to ask me if she might presume to send me a bit. I seldom declined, partly because I should have given pain, partly because I was generally disposed for luncheon about the time of their dinner and partly because my man John was at hand and his rations barely furnished him a constant table. John however was free of the house and I should be depriving my readers of a great deal of honest entertainment and all officers and military servants of a most distinguished exemplar, did I not make him the subject of separate notice, if not even of a separate chapter; but this is a question to be decided hereafter.

The whole family were peasants in their aspect, but of an order quite superior in their ideas and manners. On Sunday they gathered their household together, not for any purpose of religious worship as in Scotland is the custom, but to eat a good dinner; and I never at this hour passed through the kitchen (which I was under the necessity of doing in order to get out of the house) but I saw John, in a conspicuous situation at the board. This perhaps, I was in some degree entitled to take as a compliment to myself; but John had pretentions of his own, he was *a character*. Upon all such occasions Pa and Ma (but never Dinah) and the sons (but never the servants) rose and asked me to take a seat and partake. Of course, there were three hundred and sixty-six reasons why this was impracticable: but there was kindness in the invitation and would have been attention beyond their ordinary habits had it been accepted.

I have already said that I spent about six weeks in this hospitable house; and in the course of that time I believe that not only my own conduct, but that of my servant, was so free from objection that we might have remained among them with a cordial welcome, for as many years. Indeed, it will be seen, as this narrative advances, that they were truly *good people*. A bad servant, particularly on active service, often makes his master's quarters intolerable and untenable; but I was blessed with one whose value I early learnt to appreciate and whose peculiarities I shall take some opportunity to describe.

---

indignant; and pushing the German sergeant aside, he exclaimed; 'Get oot, ye stupid bitch, the doctor can speak as gude German as that himsel'. I afterwards consulted some officers of *the legion* and they assured me that the affinity of the queries in the two languages was so close, that they must have appeared to be identical to an uneducated mind.

# Chapter 3

# Preparations for War

This was our last move, till we took the field on the 16th of June. A few events however, occurred, which I may record by way of preliminaries to this important change in our position. Leaving therefore, the household *goddesses*, I shall remark that our colonel was most indefatigable in keeping the regiment in the most effective possible state. He was the mildest of men, while he was the best of officers. I shall never forget a punishment that took place at a watering parade.[1] The surgeon had gone upon leave for a few days to Brussels and I had strolled into the headquarter village, to give a look at the hospital, (where there was not much to be encountered in the shape of sickness) when a sergeant hailed me with a peremptory order from the commanding officer to repair to an adjacent wood, where part of the regiment was assembled and a punishment was to take place, if a surgeon could be found. We rode fast down several flights of steps formed by the entangling roots of the trees, as they interlaced themselves across a very precipitous footpath. I gave up my neck as a likely forfeit; but the sergeant rode like Mazeppa[2] and for fear of losing the way, as well as of being late, I was fain to follow: indeed, I do not believe that I could have pulled up the fury I was mounted upon, with the example she had before her. However, we arrived safely in a glade where everything was ready, the drumhead court martial over and the result only waiting our arrival. It was the only occasion upon which I ever saw the colonel present at a punishing parade. He never *flogged*; but several men had come drunk to their duty and being daily exposed to the chance of contact with the enemy, an example was required. He stood close to the culprits, refused all solicitations on the part of their captains

---

1. Note by Smith – Every dismounted reader may not understand by this, a parade or assembly of the horses (going to drink) without saddles, there being nothing on their backs but a folded blanket. This is a cavalry custom, observed everywhere, at home as well as abroad and it affords an easy opportunity for the officers to ascertain accurately the state of the animals, whether they have sore backs &c.
2. The hero of a romantic poem written by Lord Byron in 1819.

(a thing that on other occasions he never failed to attend to) and seemed as anxious that every lash should be well laid on, as if the whole safety and credit of the British army depended upon it.

For my own part, (while on this painful subject) I beg to say, that during the period of my connection with this admirably managed corps, I attended the great majority of the punishments, from my being generally stationed at headquarters. When I joined the regiment, I was not quite a novice in matters of military professional duty and had seen something of this kind of service. *Taking a man down*, who could have endured the award of a court martial, is a thing out of the medical province; and the delinquents soon found that appeals went for nothing unless they could be reconciled to my duty as an officer. I have been obliged to take men down before the infliction of a *hundred lashes* and I have seen *a thousand* well laid on without injury to the prisoner. If, after touching his hat to the commanding officer and stating that in his judgement the man could not receive any further punishment at *that time*, the punishment should be persevered in, the surgeon would be warranted to turn away and protest that he cannot be responsible for the sequel. But in this corps, no such thing was ever imagined; and never was a man during my knowledge of it, held under a threat of a renewal of his punishment. The men at the same time, knew these matters to be conducted by rules both of duty and humanity: they felt assured that there would be no danger to their lives or ulterior safety and submitted to the *pain* of the chastisement as well as they could.[3]

---

3. Note by Smith – I am unwilling to introduce irrelevant matter either into the text, or in the form of notes; but as the question of military punishment is one which has excited a good deal of sensation, both in parliament and elsewhere, I beg, as a person who has seen much of it and considered the merits of the affair with some attention, to add an observation or two.
   a. Soldiers are not subjected to the passions and caprices of individuals. An officer dare not strike a soldier; a commanding officer has no power to inflict anything in the shape of corporal punishment; that must be awarded by the solemn sentence of a court martial, every member of which acts under the moral, religious and *legal* responsibility of *an oath*.
   b. The punishment is confessedly *painful*; but what punishment is intended to be agreeable? It is said to be *degrading*, ought not convicts *to be* degraded? It has been argued that such measures break the spirit of free-born Englishmen and lower them to the level of the beasts. Now I will take license to say that in the best regulated corps in the service there are *mauvais sujets* [worthless individuals], perfectly insensible to the calls of honour or the feelings of delicacy which operate upon the generous minds of the majority of their comrades. Besides, during war the recruiting resources of our

The cavalry, as all the world knows, was commanded by the Earl of Uxbridge, whose gallant conduct obtained for him his present elevation in the peerage.[4] The first time we saw him *in officio* was upon a large meadow, shortly afterwards the scene of a very brilliant display. Here we were assembled a few times to rehearse for a review, which was to take place by Prince Blucher and the Duke of Wellington, of all the *mounted* troops of the British army. The meadow or field, was called Schendelbeck [Schendelbeke] and though of such extent that the crop of grass was said to have been bought at Lord U[xbridge]'s private cost for five hundred pounds,[5] the cavalry were drawn up in three lines, with the horse artillery between them. The day of the review was remarkably fine and the scene altogether extremely imposing. Blucher, till now I had never seen and although there was nothing surprising in the circumstances, I was struck with the contrast between his plain aspect and the brilliancy of his cortege. He wore the general's hat and drooping feather, a green coat (which at the time we thought looked old and threadbare) with one star, the only decoration. But there was an eye under that brow which looked us through and an illumination upon that veteran countenance which anticipated the glorious results that were shortly afterwards realised.

---

country are so limited by legislative enactment and by jealousy and prejudice, that the best characters in the realm do not offer for the ranks of the army. For the present it is confessedly different; but let a war, like that of the Peninsula break out and see then what sort of volunteering recruits we shall have.

c. It has been argued that there is no flogging in the French army. I dare say not; but is there no capricious exercise of authority? No vindictive feelings between individual officers and individual men? Look to their discipline and a striking proof of their inferiority of system is obvious. And do they not *take a life* for what would be a venial crime in our estimation?

d. In England this ordeal can be dispensed with; there are treadmills and solitary cells, to which by the Mutiny Act, courts martial can sentence delinquents. But on active service what can be done with such? Keep them constantly in arrest? March them about with a second set of prisoners in the shape of a guard? Absurd! Flog them off and hand them over to the surgeon to be placed upon low diet and under stoppages, which these gentry like worse than the cat-o'-nine tails.

Some years ago a discussion was raised in the House of Commons upon this question and an instance was adduced of a soldier having died in consequence of receiving a punishment of this nature; but the truth of the matter was that the coroner's jury returned an absurd verdict. The accident which occasioned his death might not have been attended with fatal consequences had the punishment not been inflicted, but this had no *direct* concern with the man's fate.

4. Henry Paget, Earl of Uxbridge became 1st Marquess of Anglesey soon after Waterloo.
5. About £25,000 in today's terms.

The two field marshals went down the ranks and the regiments then marched past. There was no manoeuvring. The king of the Netherlands and the Prince of Orange were among the spectators but took no part in the ceremonial. The shew [*sic*] we understood, was got up for the Prussian hero; and I suspect he considered he had a treat.

According to the etiquette of our army, the *wooden* officers (viz the non-combatants and the Staff collectively), are more politely accommodated in the cavalry on such occasions, than are their brethren of the infantry. We are placed on the right flank of the regiment, next to the music and in the front line, so that we have in fact, the very best place for gratifying curiosity; and when the marching past commences, we are expected to get *out of the way*. This getting out of the way commonly consisted in moving as near to the reviewing general as possible, so that the poor doctors, if they managed well, might get into conversation with some very great man in the train.[6] My clever friend, Jack B [James Castley], had a particular knack of hooking himself to *a prince*. I believe that on a subsequent occasion, of a corresponding nature, he spent great part of a morning comparing notes with Schwartzenberg.[7] No man was better able to furnish the information such people naturally wish to have, for he knew almost if not quite, as much about the character and economy of the army, as if he had been the commander of the forces. Jack and

---

6. Note by Smith – The surgeons, farriers and the band, having no manoeuvres to perform, dispose of themselves the best way they can till the drill is over. One day an accident occurred and no medical assistance being visible, the commanding officer (rather a dry humourist) shouted, 'Where are the physicians? Playing cards I suppose with the farriers in the ditch.' I beg to add however, that this did not occur in *my time*. The brigade drills, during the greater part of our stay in France (and of which I shall have anecdotes enough to relate hereafter) took place twice or thrice a week. A medical officer from each regiment was always present. The *stick*, or Staff of the whole field, was in the habit of congregating and talking nonsense, or listening to the united band. Long and wearisome as sometimes were our marches to and fro (for fifteen miles or five leagues, went for nothing) I refer to these occasions as some of the most agreeable among my 'hours of *idlesse*.' Upon the days in question I had either to rise early or ride hard. The surgeon seldom went; so Murphy [Egan] and myself had to attend alternately. It would frighten a holiday field of spectators at Hounslow from their property, did such a sight present itself as forty or fifty men and horses tumbling and rolling over one another in a charge. But this I have seen and been alarmed enough, though it turned out that there was no real occasion. On proceeding to the spot I have found all parties safe and sound; and I will venture to remark that the casualties are in the inverse ratio of the accident. The more falls the fewer fractures.
7. Austrian Field Marshal Karl Philipp, Prince of Schwarzenberg.

I spent a great deal of our time together; and I used to be amused and edified beyond expression with his details, after returning from a grand review. He was always close to the general's tail; in fact, he had nothing to do while occasionally a job fell to my share, through a tumble or some other casualty and I was on all occasions, obliged to be within call of the regiment. The day of Schendelbeck [Schendelbeke] passed over and we returned to our busy note of preparation, to sharpening sabres, to the cultivation of *moustache*, &c.

Here let me deprecate of all gallant soldiers, if I record an act of absurdity on the part of the wooden gentlemen already quoted. We now turned our attention to our upper labia; and in a few weeks there was as inconvenient an appendage to my own mouth as I could well have devised: however, there were these things to be said for us;

1. We had, at that time, no distinction of uniforms; the cocked hats, long coats and bare shoulders[8] were introduced two years afterwards; at the period of which I am now speaking we had the chaco [shako], the pelisse, the dress jacket and epaulets, and in short everything but the pouch-belt, like the other officers; consequently, as the adoption of the *moustache* by one set and the omission of it by another, wearing the same garb would have looked ridiculous in the eyes of the strangers we expected to come into frequent contact with, it was better as it was.
2. The vanity of human nature might be pleased, but.
3. The new fashion superseded the regular daily use of the razor, of which for one, I felt the benefit, when barbers were scarce. Things are odious (as they are otherwise) by comparison; a long beard at Almack's[9] would have been a short one at Waterloo and this is a word which ought to cover a multitude of transgressions.

---

8. Smith's comment: The epaulets have been recently restored. The doctors, the paymaster and the quartermaster, were at this time *put into* long coats and cocked hats; but there were distinctions even among *these*. The lordly *payeur* was allowed a *star loop* upon his hat and gold rosettes at its *gutters*. The *quartermaster* was the only person to whom was permitted the distinction of a *feather*. We the masters of health, had plain hats, black rosettes and black loops. If the authorities had even left us the *black* feather, we should have cried a *peccavi* [a cry in acknowledgement of sin] less; but they left us nothing whatever 'to flout' withal.
9. William Almack's Assembly rooms in King Street, London, became the most select of London high society.

*We* (the wooden ones) wore the bristles through the active part of the campaign and for some months afterwards; when upon the pleas that we were mere *lookers-on* and not performers, we were allowed to apply the scissors. Larry Murphy [Patrick Egan], who was not one of the original *moustaches*, held out for years, but the girls at Canterbury wrought his reformation at last and I was surprised to see him one day properly shaved.

It is my professed purpose to introduce the reader to a knowledge of *little* circumstances, which transpired behind the grand and magnificent scenery already so often and so ably exhibited to view. I decline saying all that I could perhaps, about the mighty operations in which I did perform a part, though considered a humble one. If any are to be benefited by my revelations, it will be those who follow and not those who lead troops into scenes of deadly operations. To such therefore and in particular to young medical officers what immediately follows is especially addressed.

As relates to the army, I never rose high in the profession; nor do I think I should have entered the service (which I did in 1811), had there been other means of seeing the world; but our country was then at war with the whole of it nearly; and my friends judged it desirable that I should pass the early part of my professional life in some way calculated for improvement. The army was decided upon, and the peninsula was my early destination. Fortune I had none and few medical officers possess that passport to ruin, I say 'passport to ruin', as regards *them* only and my reasons for saying so require no explanation. During several years' service in Portugal, my opportunities of acquiring professional tact and experience were almost singular; but at length the war even there came to a close and I settled down as the reader is aware, into a regimental medical officer, where there was little indeed to do.

The army is a useful school, and there was a time when any diligent and zealous officer, of whatever branch, had it in his own power to become distinguished and to gain for himself valuable friends. If, under a state of matters so much happier for general society, the encouragement has abated, there is nothing to regret. The demand for medical officers is less; let the supply diminish accordingly and all will be as it should be. The profession is glutted and its respectability is thereby necessarily lowered.

I speak however, of the civil branch and not of the military; for well am I aware, that the existing medical officers of the army, are fully entitled to carry their heads to their height.

One of the *little* circumstances I wish to introduce, relates to my own economy and proceedings. I may do this with the greater consistency, perhaps as I am engaged in a merely personal narrative. About the period of the transactions last described, my best horse fell lame, 'Fury', to wit. Another, the very contrast of this creature, I had sold to Growler [William Otway], intending to replace him with two inferior brutes and had made some progress to that effect, by purchasing a baggage animal, which was no sooner seen than coveted. Him therefore, I was urged to part with, rather advantageously as to price, but unfortunately for my own convenience, at such a juncture, I was now absolutely dismounted and although it is the fashion in the cavalry to say that any horse will do for a surgeon. I beg to observe, that this is neither correct nor considerate. The figure and the attitude may be of comparatively little consequence; but the man must be mounted so as to be able to follow the regiment. If they once get away from him, he may find it a hard matter to overtake them, if set upon 'a sorry hack.'

For the present, I was therefore obliged to avail myself of the kindness of a friend, who had a supernumerary on his establishment, with which I contrived to get through my duty, but which was by no means a desirable article to be called one's own. It was a Belgian cob, gifted with the dangerous and abominable accomplishment of rearing.[10] Upon one occasion, he rose to such a perpendicular at the sight of a water wheel, that I slipped out of the saddle, over his tail and before I knew what was the matter, found myself standing on my own two feet behind him, with the reins in my hand. I might have seized the opportunity of attempting a cure, by what is called checking him over; but we were upon a paved road and the beast was not my own. It is said that this trick is an effectual remedy for the vice in question; but it requires considerable coolness and

---

10. Note by Smith – An accomplished cavalier told me that the cure for *rearing* is not generally known, that checking over, hitting between the ears, even breaking a bottle of water upon a horse's sconce, will all fail; and that the best scheme is to be provided with an acute pair of rowels. Being so, let him rise, hang on the best way you can and (as he cannot rise a second time till he touches the ground) just before his feet reach terra firma *ram the spurs into his flanks*, and give him a burst. He is thereby both astonished and defeated at once.

presence of mind for its performance. In doing it the rider runs no risk after being dismounted: but to get clear of the saddle, in the necessary manner, is not always a certain thing.[11]

---

11. Note by Smith – It consists in the simple act of pulling the animal over by a sudden and sharp jerk of the bridle: he falls on his back and is so much surprised that he is reluctant to place himself in the way of meeting with a similar accident again. There is nothing of which horses have more dread than falling; and it is said that no horse will fall, *if he can help* it. The check, or *chuck*, in question, can only be done when mounted in a common saddle, over the cantle of which the rider is sure to slip if he takes his feet out of the stirrups. The danger from a rearing horse is great, when a hussar saddle is used for then, if the reins are not dropped, the animal may be pulled *upon* the rider, as he cannot slip over that sort of saddle.

# Chapter 4

# War Clouds Gather

I must proceed however, to matters of more general interest, lest I be accused of twaddling. Pleasant as my domicile may appear to have been, I grew weary of its monotony; and having dined with the officers belonging to a collected squadron within my district, upon the 15th of June (Thursday) I resolved to take up my abode among them; for the village was lively and the mess afforded society. Upon this occasion, bets were for the next six weeks; we considered ourselves to be merely an army of observation to keep off intruders till the Austrian and Russian forces should be able to retrace their steps. Bonaparte however, viewed the matter in another light and had that very day shewn our allies of Prussia, that he was neither asleep nor paralytic.

Early on the following morning,[1] my servant entered the room while I was yet unconscious and announced that [Cornet Lockhart][2] had sent for the horse, as there was an order to march immediately. From that hour one trouble assailed me after another, for a series of many weeks, a crowd of difficulties immediately presented themselves to my imagination. A lame charger and no baggage animals, literally *caught napping*, what was to be done? Having repaired to the quarters of the senior officer (which were nearest my own) all I could learn was that we were to remove with the baggage to Enghien, where further news would in all probability be obtained. In the meantime, we conjectured that the object was merely a shift of quarters.

---

1. Lieutenant William Hay states that the order was received at Vollezele at 3 am. Lieutenant Colonel Frederick Ponsonby had attended the Duchess of Richmond's Ball. Hay states that he was also invited but did not go, but his name does not appear on any invitation list.
2. From further comments made later, it is clear that he hoped to ride a horse belonging to one of the two subalterns who were subsequently killed at Waterloo (Lieutenant Bertie and Cornet Lockhart). He also describes him as 'young man' making it far more likely that he was talking of Cornet John Lockhart, the only Cornet serving with the regiment at Waterloo.

Returning to the farm and fain to believe that things were really as they had been surmised, I announced the event thus to my host; requesting that he would lend, or let upon hire, two of his husbandry horses to convey my servant and baggage to the nearest town, where I could deposit the latter in the track of further conveyance and manage as the case might require. For, although my stud was thinned, my purse was far heavier than usual, having the price of the animals disposed of still in possession. The honest fellow accommodated me not only with the beasts as an act of kindness, but with his oldest son, who was to bring them back when the job should be concluded. As to myself, I resolved to do the best I could with the lame mare [Fury] and had her caparisoned accordingly. I certainly did mount and rode about a furlong[3] in the course of which I had so many escapes from broken knees on her part and a broken head or neck on my own, that I was fain to get down again, being convinced that, only for the fashion's sake it was pleasanter walking. Walk the residue of the march to Enghien[4] I did, holding the bridle and dragging myself and my charger as well as I could, after a regiment of light dragoons.

At Enghien, the brigade assembled[5] and on the countenances of most there appeared to be an impression I had not seen before. Here the news reached us of the defeat of the Prussians the day before, at Ligny;[6] and as the report of the disaster had not been diminished by a journey of thirty or forty miles, it was remarked that 'things looked very black'. We went on and as we advanced, other parts of the cavalry joined the line of march, till at length the whole mounted force was brought together, including of course, the troops of horse-artillery attached to the various brigades. Still toiling on with the lame animal, which I found it impossible to ride, I was told by a fine young officer to whom allusion has been made[7] and who was about to perform one of the last kind actions of his life, that his servant was coming up with a led horse, which I might mount. Grateful

---

3. An eighth of a mile.
4. Note by Smith – Perhaps it may be right to observe, once and for all, that where the *names* of places appear, as connected with the busy affairs we were now entering upon, they were generally obtained afterwards. At the time we were often under mistakes and sometimes did not learn names at all.
5. Lieutenant William Hay states that the regiment arrived at Enghien at 9 am, when the horses were fed corn, and they remained there until 12 am.
6. He must mean Charleroi as the Battle of Ligny had yet to commence that day.
7. As having been of the Bromley party.

and joyful, I halted for the arrival of the baggage. My own servant and the young farmer came up and I stopped them, as a matter of precaution, as well as for the purpose of handing over the mare to my man as soon as the other horse should make his appearance.

This occurred in the village of Steinkirk [Steenkirk], celebrated in the history of battles.[8] I took my place at the window of an auberge, where for several hours, the troops continued to pass without the arrival of the relief I was so anxiously expecting. The landlord was a veteran soldier: he told me that he had seen the finest troops in Europe, but nothing to compare with what he now beheld. He particularly complimented the horse artillery and who can look at them without admiration? The horses, the men, the *materiel*, the celerity of their movements and the beauty of their discipline, amount at all times to an *ensemble* of attraction, even where everything by which they are surrounded is of itself wonderful.

At length my patience began to diminish with great rapidity, and my anxiety to increase. By this time there were miles between my friends and myself, as well as thousands of other troops, whom it was impossible to pass unless I had happened to be acquainted with some bye road or near cut. As neither led horse nor man came in view, the alternative was to mount one of the plough beasts and proceed onward in reliance upon some change for the better arising out of the chapter of accidents. A change of saddles having been effected, I set forward upon the principle that 'they must be far behind who cannot follow;' but in the present instance there was a full illustration of another proverb, 'the more haste the worse speed.' The unwieldy brute proved so unmanageable among the brilliant company to which he was introduced, that to avoid putting the whole line in disorder, I was compelled to take the instruction of the commanding officer of a heavy [cavalry] regiment and let all the remainder pass. This rendered joining the front quite an impracticability, even under circumstances of the most favourable description. Situated as I now was, without knowledge of the country or any source of information, I might have wandered about all night and found myself no one knows where in the morning. Evening began to close in and at Nivelles I learnt that the cavalry had passed through at a quick pace, though too late to be concerned in the operations that had distinguished the memorable day of *Les Quatre Bras*.

---

8. Fought on 3 August 1692, a French victory in the Nine Years War.

Upon arrival at Nivelles I was told that many horses captured from the French, had been sent into the town in the course of the day; a hope accordingly darted through my mind that I should be able to get myself effectively mounted, for in my then situation I was an incumbrance in every respect. Some people whom I found at an auberge promised me relief without delay, but I either saw no more of them or met with excuses. Such was my desperate feeling at length on this subject, that I verily think had an opportunity offered, I should have borrowed an animal without leave of the owner. But every horse as well as every man, had his own business to perform and daylight found me in the same plight as it left me in: literally *saddled* with a Flanders' brute, at a time when it was likely that the best broke horse in England would not have been too good.

There was nothing for it but resignation and the chance of finding a spare animal with the regiment, provided I could find *it*. My distress was mainly enhanced by separation from my servant. When the time arrives for introducing this singular character to more particular notice, it will be seen how much my chances of success in horse dealing would have been increased by the aid of his experience and activity: besides which the bag of dollars[9] was in the canteen and in his custody. John[10] however, shifted for himself and company that night the best way he could; and with the exception of a transitory glimpse on the following morning, I saw nothing more of him for a month, during which, excepting always the few fighting and panic spreading days, he was snugly deposited with all the cattle and mein herr's son in the old farmhouse under the care of Dinah, Dinah's mother, father and the neighbourhood at large. There he wisely remained (he and the boy the wonders of all around them, in consequence of the highly important part they had performed during the campaign).[11]

---

9. Note by Smith – Five franc pieces rather.
10. His servant.
11. Note by Smith – The neighbourhood flocked to the farmhouse to contemplate these adventurers and hear the story of their 'hair-breadth escapes.' The young farmer, my man afterwards told me, would have left him in possession of the horses, if he could have provided for himself, but Chiswick would not part with him. To the honour of the people, I think it right to add, that none who came for news forgot to pay for them. A loaf, a lump of meat, a feed of corn for *Fury*, or a bottle of Rhenish [wine], was generally Chiswick's *douceur* for 'spinning his yarns.' He remained about three weeks there, till the mare recovered and an opportunity offered of their coming up with a detachment to Paris.

At an early hour next morning [17 June], I proceeded onward and soon found myself [at Quatre Bras] in the midst of a scene of which many descriptions had failed to convey to my own mind, anything like an accurate idea. Vast numbers of men were lying about in all directions and here and there inconsiderable groups. Some were employed in the melancholy office of carrying a wounded individual away in a blanket; others were digging graves and interring the dead. Some again were collected round a little column of smoke and were apparently engaged in cooking. There was no particular or general object going on and notwithstanding the multitude spread over the ground, there was little noise or bustle, but on the contrary, a marked air of desolation.[12]

The first object I recognised was an infantry officer of my acquaintance led from the field by a soldier, with his head bandaged and his face partly covered with clotted blood. It was not till afterwards that I was made certain as to his identity. I stumbled almost at once upon our brigade, they had sustained no casualty and though drawn up in line, seemed to have nothing of a precise nature either to do or to anticipate.[13] There was no one to be seen in the shape of an enemy, excepting the corpses of those who had fallen on the previous day; and about one spot it was estimated that not less than 1,000 cuirassiers were lying together. The British were masters of the field and the French were understood to occupy a wood in the front and to the left of our army.[14] The intermediate space (the arena of the contest) was an expanse of corn-land covered with a promising crop.

Upon the flank of our regiment was a farmhouse, close to the point where the roads by crossing each other, given the name of *Les Quatre Bras* to the place; but this was deserted and much dilapidated. It was now a temporary asylum for the wounded; and into one of the desolate apartments I was taken by some of our officers to see a captain of highlanders who had been mortally wounded by a musket-ball. His sufferings were so great, that to remove him would have been cruelty and

---

12. Note by Smith – Such was the *first impression* on viewing a field of battle, which the combatants had not yet left: it was a scene of silent but busy interest; and such as few have *stumbled on*.
13. The regiment had arrived at the battlefield in the late evening when the fighting had ceased. William Hay states that they had marched some 52 miles, but the route they took measures some 52km or 33 miles. He also states that the last ten miles were completed at the hand gallop (a fast canter or moderate gallop).
14. The French had retired to Hutte wood overnight.

yet to leave him was to the last degree painful. Professional aid could be of no service and we were taken out of the dilemma by his death, which relieved him in the course of the morning.

At an early hour a friend (of whom I shall have occasion to make repeated mention) presented himself in *mufti* and in search of surgical aid. I was rather surprised at his appearance; more so, as I knew he had no business to be where I found him. His appointment was *pro tem* of a civil cast and his station Brussels.

I asked of course, how he came to be there? He told a curious story of his having gone out for a ride, on the day preceding; but having heard there was a fight, he could not keep away; and rode out to Q[uatre] B[ras] from sheer curiosity. His commanding officer had caught him in the thick of the affair and ordered him to return; but through the friendship of the Quarter Master General[15] he had been permitted, as a matter of especial favour to see the show. He had met with a bruise from a tumbril and on account of that accident sought me out. On a future occasion we talked over this adventure and he related to me the following, among other circumstances of an interesting nature.

During the Quatre Bras business he never lost sight of the Duke; and once he observed His Grace lie down upon the ground, with the back of his head resting on his hands and his eyes fixed upon the heavens: aides de camp and others brought him intelligence incessantly and in that quiet posture he gave his orders. The coolness and self-possession manifested by this little *trait* admit of no illustration. Those however, who imagine that in order to command an army at any time and (among others) during an engagement, it is requisite to be in a fuss, flurry or filibuster, have no idea of the nature of events.

The other thing my friend informed me of, bordered rather on the ridiculous, (as the world may have been in the habit of receiving impressions on the perturbed state of Brussels at this critical period). I advised my patient to get home with all convenient speed and to apply certain remedies to the injury. He accordingly found his way back to Brussels and that same afternoon (Saturday the 17th) he deposited himself in a back street in this frantic town, where he was so fatigued and exhausted

---

15. The most senior officer in this department present was Deputy Quarter Master General Sir William Delancey.

that he sought repose. A profound sleep overtook him and he never heard a syllable about Waterloo, till Monday morning, when the *development* of the matter came in an authentic shape before him. The uproar and confusion which prevailed in the great thoroughfares of the capital do not seem to have reached the more recluse quarters; but the circumstance of an officer having remained undisturbed in such a situation is almost a pleasantry. The people of the house must either have been *super-Belgically* stupid, or supernaturally cool.[16]

---

16. Note by Smith – I find that I have been inaccurate in stating that my friend slept from Saturday till Monday. The fact *is that he enjoyed a sound nap, from Saturday night till the morning of Sunday was considerably* advanced; that he was up however, in good time to witness the commotion caused by the *panic* in Brussels; that in consequence of the rumour of defeat, he despatched his servants and baggage to Antwerp with the crowd and immediately sallied forth himself, armed *cap-a-pie* [From French – from head to foot] to join the British army. But from the way in which the road was choked up, as I have already described it, he could not possibly penetrate further than the valley, a little way beyond the *Porte de Namur*.

## Chapter 5

# Retreat

As the day advanced the serious business of the occasion began to develop itself. The infantry had commenced a regular march along the high road, in the direction of Brussels: and it must have been impossible for the enemy to decry what was going on. The cavalry were stationed across the field, (the road as is well known, forming part of it) in three lines[1] and (what has always appeared to me to have been a very curious and even beautiful arrangement) in the following manner. In front was a line of hussars and light horse: the second line was composed of heavy cavalry, the whole of which in the English service wear scarlet uniforms, with the exception of one regiment.[2] The third line consisted again of light dragoons, whose uniform is blue; and upon the left of this, *our* brigade was placed. Where the second line stood, the ground dipped, so that screened as the troops belonging to it were by the hussars in front, the red coats only could have been visible to the enemy, who not seeing the horses, must have been unable to tell whether they were cavalry or infantry, while this part of our force was steadily retiring to take up the position in front of *Waterloo*. The cause of this retreat I have nothing to say about, wishing and proposing as much as possible, to avoid entering upon matters out of my province. I merely witnessed that act of the performance of which I have spoken and merely what I have witnessed will I presume to recount.

The operations of a bloody field were to me quite a novelty; the whole of my service in the peninsula had been at General Hospital stations; but now I had new cares and novel sensations. The 17th of June was one of the longest days I ever passed. Expecting to find that evening was approaching, I took out my watch, and found it was not yet 12 o'clock.

---

1. Lieutenant William Hay states that there were four lines, the 12th being in the fourth line.
2. The Oxford Blues.

The horses were all in their places and merely linked together, every man ready to mount and the officers lying among the corn in front of them.

No one among us had anything to do; and the day passed on amid listless and wearisome repose. Towards the afternoon, attention was drawn to the wood in front; behind which at the apparent distance of two or three miles, a collection of little flags began to shew above the trees, which indicated the arrival of lancers; and to the best of my remembrance, about 4 pm,[3] the order was given to mount and then to draw swords. This was followed by a salvo of artillery in our front and the passage of the front line of cavalry through the intervals of our squadrons, the third line now becoming the second. An advance took place for a short distance and then came the heavy cavalry through in like manner. The French were coming on in strong columns and though the business of the English, at the moment was to have followed the infantry, the third line of our cavalry, now placed before the enemy, would have been involved in a dreadful scene of carnage had not heaven itself seemed to interpose for its prevention.

There came on at this juncture a most tremendous peal of thunder. I have no doubt that the discharge of the artillery gave the clouds a concussion and threw them into a state of agitation.[4] Whatever was the exciting cause, the effect was no doubt the saving of our brigade in particular, for they were formed up to check the enemy, who (finding the field abandoned by the main body of their foes) calculated on nothing more than a smart ride to Brussels. To the thunder succeeded the heaviest rain that clouds could discharge, which with the aid of driving wind, battered the faces of both men and horses to such a degree, that the advantage on the side of the enemy must have been incalculable. They had the storm in their rear; and our animals were unable to confront it. Instead, therefore of a charge, the whole wheeled about and made for the bye-road, over which we were to retreat, in order that the French might not turn the flank of our intended position and cut us off from communication and co-operation with the Prussians. I apprehend (though I did not see it) that there had been a little misunderstanding or confusion at this moment; for a squadron of one of our regiments retreated by the high road and had some fighting, while

---

3. It was nearer to 1 pm, according to Lieutenant William Hay.
4. A prevalent belief at the time.

the rest went at a quick pace through narrow cart-tracks, where fighting was out of the question, though the enemy were so close at our heels, that the front could hardly get on fast enough for the convenience of those in the rear.

Our pace, I have said was quick and the distance by this circuitous route was considerably greater than that along the chaussee, by which the body of the cavalry retreated, as the infantry had done in the course of the day. The consternation of the peasantry as we passed through a rich and rather interesting corner of the country, was distressing. One woman in particular, attracted my notice; she had gone out for the purpose of bringing two calves from a field and on her way home was surprised by our approach, the calves were scared and ran before us for a long way, the poor frightened and wearied female following in despair, as fast as she could. At length they got into an enclosure, where in all probability they furnished the materials for a supper to those who were coming after us. The officer who had been sent to explore our intended line of retreat, did not re-join the brigade. I believe he lost his way in returning and got upon the high road, where he was obliged to accompany the troops he found going off in that direction. In consequence of this we were compelled to take guides, and one peasant after another was pressed into this service and forced to lead the way, the front however, being on the occasion in question neither the post of honour, nor of danger.

During this movement, I was still compelled to bestride the gallant Belge of farmyard, or plough and harrow celebrity. He, or rather I believe, *she* liked neither the guns nor the thunder at *Les Bras*; but when the rain came on and I was making an attempt to unstrap my cloak, past came the brigade and away started my steed, fortunately in the right direction after them.[5] I had a double bridle in her mouth, but I should have had as much control with a piece of packthread round her muzzle. Fear lent an irresistible spur and away ran she. I was in the centre of the regiment in no time and ours was the rear of the brigade at starting. The men, who could hardly move in double files, begged of me to get out of the ranks, as in case of their having to form up, I should find myself in danger. It

---

5. Note by Smith – Had a gun been discharged in the quarter we were bound for, I am confident the beast would have started for the enemy; seeing a charge made upon their front, even by a single individual, must have insured my being cut to atoms before any sort of explanation could possibly have taken place.

was more easily said than done. The road was hollow and the banks were so high, that it was only here and there that one could pass the files in front; besides, I felt my situation so painful, that as my *charger* had got again into a trot, I shrunk from the risk of once more finding room for a gallop, not knowing where it might end and apprehensive of exciting some amusement in the meantime. Besides, in the event of a charge, I stood every chance if at hand, to get a nice French horse. Upon what strange circumstances do our comforts occasionally depend! I had had no food that day; I was wet to the skin; I had little to gain, but a good deal to hazard, by the upshot and yet I would have come under any obligations merely to have been allowed to ride a manageable nag. The sorry grey pony of Larry Murphy [Patrick Egan] would have been a treasure and had I lost my dung-carter, thirty pounds would not have paid for her.[6]

As we drew near the position of Mont St Jean, we approached the chaussee, from the pavement of which the rumbling of the gun-carriage and tumbril wheels reached our ears. Intermingled with this noise was a considerable one of firing. Officers rode over some rising intervening ground to ascertain the cause; and reported that the French were taking up a position close to where, for a few minutes, the brigade had halted. We moved off and from a turn in the road, we suddenly obtained a sight of the ridge of *La Haye Sainte*, upon the summit and front of which, the army in general was already formed.

A train of Belgian, or Dutch artillery, had been so planted as to command the hollow way in which we were at the moment, and had expected the arrival of part of the enemy in that direction; for no sooner did we catch sight of *them*, than they commenced preparations to give *us* a salute we were by no means entitled to. One of our officers rode forward, waving a handkerchief and being met by one from the other party, a salutary explanation was made.[7] We passed the left of the position and

---

6. Note by Smith – She performed one feat which I must record. As we went along at this '*slapping pace*?', we came to a deep trench across the road, now flooded with water. The English horses leaped it. The Adjutant, who happened to be close to me at the moment, exclaimed, 'God help you doctor, what will become of you?' Before I had time to think of an answer (indeed I am not sure that I was not putting up a mental prayer) my heavy-heeled animal was clear and clean on the opposite side, like a first rate hunter. The feat surprised everybody, the rider not the least.
7. Lieutenant William Hay makes it clear that he was the officer sent to stop the Dutch (his identification) artillery firing on the regiment.

bivouacked in open clover fields, close to and somewhat in the rear of the farm of *Mont St Jean.*

When we reached our halting place, it was probably about seven in the evening and still daylight. The position of the general army was a short distance in front of us and the red colouring of the scene, owing to the uniforms of our troops exhibited an imposing sight. The ground rose in front of us, but a considerable part of the force was stationed on our side of the hill and consequently invisible to the enemy. A heavy cannonade took place from both sides and lasted till dark, until which time, not one of our men was at liberty to think of his own welfare or to go from his horse's head. The bits were slipped from the animals' mouths, in order that they might be refreshed with some of the herbage from among their feet. At last, the departure of day closed all hope and anxiety about any further operations taking place for the present; and the general opinion was, that we should not see the French in the morning. I believe they amused themselves with a similar expectation with regard to *us*, imagining that we were off for the other side of the Scheldt, there if possible to keep them at bay till the allied armies should come to our reinforcement.[8]

Now commenced a series of operations that, under all the circumstances of privation in which we were placed, were excessively amusing. We were to pass the night on the spot we already occupied, but the officers were in want of food, drink and fire. Of the first, our men had received a supply; the horses had also been, at least partially cared for, but water! There was a draw-well close to the village, or hamlet of *[Mont] St Jean* and that was the only resource to which thousands of thirsty ones had access. The first attack upon it was the last; for snap went the rope and down fell the bucket, to a depth from which it could not be recovered. Disappointed in the article of water, our attention was drawn to that of fire, in procuring which we were eminently successful. The adjoining village furnished fuel in abundance. Doors and window shutters, furniture of every description, carts, ploughs, harrows, wheelbarrows, clock-cases, casks, tables, &c &c were carried or trundled out to the bivouac and being broken up, made powerful fires, in spite of the rain. Chairs were otherwise disposed of, officers were paying two francs each for them and the men seemed at

---

8. This is again confirmation that Wellington planned to retreat towards Antwerp if beaten at Waterloo, rather than Ostend.

first, to be very well able to keep up the supply. This at last failed and for one, I was fain to buy a bundle of straw.

In front of the field which the horses occupied, ran a miry cart-road, (upon which the officer's fires were kindled) and by the side of this road was a drain, or shallow ditch. Here a party of us deposited our straw and resolved to establish ourselves for the night, under cover of our cloaks; but such was the clayey nature of its bottom, that the rain did not sink into the earth, but rose like a leak in a ship, among the straw and we were in consequence, more drenched from below than from above. During the evening and early part of the night, there had been an intermission of rain, which induced some to try to get their clothes dried. Two subalterns in particular, with the greatest good humour, had made this experiment in such a grotesque manner, as excited a good deal of laughter. In fact, for some time they kept all around them in a state of merriment: but they fell early on the following day,[9] one of them was the friend, whose horse I had hoped to ride. The rain recommencing, fell heavily during the residue of the night; and to troops fresh out of excellent quarters, perhaps a more unpleasant initiation could scarcely have been offered. Sleep was out of the question, all wearied as we were and a few little amusing incidents, such as a quarrel about a chair &c might be recorded, but it is better perhaps to omit them.

---

9. This refers to Lieutenant Lindsey James Bertie and Cornet John Elliott Lockhart, the only two subalterns of the 12th Light Dragoons to be killed at Waterloo.

Chapter 6

# The Day of Waterloo

Day dawned very early upon us, for we were within a few hours of midsummer and found us in miserable plight enough, wet, cold and hungry. The colonel passed the night in the exposed situation occupied by the regiment, although urged by the general[1] to share his sheltered quarters in the village, of course our chief was a participator in the common lot. When we began to look up, we found the clover field of the preceding night had become a bog and that the horses were 'fetlock-deep in *mud*.' The first thing to be done, was to move them to another spot. The fires were going out too and the supply of fuel was exhausted. I recollect wading through the mire to get a lump of wood we saw lying in the *ci-devant* [former] clover-field. News came that there was a pond not far off: to this the horses were led and the men's canteens forwarded. But at length, up came the Quartermaster Sergeant, from the rear, ie the wood of Soignies and he reported that the sutler had handed him a sack, containing bread and cold meat for the officers; besides which, the commissariat waggons were abandoned and remained unprotected in the middle of the road, loaded with bread, corn and spirits. Ten men per troop were instantly ordered to proceed upon a plundering expedition, equipped with all the haversacks, corn sacks and canteens they could carry, under the command of my young friend already spoken of. In the meantime, placing the sack between his legs, the colonel seated himself on a bank, called all the officers to him, waited for those who were not at hand and when all were assembled but not till then, like the father of a family, opened his wallet and distributed its contents among us. The cold beef, mutton and veal were luxuries of the highest order; and we thought we were the better entitled to avail ourselves of the Godsend, as we knew the wants of the regiment would soon be supplied also; that neither man nor beast would go without an ample breakfast. We had not concluded, when back came the plundering party, laden with

---
1. Major General Sir John Ormsby Vandeleur commanding the 4th Cavalry Brigade.

provisions; and never shall I forget the look of satisfaction that beamed on [Lockhart]'s countenance when he pointed to the sutler's cart. He had found it among the confusion which had already taken place in the rear and cleared a way for its owner to drive up to our bivouac. Here there was an additional store of solids and a supply of fluids of a stimulating nature, very acceptable indeed under such circumstances. The sutler was a native of Ghent, but one of those bold and dexterous fellows who had belonged to Napoleon's Guard and had returned from the expedition to Moscow.[2] The non-commissioned officers and even the privates, were admitted to his hospitality after the officers desisted; but not one of *the officers* even of the other regiments, could obtain from him a supply at any price, as long as the regiment he was annexed to remained unsatisfied. Having swallowed all I required at the time, I called a dragoon and filled his canteen with brandy as a precautionary measure; but the following day, when we met again, there was a void. True I told him, in the event of separation or necessity, to do as he liked with it and he pleaded many occasions of that nature, truly enough no doubt. It is but fair to add that the sutler never made any charge for our Waterloo breakfast and remained for years afterwards under regimental patronage.

After this the serious business of the memorable day commenced. I recollect several of us feeling drowsy after so very solid a breakfast; we accordingly retired to our damp straw in the hope of snatching a few winks, but had not been long there when Lord Uxbridge came past. We rose at his approach, but he kindly exclaimed, 'lie still gentlemen, lie still, take all the sleep you can get, you will be wanted presently.' About this time the general of our brigade [Vandeleur] came out of the village and informed us that there would be a famous day; for the Prussians would be up by eleven and that an overwhelming attack would then be made upon the French, who were considered to have committed a great mistake in waiting where they were till morning. Did not Buonaparte think we had done the same on our side? I believe he is reported to have said, when he discovered our army in the same position as he had followed them to on the previous day. '*Ah, je les tiens, donc, ces Anglais.*' [Ah therefore I have them, these English]. However this may be, all the world knows that the object of the Duke of Wellington, in falling back upon the position in question,

---

2. Lieutenant William Hay says that the sutler's name was Mr Francois.

was to form a communication with Blucher, who had been obliged to retreat to new ground not very far from our left; and that a coalition had been agreed on between the allied commanders, which would have been effected without difficulty had the country not been bogged by the rain of the preceding night. This unforeseen and irremediable obstacle caused the whole of the objection that has been urged against the English army being placed in such hazardous circumstances. But it was impossible to say how soon our allies might arrive and after the understanding that had been established, would there not have been a breach of faith had the English general left his position, when there was a fair chance of maintaining it even for a time? Another most absurd complaint has been current among the vulgar, that the Duke was surprised, that he was not at his post &c when the enemy broke into the country. I am very sure that if His Grace were to speak candidly on the subject, he would say that he *expected to be surprised*.

Napoleon was not a likely man to send his compliments with a message to inform him when he would enter upon active operations and where he purposed to commence; and as to '*the post,*' where would these wise folks have assigned it? Do they think it was either fit or necessary for the commander of an army to be performing the duty of a vidette, or at most of an officer on picquet? His proper post was precisely where it was and where on all corresponding occasions it has been, at the headquarters of the army, the most convenient place for receiving information, conducting the general business of a large army as connected with the very existence of a nation and for issuing orders. 'Oh, but he was at a ball when the news came!' What then? Did it signify which street or which house of Brussels he happened to be in? It has never been hinted that when he went to this ball he desired that no news might be communicated to him. Where would they have had him? In bed, fast asleep? In which of these two situations was he most likely to be on the alert? I wish John Bull would say nothing about what he does not understand, or talk sense. The Duke of Wellington did his duty and the British nation know not their obligations to him. If this country were the seat of war for one month, there would be a very different feeling towards those who have fought her battles upon other soils and kept an enemy from ravaging her own.

I have no correct memorial of the hour at which we left the spot where we had passed the night (for I never till now committed any of these matters to writing), but I think the regiment had been told off and moved to their position about half past ten. The brigade was now posted on the brow of the extensive ridge along which runs the hedge that gives name to the farm of *La Haye Sainte* and between the centre regiment and our own (which formed the left wing) was a knoll surmounting all and commanding great part of the English line.[3] To obtain possession of this was the object of the first attack made by Count d'Erlon; an attack which has been commonly reported to have been a feint.[4] In our immediate front were some Belgian infantry;[5] and these fellows, who had passed the night on the spot, had formed wigwams of the standing corn by tying the heads together and I dare say had enjoyed drier quarters than had fallen to our lot; nor did it appear that they had suffered very sorely from hunger, for there was a profusion of cooked potatoes lying about. I had changed my plougher and harrower for a horse belonging to the Surgeon [Benjamin Robinson] and had seen the surgical paniers placed on her back prior to these occurrences and finding myself still weary, though divested of much anxiety, I laid me down in one of the wigwams, while the French were manoeuvring upon the opposite hill and the shot were flying over our heads.

After some time, the Surgeon [Robinson] despatched me to the panniers for a supply of materials, as well as to give the man orders about the situation in which he was to be found. I discovered him just within range of shot and during the time occupied in getting what was wanted, they were falling tolerably thick about us. Considering the place I had come from to be safer than this, I directed the hospital orderly to move back far enough to be out of the reach of the balls; but to be within sight, lest I should have to come again. I was proceeding at a canter up hill to the regiment, when I was assailed by several cries from wounded men dressed in its uniform, some of whom were so disfigured that I could not recognise them. One hailed me with, 'Oh doctor, my thigh is broke!' A second, 'I am wounded in the head!' A third 'My arm is cut to pieces!' A

---

3. Lieutenant William Hay states that the regiments of the brigade were formed in column of squadrons at quarter distance. The men were dismounted but the horses were kept in hand for immediate use.
4. He is mistaken here. The preceding attack on Hougoumont was claimed by many to be a diversionary attack prior to the serious attack made by Comte d'Erlon's corps, which aimed to punch through Wellington's left and capture the village of Mont St Jean.
5. The division of General Bijlandt lined the crest of the ridge on the left, with General Picton's division in the second line and the cavalry to their rear in the third line.

fourth 'I have got a stab from a lance!' &c. Another bawled out, 'I have a horse for you, which Sergeant [?] has sent;[6] but mine is killed.' 'So is mine,' said another, 'and I am wounded; but you may have this horse, Sir, if you like: there is a nice French kit upon him.'

My first enquiry was the offspring of genuine astonishment, 'What! Have you been engaged?' I was now told that they had made a charge,[7] in which they had suffered severely; that many men and most of the officers were killed, naming some in particular, whom I afterwards had the pleasure of finding unhurt; but in the confusion, these poor fellows could not obtain more accurate information.[8]

The next point for consideration was the dressing of their wounds. We turned off to a corner of the field, (the nature of the ground being such as to cut off all possibility of seeing and therefore judging for ourselves of what was going on in front) and there I proposed to commence my operations. We had scarcely reached this spot however, when some fugitives came past exclaiming that we had better not stay there, as in a few minutes we should be disturbed by the retreating army. Could we have seen how things actually were, the falsehood of this report would have been instantly apparent; but a hill intervened between us and the scene of contest. We accordingly moved on a little further and got into a farmyard [Mont St Jean], where I hoped to have time to pay attention to the most urgent cases at least; desiring the slighter ones to keep their horses and get onto Brussels, where they would be admitted into hospitals

---

6. Note by Smith – A particular request had been made on my part to the sergeants, to secure me a horse or two if an opportunity occurred; a request to which these brave men carefully attended. I am happy to add that the particular individual now alluded to has been always much respected in the regiment and very prosperous in the matter of promotion.
7. The regiment consisted of three squadrons, the senior on the right, the second senior on the left and the junior in the centre. William Hay states that the squadrons numbered 54, 53 and 48 files (a file being two horsemen behind each other) before the charge and that the regiment was reorganised into two squadrons, numbering only 24 and 23 files after the charge.
8. It would appear that the other two regiments of their brigade had moved out to try to protect the disorganised Union Brigade after their successful defeat of Marcognet's Division. Finding the 12th Light Dragoons alone, Ponsonby took the regiment forward and attacked the formed columns of Durutte's Division which had escaped the charge of the British heavy cavalry. Many historians mistakenly believe that Durutte's troops attacked Papelotte instead of advancing on the allied ridge, but this is refuted by the testimony of Durutte's son.

and be saved the pain and inconvenience of moving again. As for my captured stud, much as I wanted it, I desired the poor fellows to request Chiswick[9] (who, I had no doubt they would fall in with in the rear), to look out for them and bring the horses up when they could spare them.

We had scarce got the panniers a second time on the ground, when some Belgian soldiers, coming past the farm in great confusion, informed us that all was over, that the enemy had turned the left flank of our army and were now coming on in great force, so that we should infallibly fall into their hands if we remained where we were. It began now to be almost a warrantable *sauve qui peut*, however my poor men and myself kept together, in the hope of finding some place or method for their relief. A crowd, such as few have ever seen (and I hope none will ever see again) now fell into the main road; and as the greater part of them were stout, hale and armed, the mischief they caused bids defiance to descriptions. The scene of the battle, dreadful as it was, must have been a paradise compared to the wood of *Soignies*. In the meantime, it ought to have been remarked, that on looking up the hill, we observed a very large body of infantry, in dark uniforms, moving down towards us; and not yet knowing the real truth of the matter, (how could we?) we concluded the report of the fugitives to be correct. In the course of a short period they came near enough to let us see that they had no musquets and that the skirts of the column were dotted by red jackets and others on horseback. The fact turned out to be, that they were a column of prisoners, who had been taken in the charge just mentioned and were marching to the rear, under an escort of cavalry. I learnt next day that their conductors had some difficulty in piloting them through the confusion, of which some tried to take advantage and were shot in attempting to make their escape.[10]

These untoward events effected the separation of my party and I had the sad assurance of being unable to do any good under existing circumstances. By this time the truth began to arrive; and I learnt that all this mischief was caused by a panic; that the army was maintaining and was likely to maintain its ground. More prisoners made their appearance; and judging as well as I could, what was my duty, I resolved to rejoin the

---

9. His servant described by him as John Chiswick; his real identity cannot be discovered.
10. Note by Smith – They knew the inhabitants to be friendly, otherwise escape would have been the last notion that could have entered their heads. Happy Frenchmen were they who in the peninsula, fell into the hands of the English. *They* never tried *to escape*.

regiment. I had got clear of the fugitives and was upon the field again, when I met the Surgeon [Robinson], coming in quest of me and the man who conducted the hospital bat-horse. At first my friend was disposed to be very wroth; but his anger subsided when things were explained. It was now discovered that the orderly was not with me and it was indispensable that we should bring him back. For this purpose we dived again into the crowd and ultimately overtook him; but by the time this was effected, it would have been as vain to have attempted a counter march against the torrent of fugitives, as it would be to row a boat up the falls of Niagara: It was therefore judged necessary, to get upon the skirt of the road and wait for some interval of a nature favourable to our wishes. This however, did not occur till night rendered it impossible to profit by it. We got into a small house and there we had no lack of surgical practice; for one wounded man directed others to us and the miserable hole soon became an hospital.

I shall fill up this chapter with a few remarks on the cause and aspect of a scene which has been frequently alluded to, but seldom described; and which perhaps, had some influence on the great and glorious event of the day. Of this I am certain, that no retreat *could have been effected* upon that road, without great confusion and slaughter; and I am not aware that there was any other channel by which the field could have been left.[11] Had the organised part of the army come off, no doubt the increase of runaway stragglers would soon have been stopped; and even as it was, the flight of these latter would have been comparatively insignificant, but for a circumstance that can hardly be imagined to have been purely accidental. This was the conduct of those who were connected with the large waggons, in which the provisions for the army were contained. I do not involve the commissariat at all in the matter, they had little or no means of control over those who were employed to conduct these waggons; but all were abandoned by the drivers and multitudes of them were overturned in such a manner and in such positions, as to make it more than matter of suspicion that neither accident nor fear was the real cause. The road was here and there completely barricaded; and this had been done before there was any certainty of a battle, or pretext for a panic. We were informed of it at a very early hour in the morning and an officer

---

11. He was unaware that a number of tracks led northward from the battlefield through the Forest of Soignes.

and party had been sent from our very brigade to have the mischief remedied and the road kept clear. These however, were tasks beyond their ability; for there was nobody present to be driven to their duty.

Among the fugitive Belgians, plunder and wanton destruction became the amusements of their progress. The road smelt most offensively of *gin*, from the staving of the casks and the evacuation of their contents. Coupled with the sight of here and there, a corpse (some of them females) which had been trampled to death, the effluence was sickening. It has been stated and I firmly believe it, that the thing had been preconcerted and intended to favour the French interests. It has been said that the news of the alleged defeat was simultaneously proclaimed in various places, distant from each other on the field, at Brussels, at Ghent, Antwerp, &c at the same moment.

The plunder, or rather (with more correctness it might be said) the useless destruction of officers' baggage, formed a distressing feature amid the horrible scene. Many of their servants had thrown away what had been committed to their charge; and where so many unreflecting individuals were left to exercise their own discretion, different results could scarcely be expected. My servant lost nothing, though as things went, he might have escaped censure had he lost all.[12] He was an old campaigner, and argued thus: – 'Why, I see nothing but a mob running away and none of our own troops among them. If it be a retreat, they will not come past in this style; we shall see something regular before the main body arrives and then it

---

12. Note by Smith – He did, however, lose an unwieldy article belonging to the king; *viz*, the pole of a tent, which had been issued from the stores a few weeks previously. There was one (large enough to accommodate half a dozen *fat* inmates) given out for the officers of each troop or company, collectively and one for each individual officer of the Staff, generally the poorest and worst equipped for such a Bristol compliment. It may be compared to a practice prevalent among the Oriental princes. When they take a pique at a courtier, they make him a present of an elephant, the expense of keeping which ruins the *presentee* and he dare not part with it, for his life. So it was with my fine tent: I was obliged to carry it about for ornament, for one would have served us all. However, they were given out in this way, upon the considerate notion that Staff officers were liable to be detached; but by that supposition our means of transport ought to have been enlarged. They would have been a surly set indeed, who would have excluded me from their tent, had I been detached, which (during active operations) never happened. Chiswick told me that he would have saved even the pole, had it been cut in four pieces instead of two; and that he found it necessary for the safety of the other things, to throw it away. The tent was afterwards returned to the place whence it came. It never was of any use to me but in the orchard at *Thollembeck* [Tollembeek]; or Dinah's bower.

will be time enough to throw away my master's property and take care of myself.' Reasoning in this consistent and creditable manner, he filed into a ravine in the forest, with young Herr Jan; but they were obliged to re-enter the stream, which carried them through Brussels and Mechlin [Mechelen], as far as Antwerp. The faithful and dexterous conduct of this man, involved as he was in peculiar difficulties, puts to shame that of many others who were furnished with superior facilities for moving and preserving what *their* richer masters had intrusted to them. Servants of field officers, of captains and of wealthy subalterns, came back with tales of danger and of plunder, which I know John Chiswick had some difficulty believing.

While we were busy in the hovel already spoken of, we learnt that a most complete victory had been achieved on the part of the English; and anxious to the last to get the particulars, the restraint we were necessarily placed under for the present, became doubly irksome. Thus closes the account of my personal proceedings on Sunday the 18 June 1815.

Before resuming my little personal narrative, (which will give the reader a *local* view of what had taken place), perhaps I may, without impropriety, make a few observations on the general events of the great day.

At what precise hour I had been despatched to the hospital orderly, I have no idea now; but it must have been towards or about noon.[13] The day was then fine and though I was wet and even weary, my spirits were high and my curiosity was eager. To the former the plentiful breakfast had contributed, the latter had been interested by the splendid and imposing panorama which had been the subject of my observation. There is something too in the sound of cannon, which excites while it surprises; and to me who had never witnessed a shot fired in earnest till now, the fact of so many balls passing harmless overhead, seemed of itself to divest these deadly missiles of all injurious properties. The fact was, the French had not yet had time to measure their range; for during my occupation with the panniers, the commanding officer of our centre regiment was struck in his place and carried off very seriously wounded.[14] A few more

---

13. Note by Smith – Upon recurring to this passage, I find I have alluded only to one errand; but after returning from the first, I was sent a second time (in consequence of the report I had brought as to the station of the orderly) to move him and convey the instructions already alluded to.
14. Lieutenant Colonel James Hay commanding the 16th Light Dragoons was so severely wounded that he was unable to be removed from the battlefield for eight days.

casualties of the same nature took place and these were all that the brigade were exposed to after the charge I am about to speak of.

When I was sent down the hill, for the purpose already excited, I left all in a state of regularity and had heard nothing of immediate contact with the enemy. An attack however, was soon afterwards made by a considerable column upon our position. This was repelled, partly by Sir W[illiam] Ponsonby's heavy cavalry, which attacked the enemy in front, while our regiment, unsupported by the rest of the brigade[15] fell upon their flank. The colonel had received *carte blanche* to employ the regiment whenever an opportunity occurred; and watching eagerly for one, no sooner observed the impression which the heavy dragoons had made, than he waved his sword for the regiment to come down the hill (towards the bottom of which he had previously repaired to reconnoitre) and led the three squadrons successively into the *melee*. The left squadron charged first and suffered severely; the centre one followed and was cut to pieces; the right was last employed and bore its proportion of the loss; but when the business was over the colonel was missing: no one had seen or was able to conjecture what had become of him and the obvious conclusion was that he must have been taken. The ground became clear, but no one could find him.

While looking about for him and others who required assistance, the sergeant major[16] found one of the officers (who had lost his horse and been assailed by a squad of lancers) endeavouring to retire on foot to the regiment and perceiving the impracticability of his doing so, in the face of two or three lancers, who were coming down to finish the little party, desired him to wait a moment and he would get him a horse. The first lancer came bravely on and the gallant sergeant major, resolved to grapple with him single handed, (ordering another sergeant who was present to stand aside, as his horse was unsteady). The lunge of the Frenchman was dexterously parried and the sabre in an instant thrust through his body. He fell, the horse he rode was secured, the officer mounted upon him and the other lancers, appalled, returned to their friends. This act was appreciated as it merited, for his general good conduct, the Sergeant Major shortly afterwards obtained a commission; and the gentleman who ran such a risk did not forget what was incumbent upon him.

---

15. This is incorrect, as the 16th Light Dragoons also advanced.
16. Regimental Sergeant Major John Carruthers was made a Cornet on 26 October 1815, but retired on half-pay in 1816.

# Chapter 7

# 19 June

The fate of the colonel was not known till the following morning, when he was found alive,[1] but severely injured, on ground that had been occupied by the enemy. Having been desperately wounded in the last charge, his horse got the better of him and broke in among the French, where he fell and lay in great torture during the remainder of the day and ensuing night, exposed not only to the caprice and insolence of the French soldiery, but to the greatest danger from the pursing army. An account of what took place has been already published; but I suspect it to be imperfect. I never had an opportunity of hearing his narrative; and the writer only picked it up as he could, the colonel was not in the habit of talking about it; though perhaps of all the adventures of the day, his was the most interesting and romantic.[2]

**Frederick Ponsonby's Account**
At one o'clock, observing as I thought, unsteadiness in a column of French infantry of 1,000 men or thereabouts, which was advancing with an irregular fire, I resolved to charge them. As we were descending at a gallop we received from our own troops on the right a fire much more destructive than theirs, they having begun long before it could take effect and slackening as we drew nearer. When we were within 50 paces of them, they turned and much execution was done amongst them, as we were followed by some Belgians who had remarked our success. But we had no sooner passed through them, than we were attacked in our turn before we could form, by about 300 Polish lancers, who had come down to their relief; the French artillery pouring in amongst us a heavy fire of grapeshot, which however, for one of our men, killed three

---
1. He was discovered by Lieutenant John Vandeleur.
2. As Smith does not explain the story of Lieutenant Colonel Frederick Ponsonby at Waterloo, I have incorporated his own account into the text.

of their own. In the melee I was disabled almost instantly in both my arms and followed by a few of my men who were presently cut down, for no quarter was asked or given, I was carried on by my horse, till receiving a blow on my head from a sabre, I was thrown senseless on my face to the ground. Recovering, I raised myself a little to look round, being I believe at that time in a condition to get up and run away, when a lancer, passing by, exclaimed: 'Tu n'es pas mort, coquin,' [You're not dead, rascal] and struck his lance through my back. My head dropped, the blood gushed into my mouth; a difficulty of breathing came on and I thought all was over. Not long afterwards (it was then impossible to measure time, but I must have fallen in less than ten minutes after the charge), a *tirailleur* came up to plunder me, threatening to take away my life. I told him that he might search me, directing him to a small side pocket, in which he found three dollars, being all I had. He unloosed my stock and tore open my waistcoat, then leaving me in a very uneasy posture. He was no sooner gone, than another came up for the same purpose, but assuring him I had been plundered already he left me, when an officer, bringing on some troops (to which probably the *tirailleurs* belonged) and halting where I lay, stooped down and addressed me, saying he feared I was badly wounded. I replied that I was and expressed a wish to be removed into the rear. He said it was against the orders to remove even their own men, but that if they gained the day, as they probably would, for he understood the Duke of Wellington was killed and that six battalions of the English army had surrendered, every attention in his power should be shown me. I complained of thirst and he held his brandy bottle to my lips, directing one of his men to lay me down on my side and placed a knapsack under my head. He then passed on into the action and I shall never know to whose generosity I was indebted, as I conceive, for my life. Of what rank he was I cannot say; he wore a blue greatcoat. By-and-bye another *tirailleur* came and knelt down and fired over me, loading and firing many times and conversing with great gaiety all the while. At last he ran off, saying: 'Vous serez bien aise d'entendre que nous allons nous retirer. Bon jour, mon ami.' [You will be glad to hear that we are going to withdraw. Good day, my friend.]

Whilst the battle continued in that part, several of the wounded men and dead bodies near me were hit with the balls which came very thick in that place. Towards evening, when the Prussians came up, the continued roar of cannon along their and the British line, growing louder and louder as they drew near, was the finest thing I ever heard. It was dusk when the two squadrons of Prussian cavalry, both of them two deep, passed over me in a full trot, lifting me from the ground and tumbling me about cruelly. The clatter of their approach and the apprehensions it excited may be easily conceived. Had a gun come that way, it would have done for me. The battle was then nearly over or removed to a distance. The cries and groans of the wounded all around me became every instant more and more audible, succeeding to the shouts, imprecations and cries of 'Vive l'Empereur,' the discharges of musketry and cannon, now and then intervals of perfect quiet which were worse than the noise. I thought the night would never end. Much about this time one of the Royals lay across my legs, he had probably crawled thither in his agony; his weight, convulsive motions, his noises and the air issuing through a wound in his side distressed me greatly, the latter circumstance most of all, as the case was my own.

It was not a dark night and the Prussians were wandering about to plunder, and the scene in 'Ferdinand Count Fathom' came into my mind, though no women I believe, were there. Several Prussians came, looked at me and passed on. At length one stopped to examine me. I told him as well as I could, for I could speak but little German, that I was a British officer and had been plundered already. He did not desist however, and pulled me about roughly before he left me. About an hour before midnight I saw a soldier in an English uniform coming towards me. He was I suspect, on the same errand, but he came and looked in my face. I spoke instantly telling him who I was and assuring him of a reward if he would remain by me. He said that he belonged to the 40th Regiment, but that he had missed it. He released me from the dying man and being unarmed, he took up a sword from the ground and stood over me, pacing backwards and forwards.

At 8 o'clock in the morning some English were seen at a distance. He ran to them and a messenger was sent off to Colonel Harvey [Hervey]. A cart came for me, I was placed on it and carried to a farmhouse about a mile and a half distant and laid in the bed from which poor Gordon, as I understood afterwards, had been just carried out. The jolting of the carriage and the difficulty of breathing were very painful. I had received seven wounds; a surgeon slept in my room and I was saved by continual bleeding; 120 ounces in two days, besides a great loss of blood on the field.

The lances from their length and weight would have struck down my sword long before I lost it, if it had not been bound to my hand. What became of my horse I know not. It was the best I ever had.

**Letter by Deputy Inspector of Hospitals Robert Hume dated 10 August 1815**
I hereby certify that Colonel the Honourable F[rederick] C[avendish] Ponsonby commanding the 12th Light Dragoons in the Battle of Waterloo on the 18th of June last, received a cut from a sabre on the outside of the fore right arm opposite the edge of the ulna which divided the integuments[3] and muscles longitudinally down to the bones extending from near the elbow to the wrist. He was also struck behind on the left side by a lance, which fracturing the sixth rib entered the chest and wounded the lungs. Besides these two severe wounds, he received several smaller cuts on his head, shoulder and left arm (which was also disabled) and different parts of his body; and was bruised all over in such a manner as to render his recovery very doubtful; his recovery towards convalescence has been very slow; he has still little or no use of his right arm and hand; his breathing is much affected, by the wound in his chest, which is still open, and his strength is so much impaired that it is more than probable his constitution will never recover the shock which it has received.[4]

About one-third of the regiment suffered on this occasion. More than sixty were killed and nearly as many were disabled, the precise numbers I cannot now verify.[5] After this they had little or nothing to do, till they

---

3. Skin and fat.
4. Despite his severe wounds he lived until 1837 and he recovered much of the use of his arm.
5. The official loss of the regiment at Waterloo (as given in Siborne) was 2 officers, 6 sergeants, 39 rank & file and 28 horses were killed; 3 officers, 4 sergeants, 1 trumpeter, 56 rank & file and 22 horses were wounded; with another 60 horses missing.

shifted ground towards evening and took part in the general charge, when the enemy fell into confusion at the end of the day.⁶

At what time the Prussian army debouched, what part they contributed to the results of the day and many other interesting details, are recorded on the imperishable page of history. My knowledge of these matters being neither derived from personal observation, nor from information at the first hand, I consider would of itself be sufficient excuse for silence. One digression, however, may be found interesting.

Among the privates of our own regiment who suffered severely, was a strong large man, who had not only had his horse killed, but was himself wounded. He recovered afterwards sufficiently to rejoin; but he never became effective again and he was ultimately invalided. One day he stated to some of his comrades, that while he was on the ground, just after the charge, he had a pole in his hand, with *a bird* at the end of it, made of metal that he thought would be worth something, if he could keep it and carry it with him, for he had taken it from a French officer; but that in this helpless state, a heavy dragoon coming past, snatched it from him and rode off with it. He was a lout of a fellow, who might have made a mistake and he certainly did not know the importance of an eagle. There were two taken upon the same occasion and the reputed captors were lauded to the skies, but does not this look as if one of them had been obtained at second hand, supposing the man's account to be true? He was

---

6. Note by Smith – A long year elapsed ere our beloved chief saw the regiment again; and when he did come, he was both unable to draw his sword in the field and to cut his meat at the mess table. It was a splendid day when he first presented himself at a brigade drill. I thought our men would have verily gone wild with unaffected joy. They cheered from the moment he came upon the ground and at every opportunity till he left it. The old soldiers saw an approved friend and the young ones saw a great man to whom they were anxious to recommend themselves by their conduct. There never *was* such a regiment; for there never *was* such a colonel; there still *is* no such regiment. When our chief rejoined us, his right arm was still comparatively useless. He mounted his horse however, by an active spring, which showed the accomplished *cavalier*, never putting his right hand out to his assistance in the slightest degree. Prior to his wounds at *Waterloo*, he wrote an indifferent and even indistinct hand; but in losing the use of his right one, the duty in question devolved upon the left and although he then wrote as Lord Nelson did for many years, his left handed work was far more distinct than had been that of the nobler; or more fashionable organ. I believe he himself became so sensible of the improvement, that although he has long regained the use of his right arm, he continues to *write* with the left hand. It was one of the finest things I have seen in a field. The Honourable Colonel [Ponsonby] marching past the reviewing officer, at the head of his regiment, unable either to draw his sword or lift his right arm to his chaco [*sic*].

making no boast at the time of his narrative, but relating the affair as an immaterial circumstance. At all events, it was too late to raise any claim and it would appear that he was not at the time in a condition to preserve his prize.

I must now enter upon very painful disclosures. The Surgeon [Robinson] and I parted early in the morning, after again changing horses and my being transferred to the back of the cursed beast already too celebrated. He [Robinson] went forward and was shortly engaged in attendance on the colonel, who had been removed to a house in Waterloo. Something delayed me with the orderly and we were yet in the horrible forest, where I was surprised to see *detachments* of English cavalry marching regularly towards the field: some had been escorting prisoners and others pretended they had been escorting the wounded; but even for these purposes, the number seemed far more than sufficient. I must not be particular as to corps; but I could be so. However, it was no affair of mine.

Having got again into the scene of action, accompanied by a few of our own men, who had been left to look about for the wounded, or were really returning from escort, I had no desire to explore the ground till I should find the regiment and obtain clear notions as to what I had to do. Proceeding along the high road, we passed many a sorry sight. There were regiments, principally Germans, yet on the field amusing themselves with a very dangerous sort of sport, firing their rifles[7] with little respect as to the objects of their mark. Even now the balls came whizzing past our ears, or occasionally fell at our feet. The peasantry too, were beginning to appear upon the dark and gloomy field; in the course of the day, they mustered in shoals (God knows where they came from) and when weary of stripping the dead, began to play with the cannon and in one or two instances, blew up a tumbril, as well as some of themselves. At length

---

7. With the Brunswick troops we had been familiar in the peninsula and their conduct was always good; in fact, they seemed much to resemble the old Highland regiments as to character. At one time I knew many of the officers and was at first rather surprised at the deference with which they treated those under their command; but this admitted of ample explanation, as there were many instances of near relatives serving, some as officers and others in the ranks, from which in many instances they were promoted. But there was a singular corps at this time on the field, called the Brunswick Yagers, or *game keepers*, composed I understood, chiefly if not entirely of such persons. They were all of course sure shots and were armed with rifles. Their dress was exactly what we see in 'Der Freischutz' [*The Marksman*, a German opera] green clothing, black belts and a broad brimmed hat, looped up at one side. They were very busy at this sort of amusement.

we reached a part of the causeway (chaussee), which was cut through an acclivity and here the bodies of the slain were so thickly piled, that our horses could not possibly pick a way among them. I presume here it was, that Bonaparte brought down the Imperial Guard, to make a last and desperate effort to retrieve the fortune of the day and where the dreadful carnage took place, both from the fire of our artillery and the tremendous charge of the Lifeguards and other regiments. In many instances the red coats and the blue (of the French) were so intermingled, that it would have been difficult to say, by looking at the sad spectacle, from which side either had advanced. Some were literally pinned together; their respective swords being passed through each other. But all were now silent, all were prostrate, for all were *dead!*

Finding it impracticable to keep the road, we got into the field and there discovered the bodies of two women lying among those of the French soldiers. In all probability, they had paid the forfeit of their lives for hawking brandy in this dangerous situation, a custom which (I have heard) is permitted in the French army but which would by no means do in ours. I shall not say that Englishmen would not be refreshed by a small supply of this nature; but the vice of my countrymen is want of self-command, whenever exposed to this sort of temptation. The French have more forbearance and may to a certain extent be trusted. As to women, I do not recollect seeing one of our nation till *after* the battle, when they came in numbers to the field in search of their husbands; and sorry am I to record that not a few, who fell under my observation, seemed well pleased with the discovery that they were *widows*. Soldiers' wives it is true, are little more than *animals* (generally speaking) and during active scenes of campaigning, lead a life of such vicissitudes that they are disappointed during any prolongation of a 'calm and even tenor,' while they look for and depend upon *changes* to make life tolerable. They are also exposed to much hardship, which their husbands have it not in their power to alleviate, or even to share, as may be the case in the corresponding humbler walks of civil life. They are frequently used harshly and are notorious for the slender nature of their conjugal attachments. Were it possible for me to relate some of the scenes that I was witness to, I might have little cause to boast of the number of my readers: but if I cannot entertain, I shall take care not to disgust.

I am unaware, notwithstanding the foregoing censure, that any acts of cruelty were committed by these miserable creatures, such as are described as having been perpetrated by the mother of Count Fathom;[8] and if I may refer to my own regiment, as furnishing by no means the fairest or the most amiable examples of the sex, I should conjecture that Moll Flaggon,[9] *et hoc genus omne* [and everything of this kind], have of late years been rejected from the ranks. Perhaps however, my knowledge of the case has been circumscribed. In the cavalry, we meet with fewer of them: women can walk as fast as a man but are not able to keep pace with horses; at the same time, if left to their own discretion, they would follow the dragoons as numerously as the foot soldiers.

But, to return from this digression. I found the remains of the regiment assembled near the famous wooden observatory which had been erected for surveying the country; and which has been erroneously supposed to have been a work of Bonaparte, for the purpose of reconnoitring. The tythe of one reflection would have shewn the impossibility of his having done anything of the sort in the course of a single night; besides which, so conspicuous an object must have been seen before the arrival of the French, by a vast majority of the allied army. It must have been remarked on their going to and returning from *Quatre Bras*; as that I cannot help wondering how such a foolish story should have remained so long uncontradicted.[10] Those in the secret (if it could be called one,) probably laughed at the mistake, and thought it no business of theirs; while those who were not, could not of course rectify it.[11]

---

8. A character in Smollet's *The Adventures of Ferdinand, Count Fathom*.
9. Moll Flaggon was a 'low camp follower' in General Burgoyne's play of 1780 entitled *The Lord of the Manor*. She killed the wounded to rob them.
10. Note by Smith – I do not mean that it has remained so till *now*. The report must have owed its origin to waggery, or presumptio, on the part of some of those intelligent personages who made a profitable trade of the silly curiosity manifested by the swarms of the [John] Bull family as visited the field shortly after the action. *Relics*, as they were styled, were purchased with avidity, e.g. buttons of the French soldiers, brass ornament, swords, straps, buckles &c &c were for some time to be had *genuine*, but after a while, the supply of these was exhausted and imitations were made for the nonce, while other things were palmed upon the strangers, which had not even the claim of resemblance to the real trophies, such as broken tobacco-pipes, pieces of old hats, &c &c.
11. The 'Observation Tower' had been constructed in 1814, when William Crann was employed by the king of the newly formed 'Netherlands' (consisting of both Belgium and Holland combined) to survey his new lands in Belgium. Despite claims to the contrary, there is no evidence that Napoleon used it. It has also been proven that from its top, it was still not possible to see beyond Wellington's ridge.

I wished much to remain with them; but as soon as I had heard more authentic accounts of the disasters of the preceding day than I had yet been able to gather, I was obliged to return to the scene of the contest, to collect the wounded yet upon the field, with instructions to see them cared for and placed in safety. There was a sergeant in particular, who had been severely wounded in the evening, about whose case several of the officers manifested great anxiety. At what precise spot he was to be found no one could tell; but a man had been left with him for the purpose of obtaining medical assistance, who would of course recognise me and take me to him. Not one of my friends had any idea of the relative bearings of different parts of the field. They had fought and bustled their way from point to point, but neither knew nor cared where they were at the present or had been at any particular moment. All they knew was that they expected to move immediately, but *whither* no one seemed to concern himself.

I retraced my steps back to the desolate and altered scene, where I had left them unscathed, but a short time before: -

> Few hours had pass'd since proudly wav'd
> O'er all these fields the ripening grain
> With brave men's blood they now were lav'd
> Now nought produc'd, save death and pain.

I returned to the heights, but they were deserted by the gallant array which crowned them but yesterday. I explored the *holy hedge* [the hedges which gave La Haye Sainte its name], but it was divested of its bright and lively ornaments. Instead of columns and lines of eager and hopeful and active and elegant warriors, I here and there found a soiled corpse, or a dying and abandoned creature, who would have blessed me with his last breath, or paid me if he could, with wealth to any amount for (what I possessed not the power to give or procure for him) *a draught of water!* Then a dumb horse in his agony, would make a stir, evidently to attract my attention and probably sickened under the discovery that one of the race to which he had been a faithful and necessary servant until his docility had led him into pain and misery, could pass by and take no heed of his wretchedness. But against a thousand, probably I ought to say against many thousand instances of this nature, I was compelled to steel my heart. Having an especial duty to perform and dissatisfied with the turn such matters had taken on the previous day, I was doubly anxious to exert myself for the sufferers of my own *family*. To many applications from wounded individuals, I could only return assurances of sympathy and prompt relief, to the horses I could do no more than cast a commiserating eye. Had Chiswick been at hand I could have secured a very good stud; for several of these simple creatures had received but superficial wounds that required only a little fomenting to have made a speedy cure of them: in the meantime, from neglect and exposure, these comparatively trifling things became stiff and the poor animals feeling pain upon moving, confined themselves to the spot and in many instances had eaten a hollow circle among the tall wheat that surrounded them.

Upon this side of the great road, I could find nobody, living or dead belonging to our regiment and returned to the chaussee in a considerable state of perplexity. I there met several other medical officers, apparently employed on a mission of the same nature; and while we were expressing our anxieties and interchanging such information as we were able to give, a dragoon came to the side of the road from among the high corn, and exclaimed, 'D[octo]r J[Smith], here is Sergeant B[aird].'[12] I replied, 'very well, I am looking for him;' but I forgot to add that he should remain with him till I could find the means of removal. The soldier, impatient to join the regiment, concluded I presume that having told me where his charge lay, his duty was accomplished. In the course of a short time, I found several men of the regiment coming through the hamlet [Mont St Jean] and halted them all, till I had collected effective assistance. My design was to have the sergeant, a very tall, stout, athletic and heavy man (fitter for the right of the Life Guard than a regiment of light dragoons), conveyed to the nearest farmhouse, which happened to be that of [Mont] St Jean. However, when we proceeded to the spot whence the man had called to me, I could neither find him, nor any indication by which to trace the poor sergeant. The men rode in all directions among the corn, round and round the place, in vain for at least an hour; and I had resolved to go to the regiment for the purpose of bringing back the soldier who had been left to watch, when one of the party discovered B[aird]. The scene which ensued my pen is inadequate to describe; but my recollection

---

12. Sergeant William Baird was the only Sergeant killed with a B in his name.

of the circumstances is vivid and I shall make the attempt, for to make it has become a duty, not the less imperative perhaps, because self-imposed.

Upon this announcement, I immediately repaired to the spot and found one of the finest moulds of manly form prostrate on the earth, with his dead horse close by, a dead hussar on one side and one within a few feet on the other, in the last agonies of death.[13] I could not refrain from tears. B[aird] was perfectly collected; but he complained, first of having been left *two* nights on the field,[14] then of the loss of the mare and next of intolerable thirst. This was the immediate urgency; and (having given the troopers who were with me peremptory orders on no account to leave us till B[aird]'s comfort should be provided for), I despatched the man who had found him in search of water, while the two others were sent across the field to drive in a sufficient number of the plundering peasantry to carry him off. 'I wanted eight stout fellows and they must lick them with the flats of their sabres if they would not come peaceably. They were not to come back without them and to be quick.' While this party was absent, an infantry soldier who had lost his regiment, came up and stated (whether truly or falsely it would have been ungrateful to conjecture) that, as he was left behind, he thought it his duty to assist his wounded countrymen. He had some brandy in his canteen, and poor B[aird] was revived a little, in the meantime by tasting it, reserving himself with great patience, for a more refreshing draught when the water should arrive. We tried the dying hussar in a similar manner, but he was too far gone to comprehend anything: so we were reduced to the painful necessity of leaving him to his fate. He was too severely injured for surgical assistance; and all my time and attention now belonged to the sergeant.

At this moment (about 1 pm) the sun was beating fiercely upon us; and poor B[aird] complained sadly of its influence. The infantryman and I unsaddled his dead charger and took a blanket from her back. This we contrived to erect into a temporary screen, by planting a few muskets in the ground and attaching the blanket to them. I now inquired about his wound and found that it had been inflicted by a round short, which, passing through the neck of his horse, had all but separated his thigh: there was still some fleshy attachment; but I already saw the advance of gangrene

---

13. Note by Smith – They were both of the 10th [Hussars].
14. The poor sergeant had only been out one night but was confused.

and had every professional fear excited as to his ultimate fate. The only difference between his case and Lord Anglesea's [Anglesey[15]] was, that the one had prompt surgical assistance and the other had not. They were both wounded in almost an identical manner, for a round shot, among the very last that came from the enemy, shattered a thigh of each of these *soldiers*. Had B[aird]'s leg been amputated immediately after the accident, I have no doubt that he would have done well, as it was, I never expected a recovery. He told me that during the *first* night (as he calculated) he had been exceedingly distressed by the moans of the poor animal which shared his fate; and that he desired an infantry soldier who passed by to have the humanity to shoot her through the head. He would have done it himself, crippled as he was, but the pistol and carbine were on the saddle; and as he had fallen about a couple of yards from her, (or rather had been carried to the spot, as all the regiment was by at the time), he could not accomplish it. He made many anxious inquiries about the fate and fare of the corps and expressed great satisfaction on hearing that certain officers and others were safe, as well as at the great and splendid victory. In fact, the heroic fellow (a Scotsman) seemed to be divested now of all anxiety about himself and to consider his sufferings at an end. For my own part, I knew otherwise; but this was not the time to reveal my sentiments.

The water bearer arrived and shortly afterwards the press-gang (if I may so call them), or recruiting party, accompanied by seven lusty Belgians – but laziness was written on their foreheads and greediness depicted on their general aspect. I conceived that I should do no good with this set, if left alone with them: so, I desired that the three mounted men would stay with us, while the seven pillagers and myself carried off their comrade. This proved to be a proper precaution; for we came to blows before the poor sufferer was deposited in the still miserable situation I had found for him. We had but a short quarter of a mile to go; but if they had been [needed] to carry him to Paris, they could not have pleaded more objections, or raised a greater clamour. One was too old, another too young, a third lame, a fourth sick and the other three had excuses which I have forgotten, but which were equally to the purpose. I was a ruffian enough, however, to disregard them all. We placed our

---

15. This is an anachronism as he was the Earl of Uxbridge at Waterloo, not becoming Lord Anglesey for a few months.

charge in a blanket, and proceeded a few yards, when excuses for inability to go on were handed in seven-fold. The rascals understood French enough to comprehend what I meant by having their sculls [*sic*] cloven, or their brains blown out, if they dared to desert; but as the burden was really more than we could bear, we rested occasionally and in the intervals the bearers asked and obtained permission, 'pour *piller* un *peu*,' [to loot a little] provided they took the nearest plunder, the dragoons keeping a sharp look out for tricks. In all probability these poor fellows would have liked to make a grab for themselves; but to their honour be it recorded, they never manifested the slightest inclination of the kind while they were under my observation. At length we got our wounded man under cover and that was almost all which could be done for him. I had previously been in the farmhouse of [Mont] *St Jean* and finding it likely to be made a temporary hospital station, resolved to gather all my own flock together there. Poor B[aird] was about the first that entered; but even then his wound was so serious that I could not decide how to act without a consultation with other medical officers; so I pacified him as well as I could for the moment, and set out in search of new adventures. One of a melancholy cast soon afterwards occurred.

I went to the gate of this farmyard in a dreary enough state of mind, knowing that there must be other men yet upon the field and unable to decide in what direction to bend my footsteps. The execrable beast, (too much execrated perhaps already) I had vowed *never* to mount again happen what would. It was alarmed at the very sight of a wounded and disabled man; as to guns and corpses and carcasses of dead horses, an epic poem might be written about its terrors when we came near anything of that sort. While standing where I have mentioned, one of the regiment came past. I stopped him and enquired whither he was going. 'To the burying party,' was the reply. 'That,' said I, 'Is the party I have been looking for all day and can't find, are you sure you know where they are?' 'O, certainly Sir: sure I am one of them and I have been down to the *town* (village) for some water and if you will come along with me, I am sure they will all be *proud* to see you, dead or alive.' 'Even among the dead,' thought I, 'there must be comfort for *me*.' So, I accompanied my guide and was surprised to find two sergeants and twenty or thirty men, at no great distance from the farm and nearly where I had encountered so much desolation in the early part of the day; but the truth was, that they did not come till after my departure and had I been allowed to remain with the regiment till these people had been despatched upon their solemn duty, B[aird] would have been more readily found and things better managed, but it is not in mortals to foresee the issue of events. Everything was intended and executed for the best.

My steps (*a pied* [on foot]) were now directed to the ground upon which I had parted with the regiment on the day preceding, just before the charge. One of the sergeants came to me and I asked if they had discovered any wounded men? 'One or two,' was the reply. I observed that there must be more, if we were upon the spot, or even near it, where the charge had been made. He *doubted*, I insisted that scouts should be despatched to look about, that the living were of more importance than the dead, that I had been unable to pick the poor men up for want of proper information and assistance, that I had with great difficulty found Sergeant B[aird] and that I would be answerable for them to the regiment, if this duty detained them; but that I could not part with them till a thorough search had been made. The sergeant then despatched two or three more in as many directions and asked me, in the meantime, if I was hungry! 'Hungry! Why I am *starving*.' 'Bless me, Sir, I do have some gin in my canteen and I believe we have now a supply of water; will you condescend to help yourself?' I *graciously* did condescend, but observed, that a razor and looking glass, with a piece of soap, would be a most agreeable preliminary. 'Can any man lend me shaving-tackle?' Half a dozen volunteers came forward. The *convenience* of a soldier's life consists in carrying all the necessary implements of personal comfort about his frame, so that the accommodation met with on this occasion ought to excite no astonishment. I seated myself among dead men, placed the mirror on a pile of knapsacks and adorned myself (such ornamenting as it was, remember the *moustaches*) amid a scene that would have shaken the hand off most of the barbers in Europe.

While this was going forward and the scouts were patrolling about, I was besought to taste some pork. *Necessitas non habet legem* [Necessity knows no law] must be my apology for accepting a dinner from a non-commissioned officer, if any apology belongs to the case. Eat of his provender and drink from his canteen I did; but I sat a very short time at a table, composed of the same materials which had formed my toilette and then we turned our attention to serious business.

The funeral process, in the meantime went on; but in the course of it several poor fellows were noted defunct whom I afterwards found well and hearty with the regiment. There was no small difficulty in recognising features; and where scrutiny could not be minutely exercised, mistakes were to be expected. The dresses being alike too, the means of discriminating could not be equal to what might be relied upon under other circumstances.

As our melancholy duties proceeded, day began to decline and some time was occupied in transporting the few survivors we could find to the shelter of the farm. It was satisfactory to be certain, that while no *living* man of the regiment was left to the miseries of neglect, no one *dead* was left to be plundered by the rapacious. All the wounded were gathered under the roof of one cow house and supplied with straw, the utmost extent of our resources in the way of bedding. Upon one of them I dressed thirteen wounds, but the economy of our proceedings, in this den of suffering, will be detailed in the following.

Before entering upon the account of what fell under my personal observation, I should be culpable in omitting the tragic event which deprived the service and the regiment of two gallant and most promising young officers, and myself at the same time, of a *friend*. Concerning this youth, something has already been said. Let me add that though not the only, he was the eldest son and heir of a gentleman, still I believe, a county member of the House of Commons.[16] He was killed outright in the charge, belonging at the time to the right squadron. The other, who, it may be remarked, had associated with him in a successful attempt to alleviate our miseries during the preceding wet night, was the only hope of a branch of a noble family, the only son of a gallant admiral.[17] He also fell in the same charge; and the death of both was prompt, if not instantaneous. They were interred where they were found lying, on the day following; and I could name the gallant owners of the tender hearts which shed tears over their remains; but I have no right or authority to do so. If these volumes bring the narrative down to a period sufficiently late, an affecting incident will be found, arising out of the fate of the

---

16. Cornet Lockhart's father was William Elliot Lockhart of Borthwickbrae, Roxburgh, who was MP for Selkirkshire from 1806 to 1830.
17. Lieutenant Lindsey James Bertie was the only son of Admiral of the Blue Sir Albermarle Bertie (1755–1824).

first-mentioned officer [Lockhart]. The year after these events, his father visited the spot upon which he fell; but he would not remove the hallowed dust, no grave could be so honourable; and there my young friend still remains.

[The final butcher's bill for the 12th Light Dragoons was: 2 officers, 6 sergeants and 39 rank & file killed. 3 officers (Sandys died on 19 June), 3 sergeants and 55 rank & file wounded. 90 horses were killed or wounded]

# Chapter 8

# Mont St Jean Farm

Twelve medical officers stationed themselves within the farm of [Mont] *St Jean*, among not less than five hundred wounded soldiers, many of whom were French prisoners; and every house in the neighbourhood was in a similar manner converted into an hospital, such as it was. I presume the economy of all the others to have been nearly the same as that of our own; and to convey some idea of what this was, must be the object of the present.[1]

---

1. Note by Smith – My especial charge was of course, the wounded of the 12th Dragoons, and these it has been stated, were collected together in one corner of a desolate outhouse, blankets and straw forming the extent of their temporary accommodation. Near them sat a prisoner, who complained most bitterly of the hardness of his fate; and as I was going in and out, the most urgent and importunate appeals were made to inspect his wound. I assured him that he should be attended to as soon as possible, but that his case did not appear to be an urgent one, while there were numerous claims more pressing to be attended to. 'Oh Sir, do *look* at my leg! What will become of me? I am not a Frenchman!' 'Not a Frenchman?' 'No I am a Dunkirk lad, if I could but write to my mother!' 'I have a mother myself I should be glad to write to, but writing is out of the question right now.' Here one of our sufferers censured his conduct in no measured terms, asking if he thought the surgeon had nothing to do but look at a bruise made by a spent ball? Advising to be thankful that it was not with him as with too many who were near him. However, as he began to weep, I desired him to remove the handkerchief and let me see what was really the matter. I have no doubt that he must have been suffering to a considerable degree, for a musquet ball had passed between the bones of his leg, inflicting a painful though not a serious wound. Having assured him that he was in no danger and would soon get well, he became *intoxicated* with the good news, threw up his cap *and cursed Bonaparte!* An observation made by Sergeant B[aird] upon the same occasion, ought to be quoted, as exceedingly characteristic. Someone had received a sabre wound on the head, which when I came to dress, I found had not penetrated the skull. B[aird] looked attentively on during the business and the wound being cleaned and fully displayed, he drily remarked, 'he must have been a weak man who struck *that* blow: it is lucky for you my lad, that it was not from *me!*' Going into one of the wards of this dreary hospital, I found it occupied by *prisoners*. I observed a *trait* here, which shocked me greatly, though the necessity of circumstances might excuse it. Two Frenchmen were *seated* on the ground (being unable to move on account of severe wounds) each with a stick in his hand; between them was another, who in the agonies of suffering had become not only convulsed, but *insensible*; and this unfortunate being was every minute rolling upon the others, whose senses were still entire and probably sharpened by bodily pain. Their whole attention was directed to the task of *beating* off, or *pushing* away, their unconscious tormentor. Thus was a

For the first day we had neither food for ourselves, nor instruments for performing any of the important operations. We were all of the rank of Assistant [Surgeons] and they are not required by the regulations of the service, to be provided with more than a small pocket case. We therefore, as a proper precaution, *en attendant* the arrival of the requisite apparatus (which was ordered from the General Hospital), bled our poor fellows all round. Towards evening the amputation knives &c made their appearance and what remained of daylight was employed in their application to some of the severest cases. Sergeant B[aird] importuned us very much to take off his leg and we at length complied, though aware that the operation was merely the infliction of so much additional pain. It was useless however, to attempt deceiving him into the belief that it would be better to delay till he got to Brussels; he was firmly importunate and we soothed his mind by yielding. Gangrene had already seized the stump and we knew too well what must be the result. Contrary to expectation, he did not die at the farm, but lived long enough to reach Brussels, where, in a few days, his fate was added to that of too many other gallant men.

We had reserved for our own accommodation, a small stable, from the loft over which we had the good fortune to obtain a sufficient quantity of hay to repose upon, when night interrupted our proceedings. It may not be improper to say that we were now among the longest days of summer, so that our bodily fatigue was necessarily considerable, not to take privations, anxieties and every description of inconvenience into account. How we managed to live I do not remember. In this respect I must in all probability, have been a severe sufferer had they not sent a soldier, whose horse had been killed, to attend to our wounded as an orderly. The man did his duty remarkably well, was exceedingly attentive to and anxious about his comrades, whom we had gathered into one group, a thing which gave them no small satisfaction in these forlorn circumstances. Some of them required two hours every time they were dressed, partly from the number of their injuries, partly from the inconvenient and uncomfortable nature of the situation we were placed in and also from the difficulty of changing

---

poor abandoned sufferer treated by his countrymen with infinitely greater barbarity, in his last moments, than even his avowed foes would have thought possible: but many allowances must be made for the influence of *the first law of nature*. Of course, as soon as this exhibition of wretchedness was discovered such relief as existing means afforded was administered.

their postures to get at their wounds. The man already mentioned, who from sabres, shot and lances, had thirteen [wounds], recovered well; but his intermediate sufferings were great.

I can hardly now connect particular transactions with particular days, therefore I must note things down as they turn up in my memory. Of myself individually, it is my desire to avoid saying more than may be necessary. I was certainly (from the causes already assigned) in worse plight than the rest; and having no baggage or servant, was compelled to wear my wet clothes till they dried upon my back and my boots, till they hardened on my legs. But there were too many claims of a more pressing nature upon our attention to admit of much commiseration for oneself.

The state of the farmhouse yard and offices of [Mont] *St Jean*, has been frequently alluded to and probably the public may be almost as well acquainted with their localities as I can pretend to be. It had been occupied by a family of great respectability and no doubt of considerable wealth, but living things except the pigeons, saw I none belonging to it. These poor creatures, secured as one might have thought them, by the aerial situation of their abode, did not escape the general doom, which the horrid necessity of the occasion had sanctioned, as to all eatable things. For the honour of the cloth, I must add that no medical officer molested them; but a party of straggling Dutch or Belgic soldiers entered the farmyard and found a ladder and sent up one of their number to pull the little innocent inhabitants from their holes. Remonstrance was vain and threats, which we had no means of executing, would have been ridiculous; but my indignation got the better of my prudence and I kicked the ladder away, leaving the plunderer like St Simeon Stylites, though on the top of a pole instead of a pillar.[2] I thought it unfair that passers-by should help themselves to what, by all the laws of war, belonged to us; but the man threatened to shoot me for my interference with what he no doubt considered a *lawful* occupation. I was fain therefore, to mind my own business. If I mistake not, this was the farm in which a woman is described as having remained during the whole of the battle in one of the upper apartments.[3] Nothing is more conceivable, though the battering and

---

2. Saint Simeon Stylites the Elder (390–459 AD) lived on a small platform on top of a pillar at Aleppo for 37 years.
3. The farmer's wife claimed to have stayed in the loft space throughout the battle.

demolition must have been appalling. Any female but a phlegmatic *frau* of Belgium must have died of fear and noise under such circumstances. Neither man, woman, nor beast was about the place when my brother *chips* [surgeons] and I collected our patients in it.

One very painful circumstance, the mention of which in the course of conversation, has always been attended with expressions of sympathy and deep interest, I must not omit to recite. During the first night (that of Monday the 19th) our rest such as it was, sustained great interruption from the most melancholy of all causes, the groans of half a thousand men in pain and the agonies of death: and although as fast as vacancies occurred, these were filled by new-comers from more distant quarters, so that the number of our charge could hardly be said (for a day or two) to have diminished, the awful sounds night after night, became more feint: some perhaps began to recover and others were removed, but I knew too well that the *grim tyrant* was also very busy in silencing them.

It has been observed that many of these sufferers were French; and generally speaking their cases were severe. No Frenchman able to take himself off, would have remained in the hands of the enemy. We made no distinction[4] as to friend or foe: and these men had probably a stronger claim upon us than our own; for to the common participation in pain and privations were added, in their case, apprehensions of a varied nature and perhaps distrust in the English surgeons. We attended to the most urgent injuries first, whether discovered in a Frenchman or an Englishman; and confident I am that, while we all felt the propriety of devoting the greater portion of our sympathy and attention to the men of our respective regiments, (to attend upon whom was our stipulated duty) not a foreigner (among *thousands*) would be found reluctant to bear testimony to the unwearied patience and scrupulous humanity (it might not become *me* to say anything of skill) with which they were uniformly treated by one and all of us. There was, it must however be admitted, a striking reluctance on the part of our captives to submit to the knife:

---

4. Note by Smith – I have observed that twelve medical officers assembled at the farm of *St Jean*, so they did; but ten only of this number congregated together. The *surgeon* and *assistant surgeon* of a certain regiment, were upon the spot; but they pitched a tent outside the farmyard and devoted the whole of their time and attention to the cases of their own men. In this they were *prudent*; but they were not *kind*. They abstained from all intercourse with us; and were, in every respect better off than the rest of their brethren. They were certainly better *fed*; for they fed *themselves*.

while we were absolutely teased out of our lives by the importunities of the English, to cut off their limbs or perform equivalent operations. Some went so far as to threaten to do it themselves if we would not. In this matter I am inclined to think that there was a strong manifestation of national character. Whatever may have been the cause, the fact was that the English never took pain into their calculation and had no idea as to future inconvenience from dismemberment. The French on the contrary, raised every imaginable objection and in several instances, we were compelled to resort to authority if not even to force. It will at once occur to the intelligent reader, that these men had an interest in saving their limbs, while our own people had a contrasted one in losing them. A crippled soldier of Napoleon had nothing to expect but what beggary or his other private resources might afford: whereas the Englishman relied on his country for a comfortable provision during the rest of his life. Granting the fact, I am convinced that my theory is well-founded. The *insensibility* of the North American savages to bodily pain has long been familiarly known; insensibility however, is not the proper term by which to designate this manifestation: it is moral indifference, or rather contempt in *them*; and this *indifference* we perceive among our troops, and even on the part of the weaker sex. Women think comparatively little of bodily pain; all sensitive as they are, they bear surgical operations better than the '*lords of the creation.*' Everyone who has 'walked an hospital' can attest this fact. I have no wish to deteriorate from the French character, for it is one which stands high in my estimation (the reasons I reserve till a future opportunity) but I think there is a sturdy resoluteness about an Englishman, which it is not in the *nature* of the mercurial sons of that happier soil to exhibit.

During occasional moments, while waiting for the return of messengers, the arrival of orders (and to do the Inspector of Hospitals[5] justice, he troubled us with very few, while he abstained as much as possible from insulting us by proffering *unnecessary* advice and assistance), we lounged at the gate of the farmyard, which opened into the chaussee, at the point where the road branches off to Nivelles and amusement was most assuredly to be had even here. Upon one occasion, when I happened to be there, I

---

5. Sir James Robert Grant was the Inspector of Hospitals based at Brussels during the Waterloo campaign.

was not a little surprised at the apathy of a squad of heavy cavalry which was passing. They halted and with something like satisfaction in their manner, pointed to a naked body, lying close to the road and said, 'that is *our colonel*!!'[6] It was so!!! Good God I thought, had it been our colonel, or even our farrier, he would not have been left there. I am convinced that our regiment was the only one of the division to which it belonged, that interred their dead.

The weather being sultry, it became indispensable to dispose of the cadaverous incumbrance, which threatened a pestilence in the country, from the circumstance of the process of putrefaction or decomposition having made considerable progress, for our own miserable part it may be said, that we abode in *stink*. The authorities therefore, pressed the *posse* into the field and large pits were dug, into which men were thrown by dozens, others being made for the horses. Many were burnt upon the surface of the field; but some of these capacious graves were close to the farm and many a gallant form was deposited in them. I am satisfied that sudden death in the field cannot be painful, for in numerous instances I saw no change of countenance in the corpse; and the difficulties of recognition, already quoted arose rather from contingent disfigurements of blood, dirt &c, than from the direct influence of death.

At the gate aforesaid, two medical officers of a highland regiment and myself, were standing on the Wednesday [21 June] (I think), when a poor looking cripple, dressed in clothes of a private of the rifle corps and a Kilmarnock bonnet[7] on his head (both his arms cautiously carried before him, as is if he desired to have them under his immediate observation, in order to protect them from injury) came up and accosted my companions, in the Scottish dialect:- 'Eh, lads, are ye here? God be thanked! I am a happy man now.' The two surgeons gazed at him for a moment, as if at a stranger. His aspect they were unable to recognise, but the sound of

---

6. Only two colonels of British heavy cavalry were killed at Waterloo. We know that the body of Colonel James Hamilton of the Scots Greys was found on the battlefield, leaving the only other candidate as Colonel William Fuller of the 1st (King's) Dragoon Guards.
7. Note by Smith – The undress cap of most of our regiments, of late years. It has many advantages over the old-fashioned cloth thing, which has not been very long exploded. It is strong, warm, durable (in the end, therefore, cheaper) and better adapted in every way for the vicissitudes of a military life. The fabric (and I believe it is a product of the loom) was originally woven at the town of which it bears the name; but probably, like cambric lace, may now be made in many other places as well as Kilmarnock.

his voice was sufficient. 'Good God, M[ackay],[8] is this you? We thought you were killed or taken!' He gave a brief recital of his adventures, the substance of which was, that he had been severely wounded and captured during the action: that as soon as they had made him prisoner they plundered him, tearing off his epaulets and depriving him of everything valuable: that they afterwards, without paying the slightest attention to his wounds, drove him with other prisoners, to the rear as far as Charleroi and behaved with the greatest brutality, making no allowance whatever for inability to keep up with the escort. By the time they got to C[harleroi] an idea of the fortune of the day had reached the place and the confusion became so great that the Englishmen contrived to get away from their guard and in several instances obtained shelter from the inhabitants. The French were so exasperated at the change in their prospects, that they resolved to blow up the town; but the knowledge of this intention coming to the ears of the authorities, they found means to wet the powder. Captain M[ackay] subsequently made his escape; I believe he had put on the uniform of a dead rifleman, because his own clothes were destroyed. We kept him with us till the following day and then found, as will be presently explained, a pleasant way of forwarding him to Brussels.

On the Wednesday morning intelligence was brought to our augean [a place of great filth or corruption] headquarters that all the patients were drunk! Five hundred men drunk!! Quite ridiculous, more than impossible. They could not find the means; they might have had money, but where could they obtain the drink even *for* money?

There was no one to sell it, nor was there enough of liquor for the purpose within a dozen miles of us, to our thorough belief and satisfaction; besides it was a *physical* as well as a *moral* impossibility that so many helpless beings belonging to so many different regiments and even to so many different *nations*, should join in one general scheme of disorder and hilarity, (their own safety being out of the question) but if it was not literally, it turned out to be in the aggregate, true. After we had retired to

---

8. Captain Robert Mackay of the 79th Highland Regiment was severely wounded at Quatre Bras and was reported as 'Missing' in the Returns. A number of records, including Dalton's *Waterloo Roll Call*, show Mackay as killed, but this incorrect, he was made a prisoner of war. He was able to escape and rejoin his regiment and was awarded a Waterloo Medal. He later went on half pay as a Captain in the 91st Foot in October 1817 and he died in October 1826. I must thank Ron McGuigan for bringing this information to my attention.

our stable for the night, a straggling party got into the farm; and directed probably by information, or it may have been fortunate or expert in the article of search, they discovered the cellar and found it well stored with wine. When we sallied out to ascertain the truth of the matter, every other man had an empty bottle at his side: the marauders had not only supplied their own wants, but with an ignorant and mistaken kindness, had gratified the importunate clamourers, who could not rise to make a search for themselves. A few bottles were yet uncorked, these we seized as munitions; and proceeding into the cellar, found the remains of the stock, which also by way of precaution, we conveyed to the stable.[9] The risk to the patients was that of inflammation; and at this stage of our progress, we should have doubly felt the chagrin of a prevalent mortality. Our cases (excepting perhaps the most desperate) did so well, that one would almost say hospitals are superfluities. In sober truth however, they can neither be too numerous nor too well appointed.

One of the most troublesome patients I had to deal with was a groom of Marshal Ney. This man said he was not a soldier and therefore, had a right to give or withhold his consent as to the performance of an operation. His right arm had been shattered by a shell; I assured him that he must submit to amputation if he wished his life to be saved and that the delay of another day might prove fatal. Still he remonstrated about his independent situation as a private character. To this it could only be replied, that as we found him among the soldiers, wounded and a prisoner, we could consider him in no other light than a follower of the army, amenable to military discipline; and that as few were responsible for his proper treatment, *off the arm must come*, no appeal could be listened to; that an Englishman would not make a word, or conceive so much as a thought against the proposal, which could have no object but his own benefit, as we subjected ourselves to great trouble and inconvenience by undertaking the operation. However, in consideration of his situation and out of respect for his master, we would give him two hours to make up his mind, hoping at the end of that time that he would see the propriety of consenting, but that we should be under the painful

---

9. Note by Smith – An account has been published, that the Prince of Orange had an interview with the owner or occupant of this farm before the action and promised him full indemnity for whatever loss he might suffer in consequence of the exposed situation of his property.

necessity of disregarding all considerations excepting his ultimate safety. At the expiration of the term we found him quite reconciled and he bore the operation with an agreeable degree of fortitude. He was a good-looking young man, possessed of all the eloquent plausibility and engaging address of the better sort of Frenchmen; but had the Angel Gabriel fallen into our hands at [Mont] St Jean, with a shattered limb, I doubt his heavenly rhetoric would have been able to deter us from whipping it off.[10]

This is not the only anecdote of a similar nature which might be related. From the puerile (after what I have said I cannot call it *effeminate*) reluctance of the prisoners to undergo operations, they incurred the contempt of the English soldiers, who amid their own agonies, could yet find abstraction of mind and coherence of language, enough to bestow upon them a few hearty curses. Our men were surprised at the solicitude we manifested for a set of thankless and as far as they could be so, mutinous creatures, who had been placed upon the self-same footing with themselves, when they had little to expect but neglect, or abandonment to the tender mercies of the peasantry, more of which hereafter. By way of contrast, let me relate that after we had been a day or two here, a short, thick-set, stout English soldier came into the farm with a cudgel in his hand, but with scarcely the vestige of a countenance! He stumbled upon me (having inquired for a surgeon) and said he would be obliged to me if I would put up his face! He had been struck by a shell and the whole integuments of his countenance had been torn off, excepting at one point and were hanging over his shoulder. These he had been resolute enough to preserve, but had not met with professional assistance. The forehead, the skin round one eye, the soft parts of the nose, a portion of both cheeks, the lips and one ear (I forget which) were literally detached and lying where I have described them. Seeing the extent of the yet remaining attachments and that the separated parts manifested no sign of putrefaction, I deemed the undertaking of replacement far from hopeless. By the aid of diachylon plaister,[11] I certainly did succeed in restoring this poor object to the possession of the 'human face divine.' No persuasion could induce him to remain where he was: 'No, he was in good health thank God, had a good

---

10. Note by Smith – I heard good accounts of this poor lad afterwards.
11. Diachylon Plaister – An adhesive plaster made from oil and the juices of a number of herbs, often called lead-plaster.

stick, the French were licked and now that he was a man again, he would go on to Brussels.' I saw and heard no more of him.

One day (probably on the Tuesday [20 June]) I felt so stiff and cold, that I requested another officer to have an eye to my men, while I took an hour's walk. I naturally directed my steps to the field, indeed our habitation formed part of it; but I mean to *the open ground*, where I met with a party of artillery. I entered into conversation with the sergeant who commanded and found him to be, as all artillerymen are, remarkably intelligent. He explained several things that had been objects of his own personal observation. He shewed me his gun, dismantled and lying on the ground, where his tumbril had been struck and also disabled; but he shewed me a far more interesting sight than all this: eighty-two brass cannon, taken from the enemy, now paraded together and all cast in *Republican moulds*!! Where they had been raked from I cannot say, but perhaps from fortified places near the frontiers. Every one of these engines of destruction bore the emblems of Revolutionary France, the cap of liberty, the inscriptions 'Liberte, Egalite, Franternite,' &c and each had some name taken from ancient history, or classical mythology. There were Jupiters and Vulcans and Brutuses and others, whose titles and designations I cannot recall.

While this inspection was in progress, my attention was attracted by some soldiers, who were guarding and conducting a heavy looking carriage (ie coach) along the road. They informed me that this was Bonaparte's own chariot, which they (Prussians) had captured on the evening after the fight and were now escorting to Brussels. This celebrated *lion* became afterwards a most profitable speculation in England.[12] I have no doubt that, had I signified the slightest inclination to that effect, I might have had a ride in Napoleon's own corner of this vehicle over the celebrated field upon which the sun of his mortal glory set for ever. But I little dreamt what was to be the celebrity of this post-chaise, when I first saw it.

Mentioning a ride puts me in mind of my personal poverty at this juncture. I found myself upon the field of Waterloo, with a single five-

---

12. Napoleon's carriage was captured on the night of 18 June by Major von Keller and his troopers at Genappe. It was sent as a gift to the Prince Regent but sold to a Mr Bullock, who made a fortune of over £26,000 (£1.8 million today) by displaying it to the public at the London Museum (or Egyptian Hall), Piccadilly. After passing through a number of hands, the coach was sold to Madame Tussaud's in 1842. It was displayed there until 18 March 1925 when it and two other carriages owned by Napoleon and many other artefacts were destroyed in a huge fire.

franc piece in my pocket. On the evening after the action, the soldier whose canteen had been filled with brandy and who had been my servant some time before in Portugal, requested I would take charge of a watch and two dollars he had taken from a French man, for the purpose of handing them over to his wife, whom I was likely to meet with before he would. The lady never came in my way before her husband and I met again, I found convenient use in the dollars; and the watch, (after having at some trouble and with some anxiety, preserved both it and my own) was returned. This man found also a note of hand, for a thousand francs, upon the person of another victim; but though made payable in Paris, we could never obtain one farthing for it, or even trace the responsible party.

On Wednesday the 21st, our supply of new cases not only ceased, but assistance of a very acceptable nature was brought to us; this was in the shape of means to convey our charge to Brussels. In many instances, curiosity to see the field brought the higher and wealthier classes out, in their own carriages.[13] They made a rule of bringing refreshments for the wounded and of taking as many as they could possibly accommodate back with them. We were now incessantly applied to for this purpose; and it was by no means, the least curious of the contrasts by which we were surrounded, to see five or six disfigured, bandaged, dirty and bloody fellows, getting into a handsome vehicle. I understand that the *authorities* sent every species of easy conveyance for the same purpose: all the hackney-coaches. To wit, spring-carts and waggons of every description, which with the auxiliaries already alluded to, cleared off the whole in the course of that and the following day. No females to the best of my recollection, made their appearance; they were busily engaged I believe,

---

13. Note by Smith – The anxieties of the *first sportsmen* (for such they may with propriety be called) who came relic and trophy hunting to the field, 'when the fight was done' were rewarded by the clothes and accoutrements, the pocket books and trinkets of the dead. Of this class of *virtuosi* it would be degradation to say more than that they would have taken the gun carriages for fuel, if they dared; and would have carried away the cargo of every tumbril, for sale in the shops of neighbouring towns; but exploits of this nature were hazardous in a variety of ways. After them came the gentry of Brussels and many of the better sort of our own countrymen; who were in ecstasies at finding, or even purchasing, a sword, or a pistol; but as time advanced, the *chandlery* spoken of, *in loco citato*, began to exhibit its claim. A reverend friend of mine seals his letters to this day with a brass button, that once decorated the throat of an Imperial Grenadier. It was picked up by him, on his return from *le Cateau*, and it is all he has to shew for his lost *sermons*.

in administering to the necessities of those who were conveyed to them, under the care of their male relatives.

Thursday [22 June] found us disengaged from our arduous and painful duties: all the houses on our side of the field were in the course of that day, cleared of their suffering occupants and we began to consider how we should be able to overtake our respective corps. Of my own I had yet heard nothing; but I had an assurance that they must be about the farthest off from the place I was then in. The Inspector [of Hospitals] now sent out two of us to scour the field, one to the right and the other (myself) to the left, in order to see if any men had taken shelter in out-houses, or other situations in which they might have been overlooked; and to report their state and numbers, so that proper assistance and means of transport might be sent to them. I now learnt that the colonel was under the care of the Surgeon in Waterloo, to which place after performing the duty in question, I was to repair and ascertain which of us was to stay with the colonel and which to set off to the army, a measure of necessity, as there was no Surgeon with the regiment. A party of the Oxford Blues [Horse Guards], which had been attending their wounded, offered to sell me a *captured* horse as they called him, for eight dollars payable by order on our reaching the army. The *plough-beast* had been put into one of the outhouses, under a decree of my own mind, that we should never more attempt to serve the king, in conjunction *personarum nostrarum* [with each other]. My purchase however, had a very distinct account of his place and station in the English army, written with red hot iron[14] on his hoof. This I saw before I mounted; but as riding *him* or walking was the alternative, I affected blindness to the circumstance till we came back, when upon

---

14. Note by Smith – Troop horses are registered as regularly as their riders; but as they do not always answer to their names, are recognised by branded marks, established in one of the following ways. On the shoulder we find the stamp of the regiment; and either under the mane or upon that part of the back which the saddle covers, the troop letter and no. of the animal are clipped into his fur; or the *regimental* mark is burnt into his hoof, which I hold to be the most humane and effectual method, though in time it grows out and requires therefore to be occasionally renewed; but the mark, which is imprinted on the *sensible* skin, remains for life. When horses are cast, they sell the better for not showing any *indelible* stamps; and it is a well-known fact that a horse which will never do any good in a *troop stable*, will often be hardly recognisable after a short abode in that of a private individual: consequently the aversion to give a fair price for a cast trooper is much diminished by the monument of his history not remaining a *permanent* disadvantage to future prospects.

announcing the discovery and pretending to be highly displeased with the folly and imprudence of these men in selling me one of His Majesty's horses, I recovered my draught and handed back the bargain, exhorting them to be sure and take care of him, till an opportunity occurred of delivering him up to his regiment. He was a fine large grey, but not a *Scots* one.

*Outward* bound, I saw nobody excepting one or two dying horses and some yet unburied carcasses. The ground was all the more desolate (as it seemed to me) from the removal even of the corpses. I presume that not less than twenty thousand had by this time been put out of sight. I met several peasants and inquired most particularly if they had any knowledge of such as I was in quest of; but upon the scene of active operations I was glad to find that no one remained, nor even in its immediate vicinity. On ascending the French side, I met two respectable looking men, whose curiosity was exercised in contemplating numerous collections of French musquets that were erected into regular piles; and they informed me that in a church a little further on, I should find a very large number of wounded, whom they conjectured to be Prussians; this was not a probable conclusion; but whatever they were, my duty was to ascertain the truth for myself, as far as I could. The church I afterwards ascertained to be that of *Planchenoit [Plancenoit]*, in the village of which name Bonaparte had established his headquarters on the night of the seventeenth.[15] Here I found a crowd of wounded men who had got together for common protection against the country people, not one of them daring to venture from the main body, to make known their situation. They stated to me that they were Prussians but had no medical officer among them and had not received any professional aid: I saw at once what they were and explained to them my errand. I stated that although I was an English surgeon, I could be of no use by staying with them then; but would lose no time in reporting their situation and that every species of effective assistance would be forthwith sent, desiring them however, to be in readiness for speedy removal. I think there were about two thousand of these unfortunate men, of whose existence till now, we had not the most distant idea.

---

15. This is incorrect, Napoleon's headquarters were established at Le Caillou on the Brussels chaussee.

My way back was by the high road, which cut through the field and upon the opposite side of which my *collaborateur de reconnaissance* was to make his inquiries. Having passed the celebrated hovel of *La Belle Alliance*, between that and the lordly farmhouse of *La Haye Sainte* I came upon a French grenadier, very much disabled, without anything upon his head and (to the best of my recollection) almost blinded by wounds. This man, whose anxiety and sufferings had in all probability, induced him to detach himself from the *Planchenoit [Plancenoit]* party, or who might not have known of them, was undergoing the most ruffianly treatment from a gang of peasants. The common impulse of humanity must have roused anyone's feelings in his behalf; but I felt quite indignant that such poltroons should take upon them to maltreat a fallen enemy, the more especially as, had the fortune of the day been reversed, we ourselves should have been subjected to similar, if not even worse usage. As all doctors as I was, I had a trusty sabre at my side and a good horse under me; the one I drew and the other I spurred; and five or six to one, as these footpads were against me and no other person within sight, they ran off, with some frivolous excuse as to the demerits of the soldier and their own zeal and loyalty. I then conducted the wretched sufferer into the farm of *La Haye Sainte* and left him safe among my countrymen and professional brethren. This instance of animosity, on the part of those who ought to have been *passive* at least, reminds me of another. While we were removing Sergeant B[aird], we passed a crippled French officer, who I recollect was in a sitting posture. He appealed to my notice and requested that I would have him *remover*; I promised to attend him as soon as I should be at liberty. My '*bearers*' however, who were all of the greedy and vindictive class of the lower orders, declared they would have nothing to do with him and *reviled* him in strong language for being a scoundrel of a Frenchman, who ought to lie there and die. We got the gentleman into the farmyard notwithstanding.

Having reported the state of the case to the Inspector, all the disposable force of physic was despatched instanter to *Planchenoit [Plancenoit]* and I should have had to accompany them, but for the necessity of the interview with my friend S [Robinson], already alluded to. I now took out my long-tailed and splay-footed charger for the last time and proceeded to the village of Waterloo, about two miles and a half on the road to Brussels; which city perhaps, I may take occasion to observe, was about twelve from the scene of slaughter to which it owed its safety. In an auberge I found the Surgeon,[16] who gave very satisfactory reasons for his remaining till he could convey the colonel to Brussels. Indeed, our commanding officer was in so precarious a state, that troubling him about any sort of arrangement was out of the question. It became therefore, my affair to make all possible haste. But the brute! We got over that difficulty through a melancholy circumstance. An officer with the regiment had a brother in the Guards, who was killed; this gentleman's servant had found his way to the auberge with two horses, to receive instructions and assistance how to get to his late master's brother.[17] S [Robinson] desired me to leave the *agriculturist* there, promising to hand him over to Chiswick, whom there was no doubt he would shortly fall in with and to mount the spare animal, taking the man on with me; he would act as my servant till we got to the regiment, where I should find myself once more at home. We intended to have gone as far as *Mons* that evening, but the crowded state of the road and the necessity of drawing rations detained us so long that we got no farther than *Nivelles*.

I was nearly pressed again into the sad duties of the last four days. At the bifurcation of the roads, there seemed to be a great squeeze[18] and the Inspector of the cavalry division[19] would still have detained and sent me back to Brussels but for the state of the regiment. On learning this he ordered me to proceed, saying he would detain the surgeon. 'Very well,' thought I, 'and welcome, let him settle accounts for himself;' and I felt, when this obstacle was removed, as if I had made a very desirable escape.

---

16. Note by Smith – It may be misunderstood if this expression be allowed to pass without explanation. The auberge of Waterloo was now the quarters of the Colonel and S [Robinson] seldom left his apartment; indeed he spent but a few minutes with me, during which he walked on tip toe and spoke in a whisper. After ordering me something to eat and making the arrangements already spoken of, he returned to Colonel [Ponsonby] and I saw no more of him. One of the colonel's servants dished me up a steak and in a few minutes, I was *en route* as was designed for Mons.
17. Captain Alexander Craufurd of the 2nd Ceylon Regiment was with the 12th Light Dragoons at Waterloo as a volunteer, his brother Captain Thomas Craufurd of the 3rd Foot Guards was killed at Waterloo. Dalton's *Waterloo Roll Call* states that Alexander Craufurd was the only son of Sir James Craufurd of Kilbirney, but Ron McGuigan has been able to prove that he had three sons, Alexander being the second son. On his death in 1839 Sir James was succeeded by his third son the Reverend George Craufurd, Alexander having died in 1838.
18. Note by Smith – In all probability owing to the arrival of the 'forces' from *Planchenoit [Plancenoit]*; though of this I am not positively certain.
19. The Deputy Inspector of Hospitals for the cavalry was William Taylor.

# Chapter 9

# March to Paris

At Nivelles we found much confusion, hurry and inconvenience. Here, while hunting up the commissary and the store-keeper, I was hailed by a voice which, though I had not heard it for a long period, was quite familiar to me. The cry came from a Chaplain to the Forces,[1] with whom I had formed an intimacy in the Peninsula, but at whom I had considered myself fully warranted to take umbrage, in consequence of too ready an ear which I believed him to have lent to a slanderous report about my conduct in a midwifery affair.[2] For more

---

1. Further evidence given later shows that this was Chaplain to the Forces Robert Tunney.
2. Note by Smith – Thereby hung a droll little tale, which this may be the most fitting time to tell; although drolleries are scarcely appropriate to the serious subject of the text. The fair apology for such mixtures is perhaps, to be gathered from the recollection that events themselves are of a heterogenous nature and we do not profess to be digesting or arranging our materials into any sort of systematic order. The story is, that the wife of a purveyor's clerk required an accoucheur [male midwife]; and as I was the only medical officer on the station, the husband sought to engage my services. They were promised *conditionally*, if no other person could be found. It was no part of my *duty* to practise in that department and I had strong reasons for reluctance. However, the *conditional promise* was construed into *absolute refusal*; and my customer repaired to the commandant for 'an order to compel.' The commandant, who always had his wits at hand (and of whom I shall have high and honourable mention to make upon a future occasion), drily replied that he would consider what could be done and appointed a time for giving an answer. Me** was punctual, hugging himself no doubt, at having turned the P[rincipal] M[edical] O[fficer]'s flank. Be it observed that of these manoeuvres the PMO had no knowledge, till long afterwards. The c[ommandant] thus addressed himself to *plaintiff*: – 'I have been considering what can be done in your case; which is a *novel* one, relative to which I am afraid there does not exist a precedent. Dr J [Smith] does his duty quite to my satisfaction among the troops and I have been searching in vain for an instance of a *soldier being with child*; so that it must be matter of private courtesy and not of military duty.' Before this decision was made, a false statement had travelled up to headquarters; and drew the censure of my respected friend the head of the department upon my character as to humanity. I soon set this to rights; the clerk denied that he had sent any such statement and that there must have been a mistake. Fortunately the *promise* had been made before another officer. I should have *deserved* censure, had I hesitated to attend in a case of poverty, or particular suffering; but this was quite of another description. Probably the *clerks*, as well as the *clergy* of the service, may find a niche hereafter. Two English officers

than a year we had not corresponded and my last letter to him had been a trimmer, which he had been rather ashamed to answer. However, his practical piety was displayed in a very amiable manner on the present occasion. 'I dare say,' he observed, when I turned at the sound of his voice, 'you will not speak to me.' 'Why not? I have no reason but to rejoice at meeting you, especially under such circumstances.' 'Do you remember the promise you gave me when we parted at Coimbra?' 'I do not.' 'That the first day we met again you would dine with me.' 'O, very likely; and if you *have* any dinner, I shall be glad to keep my word, for I run a chance of starving here, in the midst of comparative plenty.' He was like myself, a mere passer through the place; but had already got a billet. We then went in search of something in the shape of a *victualling office*, or restaurant. We found a café with no very great difficulty; but *café* was literally all they had to give us. However, though I wished for something of a more substantial nature, we exchanged explanations about the old grievance and resumed our former intimacy. He was to proceed towards headquarters on the following day, in company with a brother priest; and I was glad to engage to be of the party. So, after making an appointment for a certain hour next morning, we separated.

My quarters were in the house of one of the magistrates. I found the gentleman sitting deep in council; and as my countenance was no doubt a letter of recommendation, he dispensed with the ceremony of making out a billet, sending a messenger with me to say that I had been selected for the lodging he in common with all the inhabitants, was under the necessity of affording and desiring that I should be suitably accommodated. I was not a little pleased to find a plentiful table set out. The master's apology for

---

were one evening walking through a celebrated fair, which at the time enlivened one of the principal cities in Portugal, when they observed a C[ommissary]'s clerk standing at a jeweller's booth, with a dashing female by his side. My friends went near enough to ascertain what was going on and saw him pay down a hundred dollars for a lady's gold chain. Upon this they drew back and the one addressed the other nearly in these terms. 'Did you see that? Here am I a captain in the army, whose pay and allowances are more than double that fellow's, not to speak of *rank*, and here are *you* at least a dozen degrees above him in every respect; and neither of us knows how to get his breakfast tomorrow morning. That fellow, who is not so high in the service as a corporal, has seven shillings and sixpence a day. I saw him this afternoon ride through the streets on an English horse, for which he boasts, that he gave a hundred guineas to a cavalry officer, his servant mounted on another, equally valuable and the *article* you see now by his side upon a third. We know that he lives in the most luxurious style gives splendid dinners and the most expensive wine in profusion. There is something rotten in *that* department.'

his absence was, being fully engrossed at the town-house, issuing billets and making other arrangements required by the troops, which would keep him from home all night. *Madame* also excused herself on the score of indisposition. This was perfectly proper and intelligible. In the absence of her husband, she could hardly do the honours to a stranger, in the capacity of a foreign military adventurer and her company would have placed me under considerable embarrassment. It was better therefore, to leave me alone. Of the luxury of a good bed, I shall not attempt to speak. Next morning my breakfast was carefully provided, in the style of hospitality characteristic of the country, and I proceeded on my journey under a heavy rain, which furnished my clerical friends with a satisfactory plea for remaining where they were, so that I had to march alone. The rain signified the less to me, as I was yet in possession of a considerable part of my share of the thunder-shower of *Quatre Bras*. Up to this time my wet boots had not been off; for had I been rash enough to try the experiment of the [boot] jack while at *[Mont] St Jean*, all the hooks of Hoby[3] would not have got them on again. I had slept well it is true, but afterwards had to un-gild the gingerbread, by putting on the wet habiliments, which were now saturated at a temperature considerably below that of animal heat.

My intention was to pass through Mons, as I calculated on meeting with a relay party of the regiment there and obtaining authentic information; but this design was altered through the following circumstance. For the purpose of resting and feeding the animals, I took the liberty to enter a large stable, where there were already two or three horses enjoying the luxuries in question. At first, I could see nobody 'belonging to them;' after a while however, our arrangements awoke a person who had been taking a comfortable nap in the manger; who putting his head over the edge of his couch, inquired what was the matter. I explained; and by means of a few courteous questions, he succeeded in making me give a proper account of myself, the sum and substance of which was, that I was a medical officer of the [12]th Regiment of Dragoons, who had been detained with the wounded and was now on my way to join. The gentleman informed me that he was similarly situated, that he was surgeon of one of the regiments of the German Legion; that he had all the hospital stores under

---

3. Mr George Hoby, of St James's Street, bootmaker to the Duke of Wellington, had designed hooks with which to help pull on the tight-fitting long boots.

his charge and a considerable detachment with him; then proposing, as our object was the same and we were brethren in a variety of senses, that we should proceed together. I was delighted at the offer and we soon resumed progress. He was an older and more knowing campaigner than me and I was glad to be under his advice and direction. He thought *Mons* would be an inconvenient route, as that road was crowded; whereas if we proceeded by *Binche*, we should stand a better chance of quarters. To this place therefore we bent our way but could not find any accommodation. We had an interview, however, with the commandant, a rough-looking Belgian, who had a most extraordinary propensity. While speaking, at every four or five words he gave two or three spits and those to whom he addressed himself soon found the necessity of keeping out of the range of this unusual missile. He asked us about the news, but we could get him to spit or sputter nothing more likely to suit our purpose than the advice to go on to a village called *Estiennes* [Estinnes-au-Val],[4] where we should infallibly get good quarters. We attended to his instructions and had no reason to repent of having done so.

My companion thought that we should not go forward empty handed: we were able to get some bread and two flasks of wine, for neither of which had we any occasion that evening. In *Estinnes au Val*, we were most heartily welcomed into a large farmhouse by two fine young men, the sons of the occupant. Him we did not see, for the simple reason that he was not there, his family having recommended him to get out of the bustle and vexatious circumstances into which events had plunged the whole country. From the commencement of operations a week before, they had neither had rest nor tranquillity, first with the French on their advance and afterwards on their retreat and then with the allied pursuers. The young men were very happy to learn that, for one night at all events, they might consider themselves in safety. They provided a very substantial supper and we were perfectly satisfied with our treatment.

Next day we passed through the village of *Malplaquet*,[5] and soon afterwards reached the little open town of *Bavay*. Here there occurred a scene which, if it could be described with even base *fidelity*, would

---

4. Note by Smith – There are two villages so named on the frontier of the Netherlands: one upon a hill, *Estinnes au Mont*; and the other in a valley *Estinnes au Val*. It was to the latter that we directed our march.
5. The battle was fought here on 11 September 1709.

furnish materials for a considerable portion of an amusing volume. The first object that attracted our attention was the motley military crowd in the little marketplace or square. This augured ill for billets and in a *town* we could not safely billet *ourselves*. There was the military chest too, under a strong escort, bivouacked in the square; commissariat and other stores, stragglers and followers, among whom was a due proportion of what elsewhere might have appeared to be the *fair* sex: and I recognised some of the petticoated soldiers alluded to on a former occasion. These ladies had found new protectors, of whom they had not had time to make husbands; though already employed in lieu of baggage animals.

The prominent feature, the grand sight, the pomp and the circumstance of Bavay at this hour, was his most Christian Majesty, Louis XVIII alias *Le Desire*, alias *Le Gros*. There he was, returning to seize the throne of his fathers; and driving (as Paddy said of the losing horse at a race) all the English and Prussian troops before him! There he sat in an open carriage, like a jolly old gentleman; I shall never forget his good-natured, ruddy countenance, nor his well-combed white hair, nor his well-tied pig-tail. About one hundred and fifty splendidly dressed, tolerably mounted and equipped and good-looking sons of the best families in France, were accompanying him as an escort; while a few ragged urchins were following through the streets, with a feint and famished cry of *Vive le Roi*! Which died away as the third word of the exclamation rose to their lips.

So far, all was legitimate, proper and even reputable. The king was going forward to *Le Cateau Cambresis*, where he remained for several days, till Wellington and Blucher were able to clear the way for his further progress. But just at the outlet of *Bavay* there was such a conglomeration, as I should suppose is to be met with only at an English fight, as formerly collected on Moulsey Hurst,[6] and now in any waste and neglected part of the kingdom. Nearly all the worthies collected on this spot were furnished with some sort of vehicle, for few were on horseback and probably none upon foot. They were not composed of the higher order and many of them consisted of persons in trade, who had committed themselves with Bonaparte, by taking a precipitate part with the Bourbons on their first return and expressing themselves with less prudence and more force than they would have done

---

6. Moulsey Hurst in West Molesley, Surrey, is one of England's earliest sporting venues, hosting cricket matches and prize fights throughout the seventeenth and eighteenth centuries.

had they not believed in the impracticability of an escape from Elba. This mob, for I can call them by no name so appropriate to their appearance at Bavay, had taken refuge in Ghent and other sanctuaries furnished by the Belgian government; but they were now most impertinently and provokingly anxious to press forward to their shops and traffic. 'Sacre!' said one of them in my own hearing, to another (butcher-looking fellow, seated with him in the same dogcart), 'On ne peut pas s'avancer pour ces Anglais!!' [We can't get forward for these English]. The very people who were clearing the road for them, to be spoken of in this manner! It is true that *Les Anglais* on the spot were much in the state in which they were themselves, viz one of confusion; but still *we* had all an object of duty in pressing forward and one necessary for their purpose. I wish to speak of them with temperance and moderation; but at this moment their inconsiderate and arrogant behaviour was, to say the least of it, *disgusting*. I afterwards saw several of these malcontents in their domiciles and understood the motives of their fight and of their haste back to have been little [to] the credit of some of them. One man in particular, a vapouring ironmonger near Azincourt, a violent ultra, had been equally enthusiastic in the cause de *l'Empereur*, had sent his only son into the Imperial Service, as a volunteer and when the lad left the paternal roof to join his corps, the father engaged a fiddler to proceed a mile or two on the road before them and prevailed on a few of his *mad* neighbours to grace the procession. He took leave of the recruit with a solemn injunction to shed the last drop of his blood for the great man who had raised the glory of France to such an unprecedented pitch &c &c. When this creature bolted after *Louis* to Belgium, the ultras refused to receive him; nor could he obtain safety among them until furnished with a certificate from the clergyman and other *notables* of his commune, that he was a harmless being, rather touched in the head.

But, to return to *Bavay* and its temporary politics. Soon after the king left the place, the chief magistrate made his appearance, dressed in gala guise, a cocked hat on his head and a broad white sash round his waist. He was '*awfu fu*', but still maintained sufficient dignity, (it is wonderful how an exalted station enables a man to carry his liquor) to find his way to the *Hotel de Ville*. What *sa Majeste* and he had been about I do not know; but I learnt that the two honest gentlemen had had a long interview and had not restricted themselves to conversation. Just as his worship reached the door of the hotel aforesaid, he was assailed by a wretch, who, if not more drunk, was a thousand times more outrageous than suitable,[7] venting the most disloyal expressions and vociferating in the most treasonable style. The mayor knew not what course to take; but some of his friends came about him, apparently dissuading him from active proceedings; and the results were, the commitment of the rebel to jail, the *cloture* [fencing off] of the townhouse and a resolute determination to furnish no more quarters in Bavay. My friend W[etzig],[8] while I was attending to our interests in the street, had got into the *chamber*; but two commissary's clerks, decorated with cocked hats and flowing white feathers, spoiled the whole negotiation, by damning the souls of the scribes, threatening to fire the town and demanding quarters for themselves, as two generals. This was *too bad*! Unattended by orderlies or servants, fobbing themselves off for *general officers*! But it would not do. So they were hooted out of the office; and for our own parts, we resolved to proceed to some village farther on, where we had no doubt we should be able to quarter ourselves.

Accordingly, we advanced about two miles and then turned out of the high road to the left. Here we found a hamlet,[9] in which we resolved to abide for the night. We had about thirty German soldiers, however, to provide with quarters as well as ourselves. For this purpose it was necessary (in order to escape the chance of a subsequent reckoning with the Adjutant-General) to apply to the authorities. Having found a house free of troops, we entered, sent for the mayor, who wore wooden shoes (the allusion to which he no doubt, thought a prime joke[10]), demanded

---

7. Note by Smith – I shall never forget a scene which occurred afterwards at Valenciennes. I was riding into the town with several other officers, when we met the Duke of Wellington with his brilliant Staff coming out to receive the Duke and Duchess of Kent, whose purpose was to review the Allied army. As His Grace was crossing the drawbridge, a drunken Frenchman gave it *us all* well, but the Duke in particular. He called the English by all sorts of abusive epithets, threatening us with another war, a good beating &c. What do you suppose was the course the Duke resorted to? Why, he passed by and took no notice of him; nor did even the English sentinel at the fellow's elbow, either drive him away or so much as attempt to silence him. A Prussian would have tried the sharpness of his bayonet.
8. It is difficult to be certain, but Gottleib Wetzig would appear to be the only Regimental Surgeon in the King's German Legion at Waterloo spelt with a W (he later mentions his Assistant Surgeons are already with the regiment). He was in the 1st Line Battalion.
9. This is most likely to be Le Trechon.
10. Note by Smith – He came in his night-cap, by no means a rare article of a rural magistrate's dress among these free and easy people. 'Are you the mayor?' 'Oui, Messieurs, dans mes *sabots*.'

billets for all parties and having ascertained that we were under the roof of the village apothecary, where there was a chance of our being made as welcome as circumstances would permit, declined the invitation of the rustic dignitary to repair to his own house, requesting authority for remaining where we were.

This being accorded, our soldiery separated to their respective quarters. W[etzig] also went in search of provender, as our means of making up a dinner were by this time miserably contracted. The house appeared incapable of giving, lending or selling any assistance. The family declared that they had been so much exhausted by our predecessors, they had nothing left for themselves. The Prussians or Hanoverians (for I ascertained that the useless outrage had not been committed by Englishmen) had broken into the old man's little laboratory, had smashed his boxes and bottles and spilled his juleps[11] and catholicons[12] all about the place. He was extremely well pleased on learning that we were medical and rightly concluded that we should duly estimate his sufferings.

While my friend was absent on his foraging expedition, a party of dismounted Belgian dragoons found their way to the house; and in spite of my representations and opposition, made good an entrance. They behaved so insolently to the poor people, that if I could have mustered half a dozen of our German friends, I should have thought it my duty to drive them out at the point of the bayonet. They remained for a very long time, demanding what the people protested they had it not in their power to furnish, '*a boire et a mange*' [to drink and eat]. They vexed and reviled the old apothecary, his wife and daughters, to a most intolerable degree. W[etzig] came back (successful), but still we could not clear the house of these ruffians, who seemed disposed to set us at defiance, although they knew us to be officers. W[etzig] now resolved to get a party of his own men; but we could not find any of them. At this juncture came in a few of the English Rifle Brigade,[13] in search of quarters, who were quite contented with the barn and straw: these lads soon sent the Belges about their business and at parting I could not help telling them that they were *deserters*, who had no business to be in the rear at all and that the earliest

---

11. A sugary syrup containing medication.
12. A cure-all or a panacea.
13. The Rifle Brigade did not exist as such at this moment, he presumably refers to men of the 95th Rifles.

opportunity would be taken of recommending them to the consideration of their commanding officer. The rogues sneaked off and we found the humble habitation cleaned and put in order for our reception. The table was set out and a trait of character which now appeared, ought not to be forgotten. The wife whispered me to have the politeness to invite *Monsieur* to sit down with us, which being complied with, the joy of the family was truly great. Madame and her two daughters attended us, both agreeably surprised at a trap door being opened in an inner apartment, from the abyss beneath which were produced bread, butter and cheese in abundance, though not an atom of any of these was to be found while the Belgians were in the house.

Next morning my intelligent associate and I called a council. We were now close up with the army, he had a heavy charge, with which he could move only at a snail's pace comparatively (had he been alone we should not have parted), whereas my *chaco* [shako] covered all my establishment and the Belge and his horse were no encumbrances. We therefore decided that I must make the best of my way, his presence being the less required, as the assistant surgeons were with his regiment.

I left him about five in the morning and pushed on till about seven, when I came upon the rear of the army, gathering themselves out of the bivouac in which they had passed the night. The first troops I encountered were highlanders; and seeing before me at the roadside, a man in the uniform of my regiment, I shouted out, 'Holloa! [12]th?' No reply, nor the slightest sign of recognition. 'Holloa! You of the [12]th?' Still no answer. Keeping my eye upon him I approached the fellow, for the purpose of admonition, when I was accosted by a mounted officer, in a general's undress uniform and asked what I wanted. I now saw the matter in its real aspect. This was the gallant Sir D[enis] P[ack][14] and the man I had seen was his orderly, employed at the moment in unfolding the general's cloak, for it was beginning to rain. I apologised for my rudeness, not having observed him at first and being very anxious to obtain information where I should find the regiment. The general asked me how the wounded had fared and what I knew of Colonel [Ponsonby]. I said that I could hardly give a correct report on the first subject and that I had heard bad accounts

---

14. Major General Sir Denis Pack commanded the 9th Brigade of infantry in the 5th Division.

of the colonel on Thursday [22 June]; (this the reader will bear in mind, was Sunday 25 June). He then had the goodness to say, 'I am happy to tell you that I heard about him last night and that he is expected to do well.' 'That will be good news for the regiment. Can you inform me where I shall find them?' 'I do not know where the cavalry is to halt today, they are of course in the front; but Sir James Kempt[15] has a list of the arrangements and will be able to tell you how to proceed. He has just gone on, you will know him by his hat and feather and he wears a blue frock [coat].' 'Do you think Sir, I shall be able to get up with them today?' 'I have no doubt you will, but apply to Sir J[ames] K[empt].' I made my obeisance and went on. Sir James I never saw, probably he had patrolled from the road; and I had nothing for it but threading the maze, in which I now became entangled.

I was glad to be among regularly organised troops again; for it had been both disagreeable and dangerous to move among stragglers. The Prussians in particular, were crowding along, every man at his discretion, with bayonets fixed and arms *sloped*. Being elevated sufficiently to form a level with their weapons, I was more than once nearly staked upon the points of them. Talking to these men was of no use for two reasons, 1st, I could not speak German, 2nd, they were not disposed to attend to me, had it been otherwise; so that the better plan was to get away from them. Such as know anything about the movements of armies are aware that the miseries to which the inhabitants of the scene of war are most exposed and which are most intolerable, are those inflicted by stragglers. The effective force is always under control and management: officers are present; but after a great battle, the disorder is necessarily considerable and the license uncontrollable. If officers happen to be among the followers, they have little or no authority, for men of other corps affect not to recognise them; and there are so many means of escaping from punishment, that to threaten is almost absurd. For one Provost[16] in the front there ought to be six in the rear, as it is there that the bulk of disorders is to be looked for.

Such a day as I now went through it is quite impossible even to make an attempt to describe. In brief, I threaded the whole army from rear to

---

15. Major General Sir James Kempt had assumed command of the 5th Division after General Picton was killed at Waterloo.
16. The Provost Marshal was in effect the Military Police.

front and several times was thrown down, horse and all by tumbrils and other overbearing machines, which came crushing against us.

I got up and on again the best way I could and somewhere in the crush and crowd, met my friend the chaplain [Tunney] coming back: there was little time and less opportunity for a dialogue; but I understood that he had got as far as *Le Cateau* (headquarters), whence he had been despatched back to Brussels, the entrepot of death and consequently the great field for spiritual consolation. This gentleman imposed upon me the task (several years afterwards) of prosecuting a claim for the loss of his baggage, including a certain number of *sermons!!* but nothing was made of it. We had him afterwards as chaplain to our brigade, in the Army of Occupation, but he never could call to mind the rencontre now alluded to. At Brussels he arrived and for some months found himself most comfortably lodged in the Hotel of the Duc D'Aremberg, an old blind man who was fond of whist,[17] which my clerical friend played uncommonly well. His son, the prince, was one of Bonaparte's officers in the Peninsular war, and was surprised in the affair of *Arroyo de Molinos*.[18] What became of him subsequently I do not know;[19] but the old duke was very complaisant to my friend the parson, while he remained in his house.

After a long struggle I cleared the infantry and between their front and the rear of the cavalry there was about a mile of comparatively open ground, occupied by the followers of the latter. Here I found our quartermaster sergeant, who was in possession of a live bullock or two and a newly purchased pony, upon which he advised me to mount, as the animal I had under me was exhausted by the thirteen hours of exertion we had both been enduring. He also relieved my personal sufferings by a supply of broken biscuits and a ration of rum, assuring me that he would be answerable for the Belgian and Captain C[raufurd]'s horse coming safely in. Where the regiment was however, he could not tell: all that he knew was that the brigade was leading in front and that I should be able to find them in the course of the evening.

---

17. Louis Engleber, 6th Duke of Arenberg had lost his sight in both eyes after a hunting accident in his early twenties. He had abdicated his title to his son Prosper Louis, the 7th Duke, in 1810 and died in 1820.
18. The Battle of Arroyo de Molinos occurred on 28 October 1811.
19. Prosper Louis, the 7th Duke d'Aremberg (or Arenberg) was wounded and captured at the battle and paroled in England, but eventually returned to Belgium. He had no involvement in the 1815 campaign.

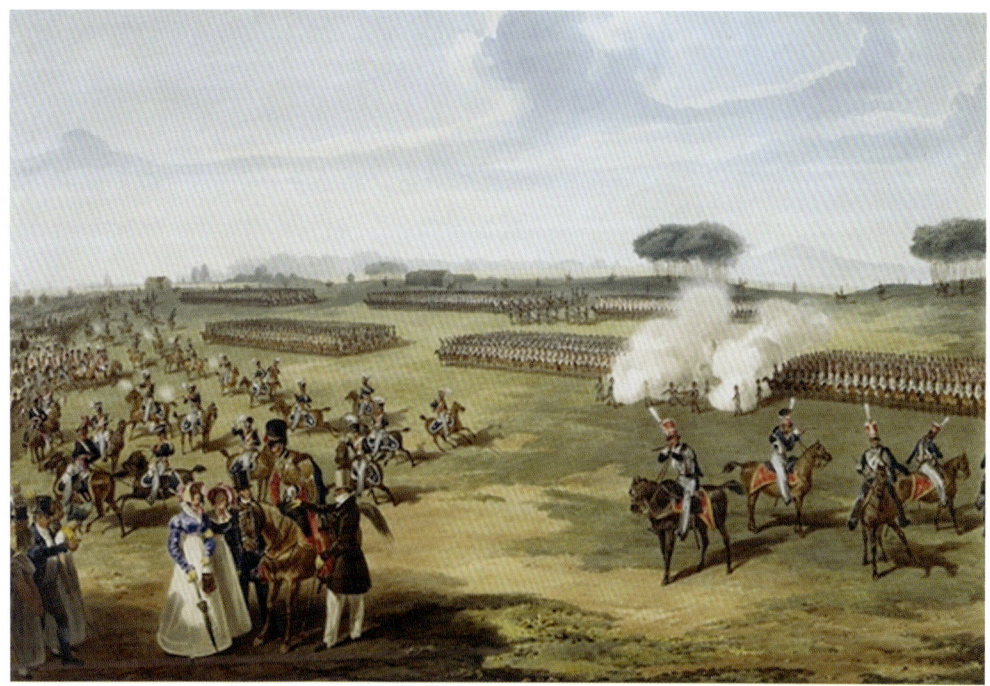

1. A Review at Hounslow Heath by Denis Dighton.

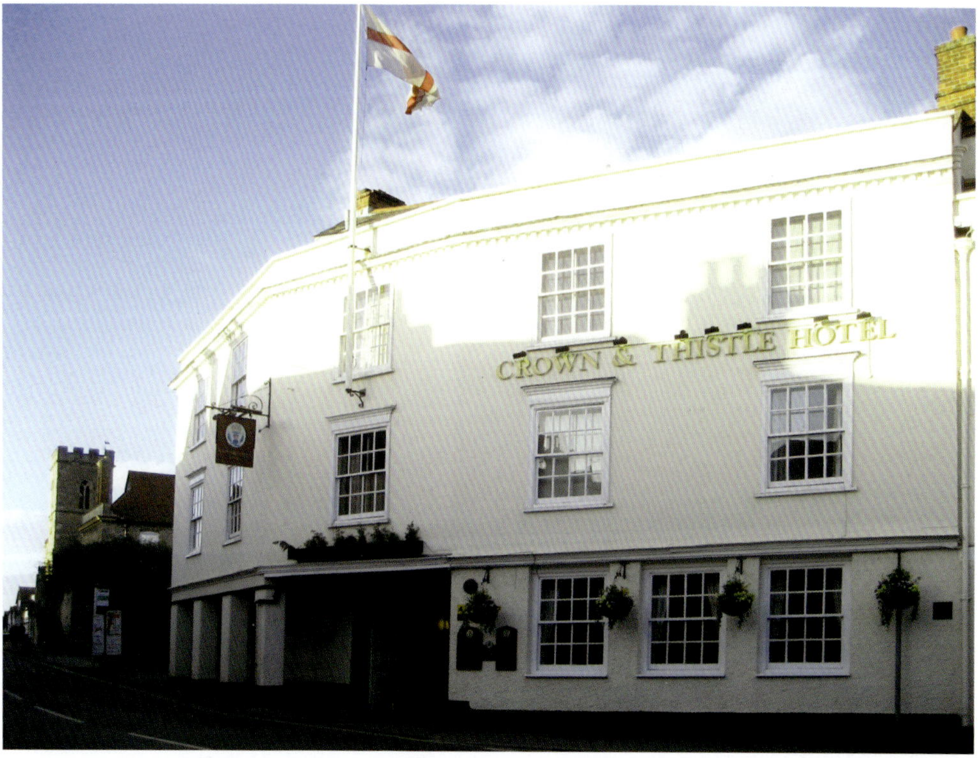

2. The Crown & Thistle, Abingdon-on-Thames.

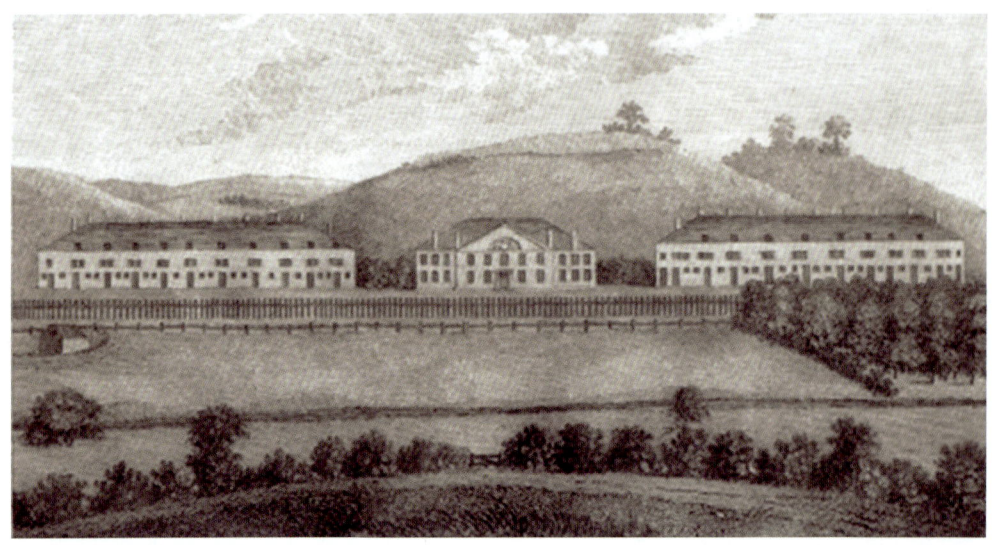

3. The Cavalry Barracks at Canterbury.

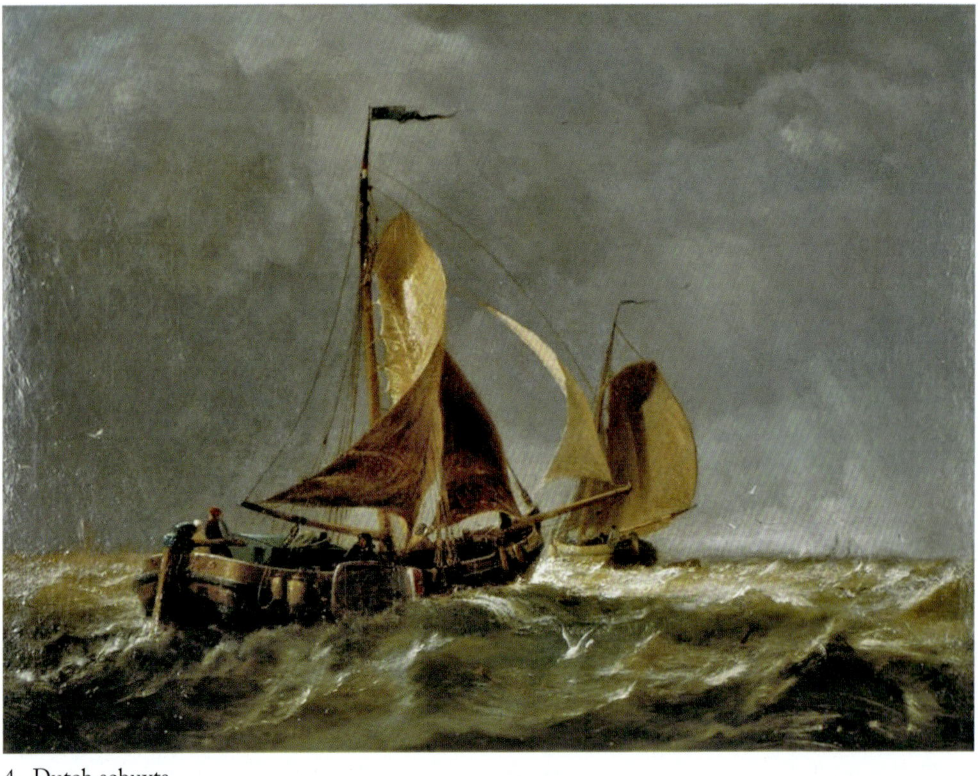

4. Dutch schuyts.

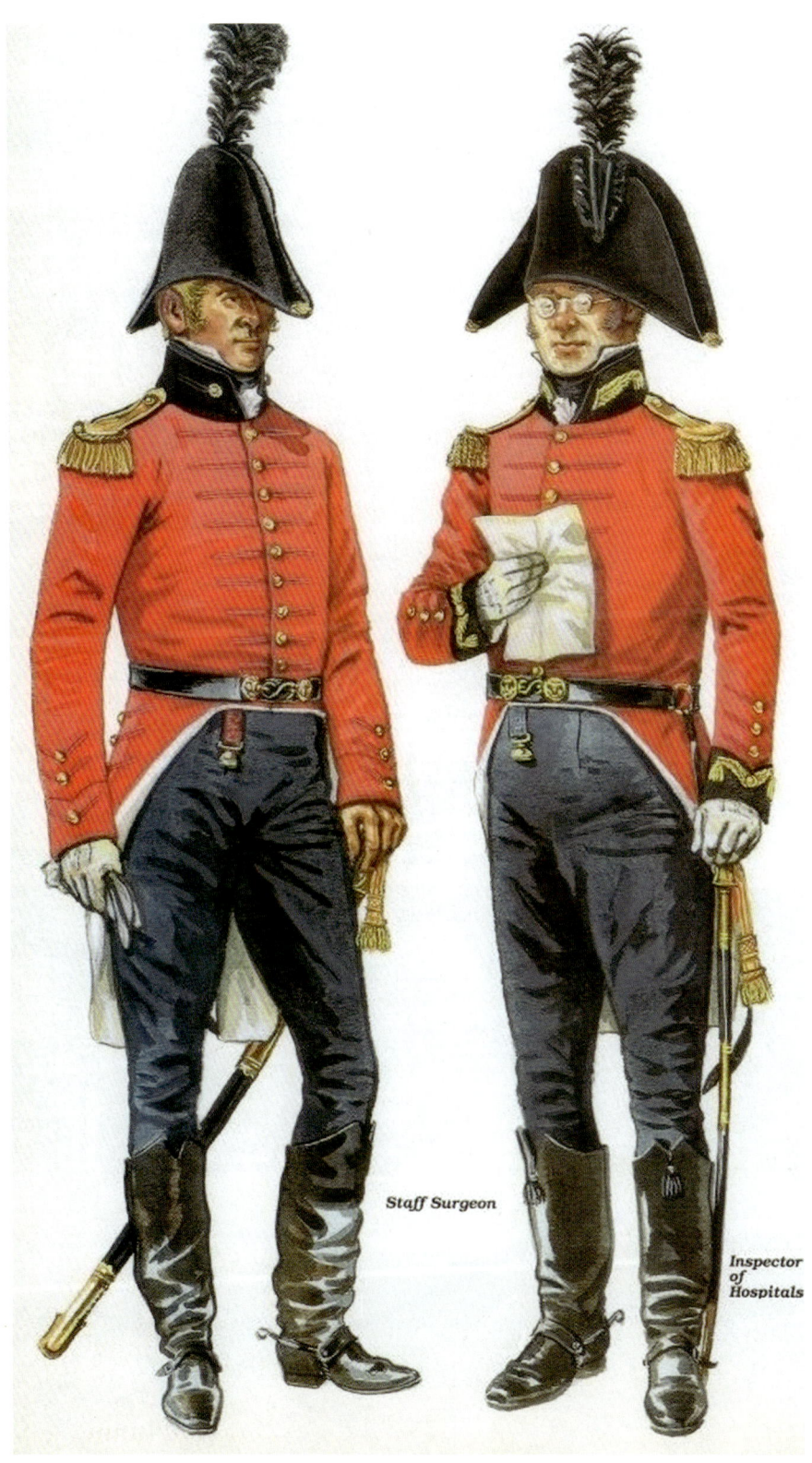

5. A Surgeon and an Inspector of Hospitals.

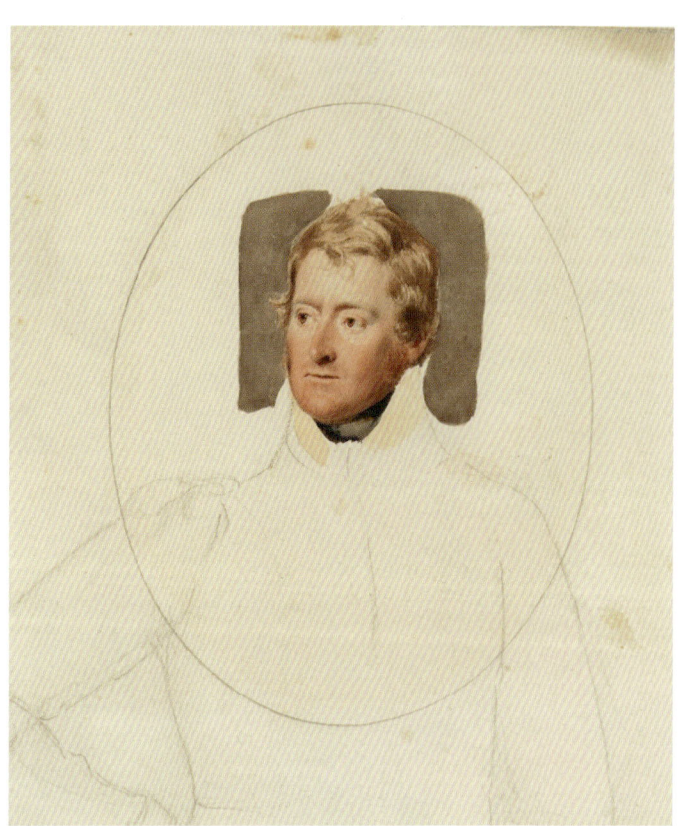

6. Study of Sir Frederick Ponsonby by Thomas Heaphy.

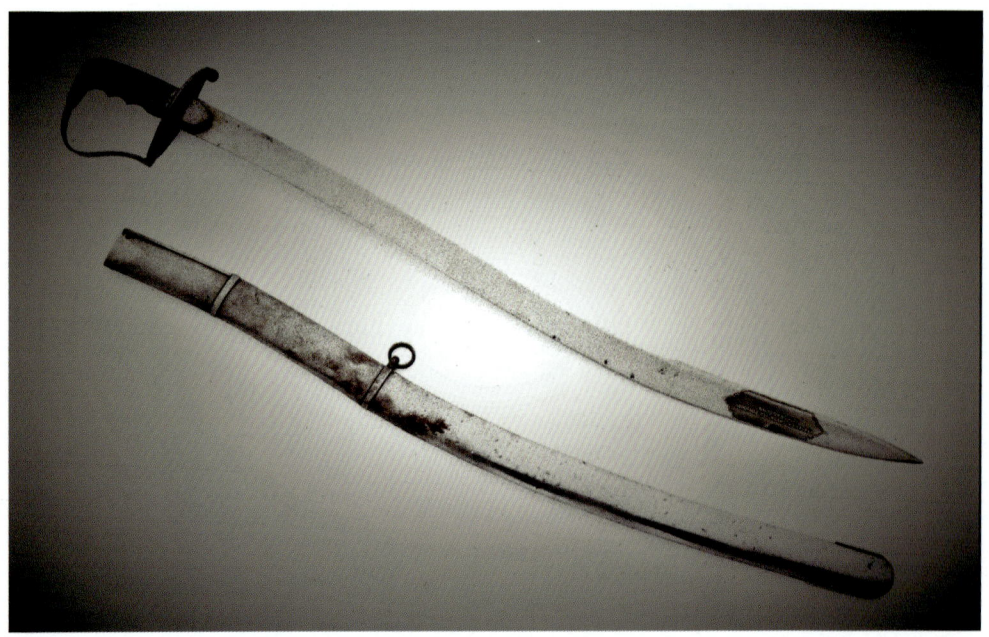

7. Frederick Ponsonby's Waterloo Sword.

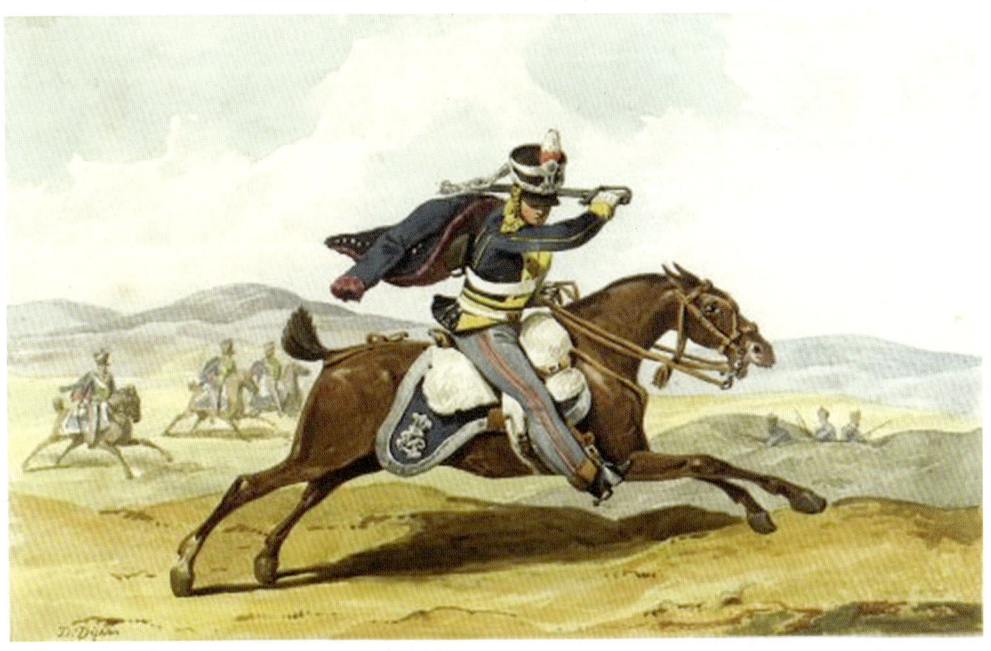

8. The 12th Light Dragoons by Denis Dighton.

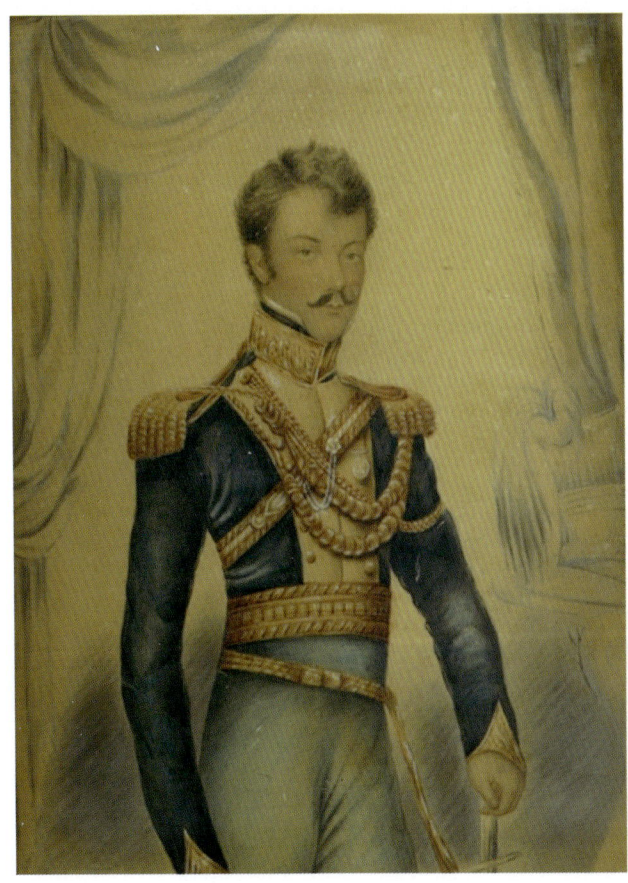

9. Captain William Hay, 12th Light Dragoons, circa 1820.

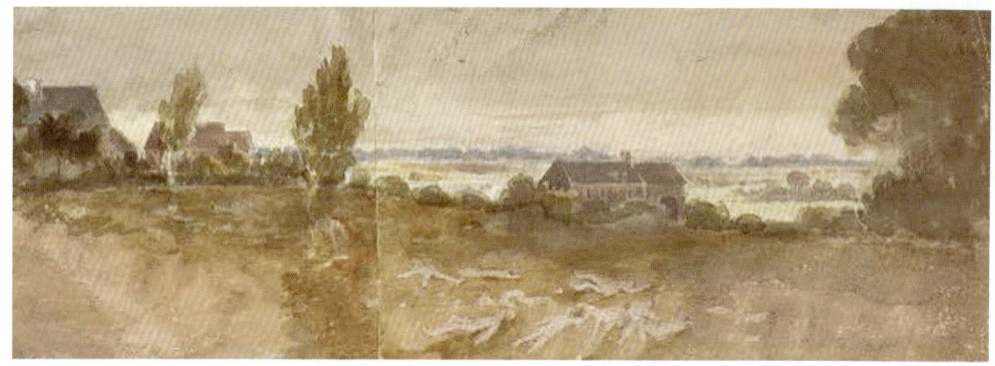

10. A view of Quatre Bras on 19 June 1815 by Thomas Stoney, with corpses still littering the ground.

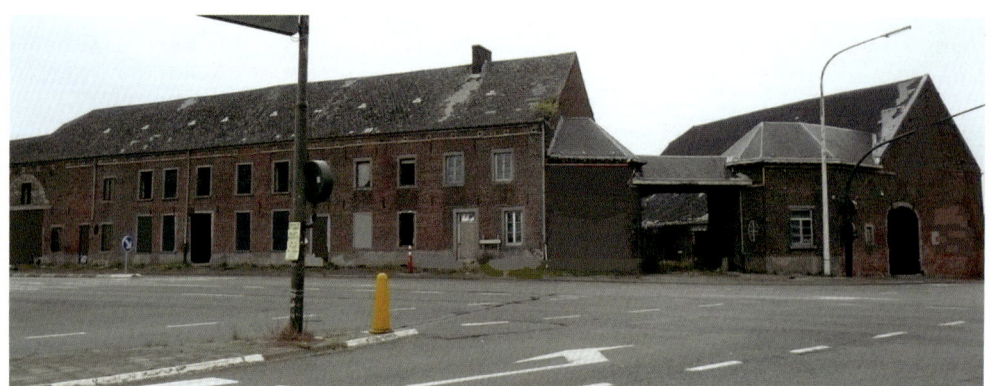

11. Farm of Quatre Bras just before it was shamefully destroyed.

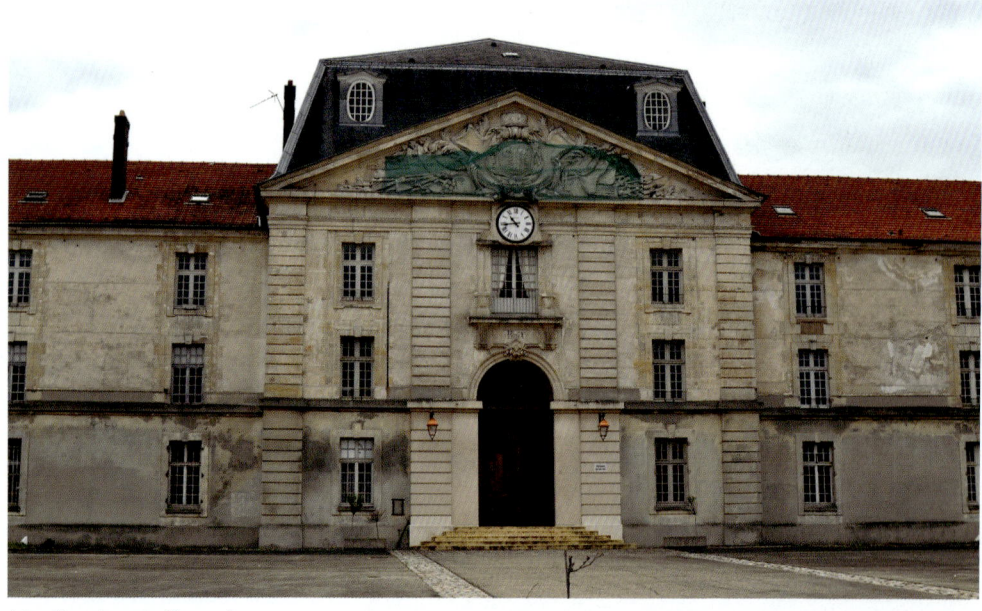

12. Courbevoie Barracks.

This Monument was erected
by the 12th L! Dragoons to the Memory of
the Officers and Soldiers belonging to the Regiment
who were killed at the Battle of WATERLOO
18th June 1815.

CAPTAIN EDWARD SANDYS
LIEUTENANT LINDSEY BERTIE
CORNET JOHN E. LOCKART

SERJEANT MAJORS
ROBERT NELSON . THOMAS SCANLON

SERJEANTS
WILLIAM BAIRD    THOMAS FINLEY    JAMES KIRBY
WILSON COX                        WILLIAM TOOLE

CORPORALS
WILLIAM HORSTON  WILLIAM MARSH    SAMUEL NICHOLS

PRIVATES
ISAAC BISHOP     JOHN GLASS       JAMES McLASHER
WILLIAM BURLEY   EDWARD GROWCOCK  EDWARD McDONALD
JOHN BAXTER      JEREMIAH HICKEY  JOHN NUGENT
CHARLES COCHRAN  GEORGE HURST     FRANCIS PERCY
CHARLES CLARE    THOMAS HALFORD   MICHAEL RAINSFORD
THOMAS CLARKE    ROBERT KELLY     HUGH SMITH
HUGH DONNEGAN    JOHN KING        WILLIAM STEWART
WILLIAM DAXTER   FRANCIS LANG     JAMES SIVELL
GUY DEVITT       DANIEL MURPHY    RICHARD SLADE
EDWARD EADIE     PHILIP MURPHY    JOSEPH WILLIAMSON
JOHN EARLY       ROBERT MATTHEWSON JAMES WIGGINS
FRANCIS FOSTER   JOHN MACFARLANE  JAMES WILMOT
JAMES FISHER                      JOHN WELSH

13. The Waterloo Memorial to the 12th Light Dragoons. One of the first memorials to include the names of all ranks killed.

14. Surgeon's Regulation Case circa 1812.

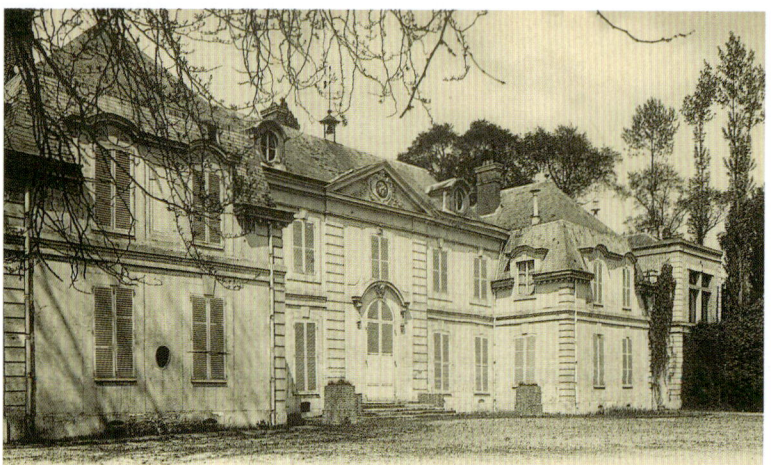
15. Chateau Marais, Argenteuil.

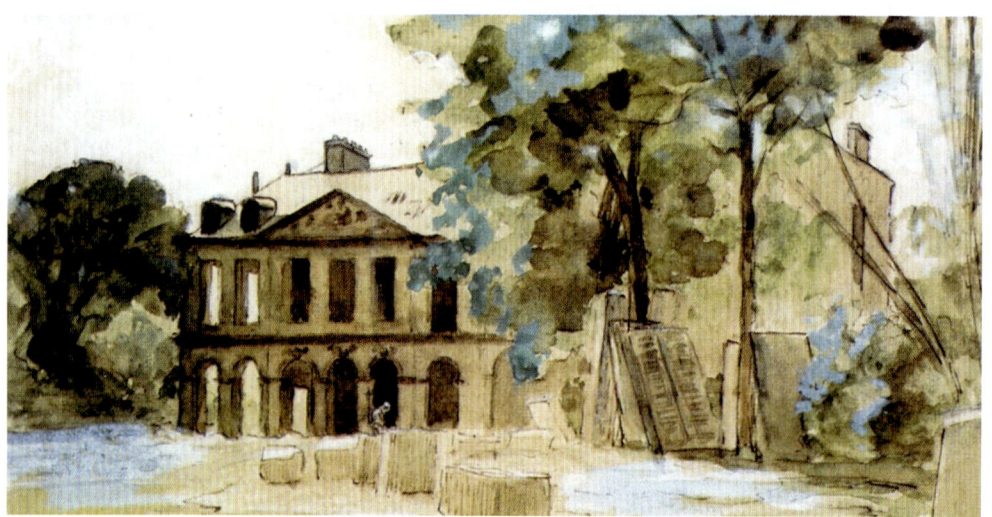
16. Chateau Puteaux before its final destruction after a fire in 1881.

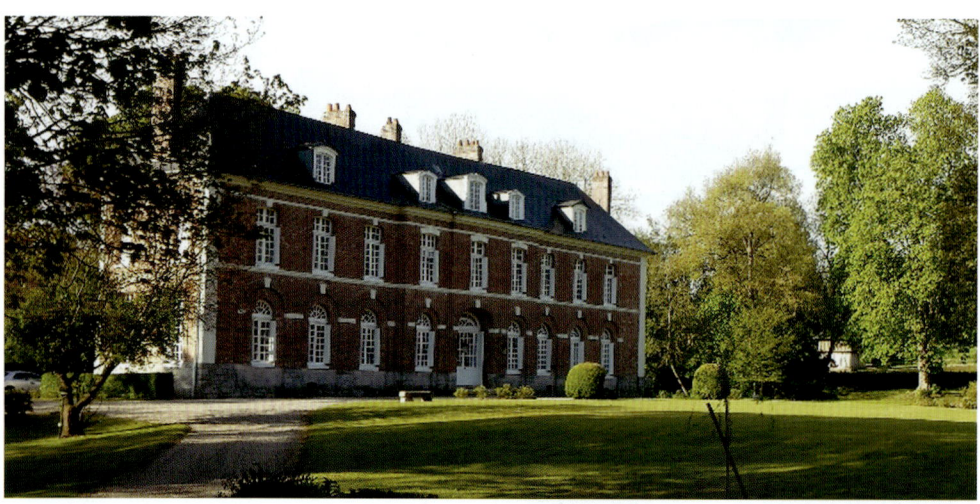
17. Chateau de Bacqueville.

Enlivened by this improvement in my personal situation, I went through the cavalry with comparative facility and finally cleared them. I then fell in with a piquet of the regiment which was coming in from a patrol and joining them, was before dark, once more installed as the professional adviser of the much loved [12]th; and placed in charge of the hospital, which had till now been for a week dependent upon the casual visits of officers belonging to other regiments. One of these came over in the course of the evening and was very glad to find the change that had taken place.

I do not know where the village in which I found my friends is situated; but it lies not far from and to the north-west of *Le Cateau[-Cambresis]*,[20] of which I had a sight when between the cavalry and infantry divisions. The night I passed there my clothes were dried before a large fire and I was accommodated in the morning with some changes that were truly acceptable. I also got a proper horse and proceeded onward in a state of satisfaction, if not of hilarity.

The march furnished no incidents that I can call to mind and we halted in and about a village on the high road;[21] where at an early hour in the evening, we were gratified by the arrival of General Thielmann [Thielemann],[22] at the head of a division of the Prussian army, which abstracted Marshal Grouchy[23] and thirty thousand men from the French. The well-known story is, that Grouchy mistook this corps for the main body of the enemy and pursued them so far that the fortune of Waterloo was decided against his master ere he could return. Bonaparte is also said to have had such reliance upon the skill, as well as fidelity of this general, that when the Prussians made their appearance in the field, he calculated on their destruction, from the circumstance of Grouchy being of course in their rear and their being thus placed between two fires.

Blucher and the main body of the Prussians were in front of us, having pursued the French army, without intermission from the field and in fact

---

20. William Hay of the 12th says they were quartered at Pommenal. This is actually Pommereuil two miles to the north-east of Le Cateau-Cambresis. Here he states that the regiment mustered with 20 officers, 31 sergeants, 3 trumpeters and 215 rank & file with 240 horses.
21. The brigade stopped in the vicinity of Bellincourt.
22. General Lieutenant Johann von Thielemann commanded III Corps in the Waterloo campaign.
23. Marshal Emmanuel de Grouchy, Marquis de Grouchy commanded a separate corps sent off to ensure that the defeated Prussians did not regain contact with Wellington's army. He failed in this, but the blame for this failure was really shared with Napoleon himself.

hunted them to a sort of annihilation; for, excepting in the strong towns and afterwards at Paris, not a soldier was to be seen. General Thielmann [Thielemann] had intended to halt for the night, upon the ground we had already taken up; but finding how matters were, he went on, summoned and took the town of Ham, which was at no great distance. The regularity with which these troops passed by was beautiful. They were marching in columns of infantry and cavalry alternately, with clear intervals between each and the men in front singing choruses of the most pleasing description. This is a custom among the German soldiery, which may perhaps be too national for us to adopt; but where the road will admit of regular formations, there can be no doubt of its beneficial influence. It does not fatigue the performers and it engages the attention of the listeners; but there must be a general taste for music where it is practised.

In the large village (*Ricquebourg*[24]) where we halted for the night, we found marked traces of military occupation. All the men had fled and the remaining inhabitants consisted of females, sick and elderly persons and young children. They were in a state of great alarm. We had great difficulty in getting possession of our quarters by *fair* means; and by *force* we had no wish to proceed.

Into a cottage however, we (*the Staff*) got and there found a woman and two children, terrified to the last degree. We had some difficulty in quieting their alarm, particularly that of the mother. Her husband had *served* and was therefore in hiding. We neither liked the *McClarty* appearance of the house, nor the vast amount of the alarm, which being perfectly unfounded, (though the poor subjects of it could not at first understand that such was the case) rather nettled us. We did not all like to be considered marauders, ravishers, incendiaries and all that sort of thing, though probably of some of these miseries they had just had a taste and must have had some acquaintance with the economy of a Bonapartean [*sic*] army when in an enemy's country.[25] We resolved merely to eat our rations within doors and to sleep in the barn, where there was

---

24. This in the book was out of sequence, as Ricquebourg is north of Compiègne and would have been passed a day or more before reaching Pont Sainte Maxence, so the editor has moved it to its correct position.

25. Note by Smith – Upon entering the French territory, proclamations had been issued, declaratory of friendly purposes, on the part of the allies, advising the people to stay at their homes and denouncing, in the severest terms, any interference on the part of the troops, except through the medium of the proper authorities.

abundance of straw. The poor woman was anxiously busy in our service; but we preferred to deal with our canteens (or rather I ought to say, with those of my friend, for mine was *neither here nor there*) in our own way. All we requested of her was to have some *café au lait* ready at an early hour in the morning. To ensure punctuality she sat up all night and on our presenting her with a five-franc piece at parting, she burst out crying and fell upon her knees in a most unexpected and unnecessary transport of *gratitude* I believe, though my droll friend Joe [James Castley] said it was *disappointment*.

Next day we reached the *Oise*, near *Compiegne* and had to pass the bridge of *St Maxence* [Pont-Sainte-Maxence]. This the retreating foe had of course, blown up; but our precursors, the Prussians, had made some temporary repairs. We were a very long time in passing, as few could only proceed by single files. However, I believe no accident occurred: and we bivouacked under a sloping wood, quite away from houses, or any other source of accommodation. Though I passed the night in a tent, as no straw could be got, I was obliged to lie in my clothes upon an oil-deck,[26] the only thing that interposed between me and the ground. This of itself would not be worth mentioning, but cold and unpleasant as I found my couch and late as I had been of steeping my senses in the oblivion of sleep, the overpowering influence of that state was such that when the bugle sounded next morning, I could not muster resolution enough to rise, though I had nothing more to do than start to my feet and shake myself. The tent was thrown down before I was roused; and that object was effected by a cup of tea. I believe that there can be and is known to be no better restorative, after a weary march than this. Wine and spirits are but substitutes and ought not to be meddled with till after the kettle has been brought into operation. The first care a campaigner should turn his attention to on reaching his camp, is a fire; the second to make tea; an hour after this he will know the comfort, such as it may be, of eating and if practicable, of drinking something more directly and diffusibly stimulant.

On the next day (the date of which I do not remember) we arrived within forty miles of the metropolis, where we fell into the track of the Prussian army, hitherto we had been marching by separate roads. If

---

26. This would appear to be an oilcloth ground sheet.

we had, up to this time, seen but few inhabitants, we had not met with '*casas rompidas*.'[27]

From *Ricquebourg* [via Pont-Sainte-Maxence] we passed by *Louvre[s]* on the great north road, to a spot whence we had a view of the towers and domes of Paris, rising about ten miles before us. It was almost incredible, though an absolute demonstration, an uninterrupted march to the metropolis of France! Undeniable! The approach to and occupation of this mysterious city (mysterious enough for nearly thirty years to Englishmen) had it is true, been realised the preceding year; but under different circumstance and in the midst of warlike operations and uproar. As regarded ourselves, we seemed to be in the very centre of peace, though our allies had not yet finished their share of bloody work.

In the course of this day's march, a deputation from Paris, at the head of which was *Regnaud St. Jean d'Angely*,[28] reached the army, in the vain hope of stopping its progress. There were three gentlemen, who alighted from a carriage, as our brigade (the leading one) entered a village through which we had to pass, and they all wore the tricoloured cockade.[29]

---

27. Note by Smith – A Portuguese term, which became a proverbial expression among the Peninsular troops. It means *dilapidated* or *destroyed houses*. Such was the general state of the case throughout Portugal that *huma casa rompida*, and *huma casa Portugueza*, became synonymous.
28. Note by Smith – Our brigade was the leading one nearly all the way to Paris; but we seldom marched upon *a road* and made a rule of keeping aloof from towns of note or consequence. We went over the open country wherever this was practicable; and generally trod our way through standing crops. We who were in front found it pleasant enough; but those who came last had something like the clover of *St Jean* on the morning of the 18th, to wade through. The infantry must of course have kept the road, for *their* moving in our train would have been impracticable. The reason for this course of procedure is obvious; had we kept to high roads and marched through large towns, the hostile part of the population might have been enabled to make reports of a dangerous nature; and it may be worth bearing in mind, that the cavalry formed a curtain for the infantry, who mustered in fearful force behind the scenes. We seldom met any of the inhabitants; here and there a few *females* might show themselves, vociferating execrations against the fallen hero, which I doubt not were sincere. It may be supposed that men were watching us (and perhaps counting us) from situations favourable for such purposes; but I rather think their sense must have shewn the danger of an interview with our patrols.
29. Note by Smith – While mentioning cockades, it may be observed, that few bones of contention have raised greater uproar, or caused more serious consequences, than the colour of a spot upon a hat. The *tricolor* and the *white*, in France, have led to more deadly feuds than ever did the red and white roses in England. All nations select some predominant colour by way of a badge. What is the cockade of England? I should say she has none; for surely the black thing worn by our military has no reference to the purpose of a cockade.

Having arrived at the point described, after a very dusty march, we filed off to the large village of *Goussainville*, which had been but half an hour in the occupation of the Prussians; in the course of which they had contrived however, to carry off everything of value that was moveable and to injure what they were unable to take away. There were many country houses in and about this pleasant place, which is probably a sort of *Hampstead* or *Highgate* to the wealthier *bourgeois* of Paris. There were no inhabitants on our arrival; and all the houses stood invitingly open. On taking possession, we found that the furniture had been much knocked about, every drawer dragged from its place, feather beds thrown upon the floors, blankets &c of course *carried off*; and everything else in a corresponding state of confusion. In the house to which we individually repaired, there had evidently been females, probably young ladies, for the tattered fragments of finery appropriate only to such, were found in some of the apartments. A poor canary bird was the only living inhabitant at first; but next morning we found a milch-cow in an adjoining paddock, vociferating most piteously for someone to come and milk her: this act of humanity there was no reluctance whatever on our part to perform.

We remained in Goussainville three days and three nights, during which we neither undressed ourselves, nor unsaddled our horses.[30] The

---

30. Note by Smith – We had hardly been introduced to our quarters ere I was summoned to a casualty. In an adjacent *chateau*, the party (quartered there) found a poultry yard and proceeded to the usually licensed business of slaughter. One of our men had brandished his sabre over many a feathered head, with great success; but at last, it fell with the whole weight of his arm upon his own knee pan, cleaving it into two equal portions. The remedy was a very simple one; but removal to the rear being judged indispensable, I was obliged to apply to the military authorities before I could prevail upon my man to go *back*. The *baits* [taunts] under such circumstances, to go *forward*, are great; going *back* is a sure deduction of tenpence a day out of the soldier's receipts, such being the charge for hospital maintenance; but it is not to be forgotten that for this slender sum, the soldier is dieted, furnished with medicine and with every possible comfort. If he requires wine, he has it of the best quality; if his case requires other expensive luxuries, the medical officer exercises his discretionary power, in ordering whatever he thinks proper; and from his judgement there is no appeal, although he may be put to some trouble, in vindicating his proceedings. Thus, *fish, fowls, eggs, milk, brandy, sago, flour* and many other delicacies (besides the *wine* already mentioned) are daily ordered, sometimes however, questioned by the supreme authorities, but always allowed if *shewn cause for*. I had a weekly account twice sent back to Weymouth from the Army Medical Board, because there was an error of a *farthing* in it; and next week came back another because we had made a mistake of *less than a farthing*. Such is the system of economy in the public departments. John Bull may rely upon it, that there is infinitely less *waste* of his money than he is told of. I have often preferred to purchase what was wanted at my

chief reason for this was the active operations in which the Prussians were still engaged. It was during our stay here that the contest took place at *Meudon*, when our allies, though victorious, lost about three thousand men.[31] After this, the convention was signed at St Cloud and hostilities ceased. But I am anticipating.

During one of the days that we were lying *perdus* in Goussainville, a discovery was made that the church steeple was crammed with bread, cheese, hams, sheets, towels and others, the necessaries of life, which I believe, some of our friends insisted upon claiming, but of which they did not obtain possession without altercation and opposition. Here let me protest against the conclusion that we were no better than the *Prussians*. Even to find fault with *their* proceedings is neither my business, nor consistent with my inclination; an apology for their conduct, on this and on other occasions, may be submitted hereafter. In the meantime, I beg to observe that, as the inhabitants (in face of the assurance, usual in similar cases and carefully proclaimed by the authorities on our entering the French territory) had shewn a spirit of hostility so far as to abandon their homes. We had no resource but that of helping ourselves and *taking* what it was their own fault that we did not *pay for*.

In the meantime, we had judged from the general aspect of the place, that the owners of its copious resources could not be far off, a conjecture which one of our party realised, somewhat to our vexation. In the course of a walk he stumbled upon a group of people who were in an adjoining wood, watching us eagerly and not in good humour, though perhaps the treatment they had received from our exasperated allies had furnished them with a plausible pretext for flight. He encouraged them to return and prevailed. Among other notables whom he brought in, was the master of the house [of] which we had taken possession. The Adjutant's office was established there; and our landlord had not returned five minutes from a scene of starvation and misery of every description, when he brought a formal complaint to the *authorities* of the regiment, against somebody who had *milked his only remaining cow* (the rest having been driven off by

---

own expense, rather than have the trouble and annoyance of a correspondence to get the public to pay for it. I have known half a quire of expensive paper used about a matter that was not worth a dot.

31. This refers to the Battle of Issy, fought on 2 and 3 July 1815, which culminated in a victory for the Prussian General von Ziethen over General Vandamme.

the Prussians) and in particular against a soldier whom he had detected carrying a pint of cyder from the cellar. The meanness and ingratitude of the fellow so steeled our hearts against him, that I believe we refused to let him stay in his own house. The cow would have perished but for us and if he wanted to save his cyder, he should have staid at home to take care of it.

This was too pleasant a life to last for ever; and accordingly, on the third morning we were started from our *comfortable* quarters. We turned *Mont Martre [Montmartre]* and found our destination to be the villa and pleasure grounds of the *Duc Des Cres* [Duke Decrès] (Minister of Marine,) close to *Argenteuil* and upon the border of the *Seine*.[32] Here a pontoon bridge was to be constructed and we had to wait its progress.

I presume the house was taken possession of by the *authorities* of the brigade; for our own parts we had no repugnance to take up with the shrubberies; and the horses were perfectly happy at the sight of many haycocks,[33] to which they were made heartily welcome, I need not say by whom. The place was tastefully ornamented, but it had been almost *created*, nature having done little or nothing for it. Some of the most glaring, if not the most costly decorations, consisted of gilded barges; emblematic of the owners' business. These were quickly set in flame and the *Prusses* [Prussians] having previously made progress in the work of devastation within doors, His Excellency's chateau exhibited a spectacle of melancholy enough, by the time we left it on the following morning.

We had not been long in the enjoyment of that position (the reclining) so much in vogue among soldiers when not required to be in a state of activity, ere we all started to our feet at the supposed sound of guns close to us. *Bang! Bang! Bom-m-m! Bang!* came in rapid succession. We waited with certain assurance the order '*stand to your horses*', but none arriving and the cannonade continuing, we began to poke about to ascertain what was the matter. Still the thundering concussions went on with little intermission and the noise directed us to the scene of action. Half a dozen Prussians (some of them intoxicated) had been previously observed strolling about the grounds and had at length stumbled upon a little mound, in the side of which they discovered a door. Here they concluded, must be a concealment of vast treasure, all the family plate at least and probably huge

---

32. Admiral Decrès, Minister of the Navy, owned Chateau Marais in Argenteuil which was destroyed by the Germans in the Second World War.
33. Conical heaps of hay in a field.

piles of money. They had provided themselves with a big log, or branch of a tree and were employing it in truly classical style against the door, upon which they were thus pronouncing a genuine commentary *a la Cesar*; sweating, sweltering, cursing and battering away with all their might and main. Some of our troopers took a turn in this fatiguing task, resolved no doubt, to have an eye to their own interests when the partition of spoil should arrive. The day was very sultry, the sun at his height and the oaken door provokingly obstinate. For a long time it bade defiance to the butts of the *ram* and the lock was about to be stuffed with gunpowder sausage, when it thought better of it and after a *warm* hour's exertion gave way. 'Now for it, stand back!' A dark and apparently bottomless pit seemed to assure the besiegers that much of value awaited a bold descent: and there being a ladder affixed to the side of the yawning and mysterious abyss, it was conjectured that the assault might be made. One of the *Prusses* volunteered to explore but had hardly got out of sight till he came up again in haste, his countenance betokening a very *cool* discovery and a *freezing* disappointment. He uttered a German execration and marched off with all his comrades. What could be the matter? Had he put his foot in water, or did he find a *bear* at the bottom of the ladder? An Englishman next had the temerity to go down; but he soon returned, exclaiming, '*Ice*, by Jove! Nothing but a lump of *ice*!' The ice however, was not unacceptable; we carried off fragments to our haycock bivouac and what liqueurs we happened to possess, were much enhanced in value and quality by the cooling which this elaborate discovery enabled us to give them.

The operations of the ensuing day were of the greatest importance. The pontoon bridge was delayed in its progress and the Duke, aware of Prince Blucher's state of exasperation against the Parisians, had exhausted his patience ere it was completed. We moved down to the river long before this took place and in passing, I entered the magnificent château, where all the dilapidation: mirrors, chandeliers, vases and every destructible thing, had been shivered to atoms. I entered the billiard room, but the Prussians had carried off the broad green cloth, which was no doubt, already in the hands of some regimental tailor;[34] chairs and tables, chiffoniers,[35]

---

34. Note by Smith – The Prussian uniform was generally green; and consequently, the cloths of the billiard tables were peculiarly acceptable and made into jackets and trowsers instanter.
35. A small sideboard.

wardrobes and armoires,³⁶ were reduced to splinters; even statues had been involved in the general fate of this beautiful retreat; and I could not help laughing at the indefatigable exertions of a soldier's Irish wife, to detach a fragment from the foot (all that was left) of what I presume had been a Cupid. Two other *fair* ones were looking on, while *Norah* hammered away with a stone infinitely softer than the marble she was venting her spite upon, exclaiming while the weapon crumbled in her hand at every blow, 'There is the *ould Napoleon*,' (pointing to a demolished Apollo of the same obdurate material): 'they've done for him anyway; and now here's the young Napoleon,' meaning the Cupid, 'and fait I'll have one of his toes.'

Shortly after noon, the bridge was rendered passable and the Duke transferred himself to the opposite end, but still had to wait upon it till the last planks were laid. A troop of our brigade, but not of our regiment crossed with him,³⁷ and then the horse artillery. This called down the censure of his Grace and even roused his anger. The men were compelled to *ride* their horses over, whereas the others found it enough to lead them in their hands.³⁸ Another troop of cavalry having passed, the Duke rode off to St Cloud (escorted by this squadron) at a quick pace, as rumour afterwards represented, to conclude a convention and prevent the Prussian general from sacking Paris, which it was universally credited was at this time, his serious intention. These are matters, however, for which I cannot vouch: I introduce the allusion to them as connected with the talk of Paris and even of the army.

---

36. A two-door free-standing cupboard.
37. Note by Smith – The brigade was composed of three regiments, by number, [11th] formed *the right* of the line; the next, [12th] *the left*; and the youngest [16th] always occupied *the centre*. One day we marched *right* in front, and the next day *left*. The regiment to which I belonged was on the *left flank* of the brigade and accordingly sometimes led the van. On the day in question the right happened to be in front; and we in consequence, were the last of them to cross the river. It was my first appearance upon such a stage. The *Seine* was rapid, the boats were unsteady and the tramp of so many horses at a time did not render them less so. We passed by two abreast, each dismounted and leading his horse. There was no parapet or balustrade; so that the slightest disorder or disturbance would have sent us off the planks into the stream; but it was absolutely edifying to observe the decorum of the animals. They set their *rational* comrades an admirable example. A horse (of common sense) never kicks up a row except on *terra firma*.
38. Note by Smith – A short time afterwards, a commissary lost his life at this bridge through an accidental circumstance. The pontoon requiring repair, a sentinel was placed for the purpose of advertising the circumstance of a boat being removed. S**. unfortunately galloped upon the bridge, and the soldier did not warn him, he and his horse were drowned. The affair happened in the dark and was much lamented.

The whole brigade having crossed the Seine without interruption, followed by two companies only of light infantry, we advanced upon the village of *Courbevois* [Courbevoie], where another turn of the river met us. Here we found a fine bridge, of which our design was to have at least *shared* possession with the French. This was the *Pont de Neuilly*, to which we were not allowed to approach without altercation and even the aspect of something more serious. It was in the possession of 5,000 troops, supported by ten pieces of cannon; and though there was already a cessation of hostilities, in consequence of the Convention of St Cloud, they refused to give up even the end of it which touched our side of the river. I heard many expressions of dissatisfaction while we were idling away the time, (under the shade of Courbevois [Courbevoie]), at this inactivity. There seemed to be no one to give orders[39] and our forces was so inadequate to a contest, that to shew ourselves and draw the enemy (for such the French still *affected* to be) out to see our inferiority, would have been preposterous.[40] They could not have known the real state of the case, or else they would have driven us back to the pontoons and killed or drowned the whole of us. Some of our brigade, who had ventured too near the bridge, had been fired at; and though (thank God) no *man* lost his life in such unnecessary warfare, *one horse* was shot, which was the only feat the covering force of the French metropolis had to boast of against the advanced guard of the British army. General Clinton[41] came up at a late hour and threatened the French officer with 'terrible consequences,' both as to slaughter and responsibility, on the score of the convention being disregarded: and then this reckless puppy thought proper to leave one end of the *Pont de Neuilly* in our possession and retire to the other. Towards ten o'clock, we were ordered to establish ourselves in a garden, or pleasure ground adjacent; where (for my own part) I passed one of the happiest nights that I can call to mind as having cheered the course of my existence.

---

39. Note by Smith – Even the officers of the other regiments loudly expressed their regret that [Ponsonby](our colonel) was not present: – 'He would have talked to the Frenchmen in a language they would have understood,' &c. But this great man was lying in pain and danger of his life, far away from the scene.
40. Note by Smith – I presume we could not have shewn eight hundred sabres among the three regiments. We had five pieces of six pounders, a howitzer and two companies of infantry, on the skirts of the large force already mentioned; but they did not know it.
41. General Henry Clinton commanding the 2nd Division.

In the first instance I missed my associates and had fallen asleep under a shrub, when a familiar voice awoke me by advertising me as lost. This was my friend the Vet's [Castley's] servant. Starting up, I asked where Mr B [James Castley] was. 'Close by sir, with a roaring fire and everything ready for supper. We are just going to fry some steaks and he wants you very much.' Of course, no time was wasted in apologies; and on repairing to the spot, I found Joe [James Castley] seated on a garden chair, with an unoccupied one by his side, smoking a cigar and watching the conflagration of a large bench which had been *massacred* for fuel, while another was abiding a similar fate. Steaks, tea, cigars, grog, all had their turn; and we crammed each other with stories, jokes, *poetry* (for we both had a touch of the disorder) and nonsense, till daylight surprised and discovered us to our brethren, whom in all probability we had somewhat disturbed. We now therefore laid ourselves down and finished with sleep.

On the following day we moved up the Seine to *Puteaux*, near the chateau of the *Duc de Feltre*, (Clarke),[42] and here we remained three days. I was billeted upon a *washer-man*; and had cause to remember my accommodation long afterwards. There had been Prussian soldiers in the house the night before and even in the bed which I was to occupy. Scrutiny was not likely, under such circumstances, to be strict; and there were no *visible* signs of my approaching fate. There however, I encountered a contamination, the real nature of which I was for months unwilling to believe in; however, it was too true; but at length, when convinced as to the nature of a malady which had resisted every application for a long period, recourse to the specific extinguished it in a few hours:- '*Honi soit qui mal y pense*' [Shamed be the person who thinks evil of it], I was not worse off than some of my neighbours.

While we were lying inactive at Puteaux, arrangements were in progress for the removal of the French army to the left bank of the Loire. These were completed on the 7th of July; and on the 8th the town was occupied by the allies. In the meantime, we were not a little amused with a trait of French indifference. At one end of the bridge of Neuilly was posted our vidette, attentively watching a Frenchman stationed at the other, each with a loaded carbine in his hand, exhibiting the usual

---

42. The Chateau of Puteaux was destroyed by fire in 1881.

indications of two hostile armies being near each other; but between them a party of dancers assembled every evening, many of whom must have experienced considerable inconvenience in crossing the trenches that intersected the road though the *Champs Elysees*, while in consequence of the bridge, or the approach to it being mined, it was literally true that they were capering upon gunpowder! How very differently would the people of London behave under similar circumstances. True, we are not a dancing people and it might be supposed that the individuals alluded to were really rejoicing at the turn affairs had taken. I question however, whether this apology be admissible, perhaps what was seen upon the 8th of the month may bear me out in this surmise.

Before that day came round, a reinforcement, or remount, reached the regiment from Canterbury[43] and among them who should make his appearance but my *brother* Larry [Patrick Egan]![44] Never was greater surprise: *Bonaparte at Ligny* was an everyday occurrence compared to this. Who had sent for him? For what purpose was he wanted? These were queries that Larry [Patrick] himself alone could answer. All the answer he gave however, amounted to this, that he *had* been sent for and that we could not do without him. Well or ill, we *had* done without him and had given tolerable satisfaction. When the party joined I was going to Courbevios [Courbevoie], to see the major,[45] whom we had been obliged to leave there in a fit of the gout, at the time we repaired to Puteaux, Larry [Patrick] leading the way in virtue of his having been at Paris before. We shook hands and held a brief colloquy. 'How are you, Murphy? How came you here?' 'Why, don't you see?' (Larry generally had a short, but not always a witty or polite answer ready, though intended to be of the former description) 'Upon a mare, to be sure.' 'Yes, I observe, you are well mounted. You are very near Puteaux and as you will not be able to settle yourself today, my quarters are at such a place and you had better take possession. There will be some ration beef ready at five and then we can have all the news on both sides.' 'Thank you,' says Larry [Patrick]; 'How did *you* get on?' A private belonging to the party, who had lost his horse at Waterloo and had been detained in consequence till

---

43. On 12 July Lieutenants Leech and Mickelthwaite, Cornet St George Barry, Assistant Surgeon Patrick Egan and five rank & file joined from Canterbury.
44. Assistant Surgeon Patrick Egan.
45. Major James Bridger.

this opportunity offered of coming up, saved me the trouble of answering the question by vociferating, 'Like *a gentleman*, he did his duty *like a gentleman*.' I conceived this remark to be intended rather for Larry's [Patrick's] annoyance than my gratification and if I did not still think so, it might be wrong to record it. Opposite Puteaux is *Bagatelle*,[46] which had been first a favourite of Napoleon and in the intermediate time, a sort of suburban hunting box of the Duc de Berri.[47] I was much gratified by a visit to it and pleased to find it under the protection of an English guard.

---

46. A large park area which still exists as part of the Bois de Boulogne.
47. Charles-Ferdinand de Bourbon, Duc de Berry, nephew of King Louis XVIII.

## Chapter 10

# Paris in Peace

On the morning of the 8th, Paris was left to the occupation of the allied armies and at an early hour we made a party to visit this celebrated metropolis, full of vague expectations, but prepared for all occurrences. One was a visitor belonging to the Quarter Master General's department, who was to establish himself in Paris (now the seat of headquarters). As we entered the gates, battalions of Prussians were pouring in from all points and they were soon in possession of the interior, while the English army halted at and beyond the barriers. At this moment nothing but tricolored cockades and flags was to be seen. One of the latter was flying over the Tuileries; and though all the citizens had declared their willingness to receive back the king, they at the same time expressed a determination never to change the national emblems. However this may have been, before my friends and I could find our way to Very's,[1] the party-coloured drapery was replaced upon all the flag-staffs, by the *white*; and when we returned to the streets again, nothing but *white* cockades, scarfs &c &c was visible. On our way out of town, we stumbled on the royal procession, or rather the *retour* [the return]. Balconies and windows were filled with ladies, dressed in *white*, some of them having *white* plumes on their heads and all their lovely hands furnished with *white* kerchiefs. The king was in the same landau in which I had seen him at *Bavay*; but of course, the style of the exhibition was elevated in proportion to the difference of local and other circumstances. If expressions of dissatisfaction were to be heard, none of them fell upon my ear; all seemed to me to be gaiety and satisfaction and a good deal of what we saw even appeared to be folly, if not madness. Old women and young girls were dancing in the streets and boisterous loyalty seemed to be the humour of the day.[2]

---

1. Very's was one of the finest restaurants in Paris, having been established in 1765.
2. Note by Smith – I was absolutely pulled from my horse by a woman old enough to be my mother, who insisted upon kissing me. She was [thankfully] not *Poissarde* [a fishwife]. She was dancing and singing with several others and the chorus was, 'Nous avons trouve notre bon Pere' [We have found our good father].

Upon entering, I had hardly got the length of the *Place Louis XV*,[3] when I was hailed from the crowd by name! a circumstance not to be expected from a Parisian, for I had never been there before and had not a single acquaintance that I knew of in the place, or even among the inhabitants of the kingdom. The person however, who thus welcomed me was a well dressed young man, who had been a follower of Napoleon in the peninsula and had the year before (as a prisoner) been under my professional care in Lisbon. He was now a private gentleman and looked to advantage. There was so great a bustle however, about the spot, that I could not hold much conversation with him.

The day after this we were ordered back to Courbevois [Courbevoie], where we passed the residue of the month, with little to do but taking our tour of duty on the barrier in the *Champs Elysees*. *Courbevois* [Courbevoie] is chiefly celebrated for containing a barrack, rendered unfortunately famous by the massacre of the Swiss Guard which occupied it in 1792. This was at present of course empty and we established our hospital in it. The village is about a league from Paris and as I have said, touches the western extremity of the handsome bridge of Neuilly, the suburb of that name being situated at the other and consequently, on the Parisian side.

To attempt any description of Paris as it appeared in July 1815, would be vain for several reasons. In the first place I saw little of it, having been indisposed during much of the time that we spent in its vicinity; the picture has also been so minutely and repeatedly drawn by those whose professed object was observation, that anything of the same kind from a pencil such as mine and at such a distance of time, would be but indifferently received. Besides this, in order to have gleaned matters of real interest, one ought to have resided in the town, instead of being a league off and under the necessity of passing most of his time where other business required attention.

Upon entering C[ourvevoie] I found my name chalked upon the *porte cochere*[4] of a small but neat looking house, which belonged to the director or leader of the orchestra at the Opera.[5] He was absent and the house shut

---

3. Now the Place de la Concorde.
4. A covered porch under which people could embark or disembark from vehicles.
5. The Paris Opera had been formed in 1669, but during the Revolution, Empire and Royalist eras underwent a series of name changes. In 1815 it was called the Royal Academy of Music.

up. This looked at first, like an act of hostility. The day was very hot and it was by no means pleasant to be left exposed to the sun in the street. Chiswick had not yet come up, but I had got a temporary stud and servant. Impatience and dissatisfaction were beginning to be expressed without much ceremony and the neighbours interfered with their advice to take possession, *by breaking in*. To this I would not consent; but a locksmith happening to pass and declaring himself to be a *vieux militaire* [old soldier], who had served in Egypt, took upon himself to force an entry, which he said was perfectly according to the *laws of war*. I found that the proprietor had left everything in such a state as indicated both recent occupation and the intention of soon returning. Drawers were discovered unlocked, room doors open and all the furniture at our mercy. In these circumstances, I placed myself sentinel on the property, put the horses under cover of the gateway and despatched a messenger to say what was the state of the case, as well as to request the owner to come immediately and take care of his interests. He came in a great fright, expecting no doubt, to find his *chateau ecrase* [crushed castle] and every moveable upon this cherished spot carried off or destroyed. His surprise was amusing when he verified the state of the case by actual survey. He was not much pleased with the conduct of the locksmith, to be sure; but thought nevertheless, he had gotten cheap off. He was a very genteel looking and pleasing mannered old man, who (as he told us) had nothing to do with politics, emperors or kings, that his business was to play, or cause to be played, the fiddle, that he had played his own to Louis XV and afterwards before Louis XVI, then for the Directory, next for the gratification of the Emperor; when Napoleon went and Louis XVIII came, he had still done his work with alacrity and so during the hundred days, just expired, while he was ready to do it for the king again. I never could accurately make out Monsieur R[ochefort]'s political penchant. He came often to C[ourbevoie] and seemed rather disposed to dwell upon the *beaux jours* [good years] gone by, when Paris had been the resort of all Europe; and more especially of the English nobility, in the advantages of which an *artiste* must have shared extensively. He was replete with anecdotes of personages and occurrences and never gave us a single cause for offence. As to his absence on our arrival, he very satisfactorily explained that by assuring us that he had no idea of troops coming, that after having been at his house for several days, he had run into Paris, to inquire for madame, who was indisposed. He was of course, pleased with the anxiety that had been manifested about his chattels and I was then put in possession of my apartments.

During the time I remained here, I presume that I might have had access to all the public amusements of Paris gratuitously. As far as the Opera was concerned, I was repeatedly urged to avail myself of my host's patronage; and urged to dine at his town-house into the bargain; perhaps it was wrong on my part never to have done so. Murphy [Egan] (who happened to by my next neighbour) was less scrupulous and Monsieur Rochefort's invitations were not thrown away in that quarter.

Murphy [Egan], it has been already stated, was not upon the present occasion, at Paris for the first time. He had been left at Talavera and had consequently fallen into the hands of the enemy: the result was a journey to the French metropolis, where for a short period he was a prisoner on parole.[6] Having shewn some attention to the wounded among the French, I understand he had been favourably reported to the government, (to the *Empereur* himself, Larry [Patrick] constantly maintained and tried to make it out, that they had been on terms of intimacy if not of friendship) through which he obtained permission to go home, with the *cadeau* [present] of a thousand francs in his purse. If ever man had an opportunity of recommending himself to powerful notice, it occurred at this time to Murphy [Egan]; but it availed him nothing. I cannot fully describe it and even a partial and imperfect account will form a digression rather perhaps too long, though the story is by no means void of interest.

Passing through Spain after his capture, he found among some Spanish women, a boy whose father had been reported killed in one of our highland regiments. How the child came under Murphy's [Egan's] particular care I do not recollect and the printed account is not at hand to refer to;[7] but they came to England in company and waited together upon his late R[oyal] H[ighness] the Commander in Chief.[8] The benevolent prince displayed considerable interest about the boy; but as the colonel of the [42nd]

---

6. This confirms his real identity as Patrick Egan, who was captured at the Battle of Talavera when Assistant Surgeon of the 23rd Light Dragoons and was a prisoner of war for some six months.
7. Note by Smith – This account made its appearance at last in the M[onthly Register], I believe in the year 1820, under the title of 'The Romantic History of Jamie M[ellis]h.' It was furnished by L.M. [Patrick Egan] himself. [Searches of the journals of 1818–1821 have failed to find it.]
8. Frederick, Duke of York.

Regiment was at the time in London, his Royal Highness desired Murphy [Egan] to convey his *protégé* to the residence of his lordship. Going along the street upon this errand, they encountered a sergeant in the uniform of the [42nd], of whom Murphy [Egan] began to make inquiries as to the boy's father, naming him and alluding to his reported fate in the peninsula. The sergeant asked his reason for such inquiries; Murphy assigned them. The sergeant then avowed himself to be the individual and turning to the child, exclaimed, 'Jamie, don't you know me?' They were all proceeding to the same house and of course the story had gathered a vast accession of interest by this accidental recontre. Lord [Gordon],[9] learning that Murphy [Egan] was about to visit Dublin on leave of absence, kindly gave him a letter of introduction to his near relative, then Lord Lieutenant of Ireland.[10] Murphy [Egan] presented himself; but neither his personal appearance, manners, nor address, could do him much good in that quarter; and this interesting adventure terminated in a thing for Murphy [Egan] to reduce to writing and read to everyone who would listen to it. We had it by heart from right to left of the regiment years before he printed it and some copies in manuscript I have heard of as having been circulated privately; in fact he generally had one, rubbed almost to tatters in his pocket, which being his chef d'oeuvre in literature, he was ever ready to produce.[11]

---

9. George Gordon, Marquess of Huntly, later 5th Duke of Gordon, was Colonel of the 42nd Foot (Royal Highland Regiment). He was the brother-in-law of the Duke of Richmond.
10. Charles Lennox, 4th Duke of Richmond was Lord Lieutenant of Ireland 1807–13.
11. Note by Smith – The regiment (in which Larry [Patrick] and I served together), many years subsequently came in contact with the 42nd. Murphy was invited to their mess along with others, and the band of the Highlanders was in attendance. The story of Jamie being 'called for' by some of Larry Murphy's [Patrick Egan's] 'ancient comrades,' and told by the author with all its prose and incidents, the commanding officer gratified the dragoons by saying that Mr Murphy's [Egan's] *protégé* was actually among the musicians at the door and should be ordered in to drink the health of his protector. In came accordingly, a fine stripling with a French horn, (or clarinet or it might be a serpent, bassoon, trombone, flute, or tambourine) in his hand. Being ordered round to the back of Murphy's [Egan's] chair, he was asked by his colonel if he had any recollection of that gentleman? The lad looked with both his eyes, but there was 'no speculation' in them. 'No, Sir,' was the answer; 'I never saw him before, as far as I know.' The burst of laughter which this statement drew from the younger officers (who knew nothing of the Jamie business but what Murphy [Egan] himself had always been harping on) was a *floorer*. The truth of the matter is obvious: the lad had forgotten the early part of his own history. Murphy [Egan] I *knew* had been a staunch friend to him; and I think I am correct in adding that *Jamie* had, through M[urphy]'s [Egan's] agency, the benefit of an education at Chelsea.

I must not, however make too much of Murphy [Egan]. He was but an obscure object during the time of the Parisian masquerade, for such was the case with the gay metropolis throughout the period of its occupancy by the allies. One more allusion in this place to my brother chip [medic], and I shall fall again into the current of affairs.

Murphy [Egan] brought out with him, from the regimental *depot*, a very fine soldier, in the guise of his servant. The man was universally known and respected throughout the regiment and all his comrades expressed their astonishment at his coming among them in the character of Assistant Surgeon Murphy's servant; not that Assistant Surgeons were less esteemed than other officers; but Larry [Patrick] had a terrible *Karackter* among them all as a master, (I shall call this man Batty, he did afterwards beat the big drum in the band) and the surprise was general. In the first place, none of the authorities, military or medical, could reconcile their complacency to Murphy [Egan] *himself* appearing. We did not miss him; but, as he had joined us in a foreign land, we were disposed to behave well. Mr Batty, however, had merely taken advantage of the opportunity to rate himself (as our friends of the Navy would say) on Murphy's [Egan's] books, in order to get away from the *depot*. He had not been long at *Courbevois* [Courbevoie] when the *soldier* shone out to the disadvantage of the *domestic* and Batty committed some crime (the nature of which I could never accurately ascertain,) that brought him to a court martial and ended in three hundred lashes.[12] This sort of occurrence might not perhaps, find an appropriate introduction here, but for the curious characteristic circumstance of Larry Murphy [Patrick Egan] taking particular care to see the punishment inflicted under his own eye. We (the other medical officers) thought this rather an indelicate proceeding. He ought to have asked one of us to attend for him and we should have done so; but no; he said his man was a great rascal (nobody else considering him so), and that he should have every lash. Murphy [Egan] at a future period, saw another of his servants flogged to the same extent, for giving *him* a right good beating. We then thought, that although the transaction had taken place in a quarter, under the medical charge of Murphy, he might for decency's sake, have asked S [Surgeon Robinson] or me to have been present for him, engaging perhaps, to do a

---

12. Details of this court martial and the real identity of this man cannot be found.

similar duty for either of us in return; but no: Larry [Patrick] was rather *just* than *generous*. He would have made an excellent monarch where no such word as mercy found a place in the national dictionary.

During our abode at Courbevois [Courbevoie], I had the benefit of my servant Chiswick's arrival. *Fury*[13] came up too, quite recovered, with all my original cash and with addition of the proceeds of my canteen, which I had ordered John to dispose of at Brussels. My baggage was of the light sort; and I have no recollection of the fact of its restoration. Trunks of clothes and books had been left in store at Canterbury, which I saw nothing of for the space of three years. I rather think Chiswick had contrived to forward my *kit* by some conveyance; and I distinctly remember being surprised at the small amount of his own pecuniary expenditure, notwithstanding I had instructed him by letter to take care of himself till he could find an opportunity of joining.

The peculiarities of this man's character merit distinct notice; but perhaps I shall do well to abridge. When I joined the regiment, it happened to be the turn of the troop to which he belonged to furnish the first servant wanted for the Staff. John came to me, therefore, as a matter of course, but with the strongest recommendation from his captain.[14] 'I give you, doctor,' said this officer, 'the best man in my troop.'

We had not been long domesticated till I heard sad accounts of him: he was the worst tempered man in the regiment, could never agree with his former masters &c, good for nothing, 'and all that sort of thing and everything in the world besides.' 'Well,' I thought to myself, 'I never had a bad servant yet, even when kicked about as a solitary individual on the Staff of the General Hospital and now that I have got *home* to a regiment, I shall be truly unfortunate if I am to begin.' I soon found that C[hiswick] knew his business to the full as well as I could imagine myself to know mine. I became therefore, exempt from what I never had any particular fancy for (but which formed the solace, if not the grand business, of Larry Murphy's [Patrick Egan's] life), giving domestic orders and directions. It has happened that Chiswick and I have looked at each other for weeks together, while a word was never uttered on either side. I saw nothing to be altered or improved and what I wanted he knew perfectly well

---

13. Fury was his previously lame horse.
14. Captain Samson Stawell.

without being told. This is a specimen of his *temper, insubordination* and *worthlessness*. Of his *minor* qualifications, I beg to say that he could physic and even shoe a horse, build a stable, cook like Eustache Ude,[15] and make clothes with Stultz,[16] or shirts with any spinster. He could starve, stand fatigue, get the goodwill of the natives, or push them about when necessary, like a Prussian, though he preferred the *suaviter* [sweetener] to the *fortiter* [fortifier]. He was acquainted with every man, woman and child in the regiment and had more influence over them than any non-commissioned officer.[17] He had a negative qualification, exceedingly rare, he never could or would drink; and during the four years we lived together, which was during the whole period of my service in the regiment, I never found but one fault with him and that must [be], from sheer love of justice reveal[ed].

The current coin of the realm, the produce of the still and all other *perishable* commodities, might have been left, without weight or measure, as articles of temptation to John Chiswick in vain: but he had a failing, not common even among soldiers, he *pryed*! I required always *one key* and that I never could let out of my custody. It was the key of a drawer for the *Post Office* department. John read everything that came in his way and sometimes carried his operations a step farther. I was much confined to quarters at Courbevois [Courbevoie], in consequence of the ailment already alluded to. I had at this time, a favourite and very intelligent correspondent at home, to whom I had penned a foolscap of descriptive

---

15. Louis Eustache Ude was a renowned French chef working in London.
16. Stultz, originally a German military tailor, opened a shop at 10 Clifford Street near Saville Row and soon became the premier tailor for gentlemen.
17. Note by Smith – There was but one man, however, whom he admitted to intimacy. He too, was a *character* and after obtaining his discharge, for a complaint, perished in one of the South American affairs. This person had a notorious *poodle*, which, like many of the breed, was crabbed to strangers. He had been taught by Chiswick and his master to take care of *my* property, as well as *theirs*. It may gratify the lovers of *animal biography*, if I relate that, upon one occasion, I was thoughtless enough to lay hold of a bone which Thomas was gnawing, and he instantly paid me back by seizing my thumb. The remorse he appeared to be immediately struck with, would hardly be credited, if described. Prior to this adventure we had not been acquainted at all, except by sight or name. But T[homas] saw his mistake and acknowledging the difference of *rank*, allowed me to give him an unlimited kick, (though I was, in fact the aggressor) and afterwards, though naturally surly, became obsequious enough on all occasions. I am certain that dogs acquire a character, or temper, from the circumstances in which they are placed; and respect to superiors being the *vis vitae* of military life, regimental dogs are generally attached and obedient to *officers*. By regimental dogs I mean the soldiers' dogs.

matter, concerning the principal occurrences to which I had been witness. Chiswick it does not require to be repeated, had been separated from me during the whole series of the operations which form the prior part of this narrative and therefore, could not describe what he had never seen. However, upon one occasion when he was from home, I made a patrol into the garden. We had fitted up an arbour and greenhouse, in Rochefort's *bijou* [small residence], for stabling; and Chiswick always passed his days and frequently his nights with the horses.[18] Poking about, I got into the said green or tool house and in the temporary manger erected by Chiswick, found a written sheet of paper which appeared to be something I had seen before. It was John's manuscript [letter]; and I read (shame to me for doing so), because I perceived the subject was not unknown to me. I had not gone far till I found that I myself was the author, wherever or however it came by transcription. It was my own (unfinished) letter to my friend, which Chiswick had gotten hold of and was concocting into an epistle for his father. Where however, the personal pronoun had been introduced (*quasi* [partly] ergo I), John had made use of a possessive and a substantive, in the shape of my master. Of course, he added, 'says' so and so, or 'told me' so and so. I looked after my compositions and correspondence a little more strictly upon this hint. How John concluded his letter I know not; mine has found its way again into my possession and the story raised a regimental laugh.

---

18. Note by Smith – I never purchased a horse during the time I was in the regiment (and I certainly bought a few *rips*), without improving their condition so much, by this man's agency, that at the end of a few weeks, they doubled their price. I was guided by my messmate's opinion (the veterinary surgeon) and Chiswick had the art of attaching all sorts of beasts to him. The horses would follow him like dogs; if they were turned loose, they would come at a whistle and what will the epicures of the club houses say, when I pledge my honour, that in a stable, fitted up by himself, he contrived to decorate the rafters with *mushrooms*. At this time I kept half a dozen greyhounds, whereby hangs the following tale, which sportsmen may do more than consider. Lady greyhound pupped and we supposed the sire to be a fine dog of the same breed. A brother officer, either from mischievous design, or through ignorance, declared the litter to be mongrels and advised their destruction with the exception of two, whose tails he recommended to be shortened. Unhappily his advice was followed; but the things grew up *genuine greyhounds*, of a remarkably fine cast, though the *docking* spoiled their appearance. It is a mistake to suppose that greyhounds cannot course if short tailed. My puppies ran to all intents and purposes, as well as their sire (*Brandy*), or two younger brothers, who kept their tails and were named *Rum* and *Gin*. *Brandy* was a remarkably powerful and knowing fellow. I got him in a present from a captain in the regiment, who went on leave. *Fly*, the dam, was worthy of him: either could kill single handed; and the pups were genuine descendants.

As I may not perhaps find another opportunity of doing justice to an invaluable, though humble and modest individual, I am confident that all military readers will pardon me for adding a trait of character, which the kind and brave hearts of British officers will duly appreciate and which perhaps is hardly to be paralleled since the days of *Trim*, though I aspire not to be a *Shandy*.[19]

I joined the regiment at D[orchester] (to the best of my recollection) on 23rd of November 1814 and left it that day four years. During the whole of the intervening period, I never was a week absent altogether, never (and that upon the occasion of a visit to Brussels) more than three nights at a time. Often have I gone ten or fifteen miles to an out-quarter and preferred sitting up till daylight to ride home, rather than avail myself of the hospitable offer of a bed. During the full length of this period, Chiswick stuck to me like a burr. We once did quarrel and I absolutely returned him to his troop, but he would not *go*. When we reached England, after the occupation business was over, I found that as junior assistant, I was *doomed* to half pay. Chiswick declared that as I was going, *he* would stay no longer, if I could get his discharge. Having served twenty years, he was entitled to one shilling per diem of pension. Discharges at this time were to be had for asking for. I put the question to my good and gallant friend his Captain (who now commands the regiment, and who may justly be *proud* of his appointment, while the whole corps is *delighted* under it[20]); and I was told that Chiswick must not go, for his character was so high, that it was the wish of the committee to make him *mess waiter*, alias regimental butler. This flattering and advantageous proposal was declined on the following plea, 'If you were to stay Sir, I would stay with you; but as you are going, I am anxious to go too.'

He got his discharge and pension, did (what his master never could accomplish) obtain a wife and afterwards lost his shilling a day by refusing to serve as a veteran during the *radical* times. John Chiswick is not yet gathered to his fathers and I have not lost sight of him.

The greatest event, of a nature interesting to us, which took place at this time, was the review of the British army in the *Champs [Elysees]*, by the Emperors of Austria and Russia and the King of Prussia. Their forces

---

19. Corporal Trim was a character in Laurence Sterne's *Tristram Shandy*.
20. Captain Samson Stawell became Regimental Lieutenant Colonel in 1827.

had not yet re-entered the French territory, but their majesties themselves, had found their way to Paris. I was a spectator on the occasion; but owing to the complaint already alluded to, which made me constitutionally ill, I could not appear in my place, that is to say I could not *take the right of the regiment*. His Grace the Duke of Wellington marched past the crowned heads, tolerably well for one unaccustomed to play second fiddle on similar occasions; and my friend Joe the Vet [James Castley], stuck himself among a crowd of German princes, with whom he held a colloquy till the show was concluded. I recollect seeing the Prince of Orange, with his arm in a sling and Lady Castlereagh,[21] whose lord then swayed our destinies, in a carriage, drawn by four horses. I also saw (besides their Imperial Majesties, and the King of Prussia) *not one* of the French royal family; but I did see J[ames] K[empt?],[22] riding hard after a vagabond who had the impertinence to cry *'Vive l'Empereur!' Which* emperor (for there were three in question) J[ames] did not give him time to specify. After a coursing match of half a mile or thereabout, the animal was seized by the *queue* and conducted in triumph by his captor, who perhaps did not receive many thanks for his pains.

In the meantime, Paris was a focus of curiosities. The Prussians held possession of every vacant space, open places, squares (as we call them in England) bridges and the like, were covered with warriors and their appliances. The marble vases of the gardens at the Luxembourg were deprived of their fish and filled with soapsuds; for they became the washtubs of the Prussian laundresses. At either end of every bridge, viz the Pont Louis XV,[23] the Pont Neuf, the Pont des Arts, Pont d'Austerlitz &c &c, were two pieces of artillery, guarded by a competent force and ready to be fired down the adjacent streets on the least appearance of disturbance. Matches were kept burning day and night and all the vigilance and jealousy.

This circumstance doubtless stirred the wrath of the Parisians; but there were other causes of grievance on the part of the sufferers. Why the Prussian army was destined to *enter* the town, I do not till the present

---

21. Robert Stewart, Viscount Castlereagh was married to Amelia (Emily) Hobart daughter of the 2nd Earl of Buckinghamshire. Castlereagh was Foreign Secretary from 1812–22.
22. There is no certain identification of this person. He could be referring to Sir James Kempt, whose initials fit, but he perhaps talks too casually of such a senior officer.
23. Now the Pont de la Concorde.

hour know. Probably (according to the reason and nature of things) the English ought to have changed places with them; but they had the fortune to arrive first; and perhaps here was a degree of dexterity on their part, in dealing with the Parisians, which the English either would not or could not have displayed. Probably Blucher and his followers would have been annihilated, had it not been for the army of the Duke of Wellington; or more probably they would never have reached the barriers in anything like order or condition, had not the Duke's army been at their heels. I think too, that had the case been altered, we should all have been better friends, though the Parisians would unquestionably have taken advantage of our *good nature*. The French never professed any animosity against the British; and on the other hand, the latter never shewed the slightest sign of triumph or superiority over them.[24] One important cause of this distinction between the acceptability of the one army and that of the other, is referable to the fact of the French having invaded and (there can be no denying it) behaved with much *insolence* (to select the mildest term) in the Prussian territory. They had also *conquered* these fine fellows and brandished the strong arm over their monarch, as well as over the people. Upon English ground, no armed Frenchman had ever planted a victorious foot, at least from the time of the conquest; and at that period the Normans were not exactly French; consequently we had no quarrels to revenge and no painful remembrances to rouse vindictive passions. Our allies however, began very soon to get into broils, through which our countrymen (the junior part in particular) were not over scrupulous in helping them. We were upon several occasions concerned in jobs of this sort at the Palais Royal and elsewhere; and a few of our friends, who got into scrapes of their own, got out of them by pleading *Prussian privilege*.

Our stay in the neighbourhood of Paris did not extend beyond the 1st of August. It then became necessary for the cavalry to retire to Normandy, which as I have already said, is the *kitchen garden* of France, as Kent is that of England. We saw and felt and tasted in the land of our ancient conquerors; but more of this in due time.

---

24. Note by Smith – The Prussians never parted with their swords. The duke could never prevail upon English officers to wear theirs, when not upon duty, till he resorted to strong measures. A French gentleman remarked one day to an officer of our German Legion, that the British were unlike soldiers, for they seldom wore their swords. 'Ah, mine dear vellow, as for de zordz, it is a bad day for Vrance ven ve bud dem on.'

The narrative, down to the present time ie 1st August 1815, contains nothing but what is *literally* or *circumstantially* true. I describe only part of what I saw, or occurrences seen by my associates. Much relating to the campaign of Waterloo has been already published; but no one of my own cloth has been candid enough to stand forth with the story of his own proceedings.

I shall here mention that an allegation was set up against some of the medical officers, that they left their duty. I know from what quarter this scandal emanated; and the party to whom the authorship was traced had better have '*cast the beam out of his own eye,*' before he proceeded '*to cast the mote out of his brother's.*' For my own part, I heard nothing of this till afterwards; but I did hear, with sentiments of sorrow, that although more skill and exertion had been displayed and a greater proportion of lives had been saved upon this than upon any collateral occasion, the surgeons had been censured. The hands of *the censor* were by no means clean; and one of the preceding anecdotes may help to prove that such was the case.[25]

---

25. Note by Smith – How came a dozen of us, as mentioned, to be left without rations, orders, or instruments for nearly two days? It must be recollected that we were not among the barren mountains of the peninsula and that the *surgical* fatigues began only when the *military* were over. And afterward we were entirely at our own discretion, a compliment no doubt, though I question whether it was *intended*, or under circumstances of better arrangement, would have been *paid*. The I[nspector] of H[ospitals] whom we had to deal with, appeared anxious only to find excuses for riding *about* and doing nothing. He ought certainly to have sent a senior or Staff Surgeon (of which Brussels contained a *brigade*) out to us. We were all young officers, without a head or a reference, in cases of difficulty; but we did our duty conscientiously, diligently and effectively. *Let us be known by our works.*

Chapter 11

# Normandy

The place of our destination in Normandy was a little, quiet, dull town, about eighty miles from Paris; situated in a very uninteresting country, but celebrated for its mineral wells,[1] one of which had the reputation of promoting the wishes of ladies 'who love their lords'.[2] We were four days on the march; and though we neither encountered difficulty nor adventure worth relating, to me the expedition was both amusing and interesting, chiefly from the novelty of the appearance and manners of the people. To the greater part of my friends this charm was wanting; for the regiment had passed through a portion of the same country the year preceding, on their long but delightful march from Bordeaux to Calais. There were very few things about, connected with or relative to *Murphy* [Egan] (my colleague) for which it was possible to envy him; but, for having accompanied the [12]th on this occasion, I was always much inclined so to feel. In the first place, after the miseries of the peninsular campaigns, they enjoyed themselves to no ordinary extent, in one of the finest towns of France for several months; and secondly at no expense, under circumstances too of the most gratifying nature, they nearly traversed that delightful kingdom, on their way to their happy homes. How large a portion of the British army was shipped off, on the same occasion to fight bloody battles in America, the history of the time has already told. This disappointment, the extent of which I did not know until I came among those who had enjoyed and were continually alluding to the treat, arose from the following circumstances, the introduction of which though not strictly in order, may perhaps be suffered.

When the General Hospital was broken up at Coimbra[3] and all the moveable sick, as well as stores, were conveyed to St Andero [Santander]

---

1. Forges-les-Eaux is a small spa town 80 miles north west of Paris.
2. Note by Smith – It was called *The Cardinal*; I cannot say why. By the Editor – It is named so because it was visited regularly by Cardinal Richelieu.
3. Note by Smith – In August 1814.

and Bilbao in the north of Spain, it was found that nearly thirty poor fellows could not be disturbed. The cases of the majority were hopeless and there was nothing apparently to be done but to let them die in peace. To leave them without a medical officer in these desperate circumstances, was not to be thought of; and it was the more necessary that one, supposed to possess some general intelligence, activity and acquaintance with hospital routine and returns as well as disease, should be preferred; for, as the usual assistance from the purveyor's department was no longer to be had, a very *responsible* duty was to devolve upon him, in the article of providing comforts for the sick.[4] I was the individual upon whom the Inspector turned his eyes, and being at the time on the strength of a regiment gone to England, he probably thought I was least likely to be ordered away before the removal of the whole. It was a great compliment to be thus selected and it was done in a very flattering manner. I have no doubt that the matter would have been greatly to my advantage had the war continued long enough to occasion a vacancy among the physicians to the forces, for I thus became *Principal Medical Officer* of a station, under circumstances of peculiar difficulty and was thrown into direct and daily correspondence with headquarters. In a short time I had above a hundred sick to look after; and as other stations in the country were broken up, detachments of sick and convalescents, consignments of stores &c, came down to Coimbra and I had to become answerable for all. This sort of thing lasted several months, one passing away after another, in the vain hope of transports arriving at Figueira [da Foz] for the purpose of clearing us all out. My soul began to be weary of a life which would have been perfectly intolerable had I not been cheered and encouraged by some of the officers. In the commandant and parson, as well as in one or two others, I found not only agreeable associates, but warm personal friends; and it would be unhandsome not to express the pleasure I felt in having for an assistant, one of the professors in the university. This

---

4. Note by Smith – Detachments also, of men in health, amounting to about six hundred, were left under a regular commandant. There was an establishment of the commissariat, a purveyor's clerk, whose stores were afterwards made available, although the accounts were said to be closed; and we had a chaplain, waiting for orders. I have spoken of this gentleman already. Most of the thirty men died, as was anticipated; others got round, contrary to all expectation. The most troublesome and thankless part of the duty, generally (though not without exception) was attending sick *officers*, of whom there was also a considerable number.

accomplished gentleman held temporary rank as a medical officer, in the English service, and from the peculiarity of his situation, could not well be moved from the station. He lectured in his black robe in the morning and dressed (for dining with us) *a la militaire*, in the afternoon.[5]

To be more minute in allusions to my situation and circumstances, at this time (upon the whole, the most arduous and most delightful of my life, possessed of at least an *official* importance, which was new, both in itself and in the circumstance of its attaching to so young an officer), would swell what is likely, *as it* is, to be an unreasonable digression, into utterly intolerable bounds. Suffice it that I had *Camoens*[6] and *Inez de Castro*[7] 'familiar in my mouth as household words;' and a specimen of the purpose my excursions with Dr A[lmeida][8] were turned to, I take the liberty to introduce.

The university session opened during my reign and the graceful costume, the joy and mischievous propensities, of the *juvenes ingenuosi* [talented young men], the peculiarities of their economy and discipline, together with other matters of a curious and unique description, may furnish materials for a future volume.

In the midst of these proceedings I was appointed an Assistant Surgeon on the Staff. I had already obtained permission from Lord Wellington to remain in the peninsula, for the purpose of exchanging into a regiment belonging to his army. I had many offers, some ridiculous and others absolutely impudent. To get to England, from the harassing scenes of the Pyrenees, was like going to paradise. My then regiment (in the light cavalry [11th Light Dragoons]) had been at home for some time. A gentleman who offered (among others) to exchange with me,

---

5. Note by Smith – He spoke English uncommonly well; was a great friend to our countrymen; understood the manners, and was well acquainted with the history of Portugal in general, and of Coimbra in particular.
6. Luis de Camoes is considered to be Portugal's greatest poet.
7. Ines de Castro was a Galician noblewoman who was to be married to King Peter I of Portugal, but was murdered by the nobles to prevent it (although Peter claimed that they had already married secretly). A myth states that when proclaimed king, he exhumed her body and forced the nobles to swear fealty to her corpse.
8. Dr Antonio de Almeida Caldas was a physician. He was professor in medicine at the university until the war. In 1810 he was appointed Primeiro Medico (First Doctor) of Coimbra's Military Hospital and was the hospital's director. He was later appointed to inspect the hospitals at Beira in 1813 and established a military hospital in Aveiro in 1814. My thanks to Moises Gaudencio for identifying this man.

very coolly wrote to say that as he understood the [12th] Dragoons were under orders for India, he desired *I would lose no time* in concluding the arrangements necessary to facilitate his transfer. The negotiation did not succeed. I applied for permission to go to my regiment; but was appointed by the present director general to the Staff, (which was never acted upon) and about the same time removed by interference at home, to the corps in which I played the part it is the purport and intent of writing these volumes to describe.

Along with the news of my transfer, came '*orders to join.*' Joyfully were they received; but I had a subordinate station, a second 'cure', a plurality of torment, down at the mouth of the Mondego, in the shape of another depot. To make some arrangements for its future welfare and to inquire about a passage to the army, were indispensable duties. Accordingly, I took what I thought but a temporary leave of my Coimbra friends and proceeded with a lightened heart, to the station alluded to.

Here in the little town of Figueira [da Foz], I found a considerable hospital, under the immediate charge of an officer, who was himself less sick than surly. He was an hospital mate; and consequently the nature of such a duty was more coincident with his appointment than with mine. The moment however that I arrived, he declared his inability to do any more work and that the safety of his constitution if not of his life, demanded his immediate removal to England, *via* Lisbon. The commandant was glad to get rid of him; and at this I do not wonder, for the military authority possessed a zeal for the service which was *unbounded*; the doctor never *felt* I believe, that there was a second person in the world. This unhappy being (and I call him so for sundry good but inexpressible reasons) would do nothing more for the king; and the commandant, whose friendship I have retained down to the present hour, laid violent hands upon me. To shorten a long story, I was impounded in this hole, expecting daily to get away for five long and dreary winter months, which I passed very uncomfortably, although in what were as thing went, good enough quarters. When at length, we were set free, instead of proceeding to my regiment I was compelled to follow my charge to Lisbon, where I arrived about the time that the troops settled themselves in Bordeaux.

At Lisbon the demand for medical officers was considerable. There were still a General Hospital, Staff and garrison of some magnitude and I was ordered to do duty among the French prisoners, amounting to several thousands.⁹ As far as professional improvement, comprehending medical tact and surgical dexterity, were concerned, my experience was equivalent to what a *life* spent at home, under the most favourable circumstances, could possibly have afforded. The benefit of this I have since uniformly felt; and my object in going into the service was neither to affect being a soldier, nor to forget that I was an Esculapian [medic]; while one of my purposes in writing these pages is to show the young army surgeon that, even under perplexing and difficult circumstances, under the greatest disadvantages, of a nature which are rather military than professional, he may perform his duty, with credit and advantage to himself, as well as to others, if he will but do his best to perform it actively and honestly. There may be in some minds, a fanciful notion of superiority, because the fancier may have a longer purse; but the balance is in favour of *intelligence*, more especially since exertions have been so successfully made by the present heads of the army medical department, to fill vacancies with none but men of the highest pretensions, both as to character and education. There is a race of medical men now in the service such as it never saw; and the results have for many years been as creditable to all parties, as gratifying in the contemplation. But lest I should incur the charge of becoming *prosy*, let me hasten to say that I was not at liberty to quit Lisbon till October 1814: and that being obliged to take a month's leave of absence, through ill health on my arrival in England, I did not join my regiment until I had been numbered, but *not* mustered among them for fourteen months. In fact, for a long time prior to my appearance at Craig's Court,¹⁰ I had been *lost, totally lost*, reported 'absent without leave,' pay stopped and I know not what all; although the duties in which I had been employed, I had on first descending upon '*the Peninsula*,' been accustomed to see discharged by an Inspector of Hospitals.

*Revenons a nos moutons* [Back on topic], this *intolerable* retrospect was introduced, upon the recollection that as we passed through the part of Lower Normandy, my associates called to mind many scenes and places that were yet fresh in their memories. We filed along a beautiful valley, between *Gisors* and *Gournay* [en-Bray], the left acclivity which bounded it, being covered with a dense hanging-wood that would have done credit

---

9. Note by Smith – My Figueria predecessor I found still at Lisbon, playing at billiards in the most free and easy manner possible; and several months after this again, I found him (on the sick-list, certainly) at Portsmouth.
10. The location of Greenwood & Cox, Army Agents.

to any English nobleman's park: above which shot here and there a church spire or tower; and the greater part of these churches, as well as of others in the neighbourhood, was said to have been built by the English.

The Normans professed themselves to be of the same stock as the English; and if a jolly appearance and an uproariousness of deportment are the points of identity, I for one will never contest the validity of their claim. This is a country in which it would be an insult to place a goose upon a gentleman's table: it is food, according to Norman notions, fit for beggars only.

Passing down the valley in question, we saw the females busily employed at their doors in *lacemaking*. Their lace is perhaps not equal to that which may be bought at *Cambrai* or *Valenciennes*, but looks as well; and when we call to mind (what was not known at that time, but which has come to light since) that most of the French lace and some even of Flanders and Mechlin [Mechelen] reputation is made in England and afterwards sold and repurchased by *the Bull family* in the places alluded to, perhaps a pleasanter journey might be made by repairing to Normandy, instead of [Cateau] *Cambresis* or *Flanders*, at least in quest of this necessary of *female* life.

The night previous to our arrival in what we expected to be permanent cantonments, we passed at Gournay [en-Bray] a neat Norman bourg, not very interesting either in history or topography, but not unintroducible here, on account of the following circumstance.

One of us had upon this occasion, been lodged or *billeted* (should the military reader prefer that *façon de parler* [way of talking]), in the house of a man, hardly entitled perhaps to call himself *gentleman*, who had treated his inmate to a good dinner in the military sense of the term. This act of attention dwelt forcibly upon T[homas]'s[11] grateful mind; and after we were established in headquarters (about twelve miles off only) he proposed, by way of *returning the compliment*, to ride over one day, with O[tway], (a good natured, rattling fellow), to take *pot-luck* with his friend at Gournay [en-Bray]. Taking *pot-luck* with a Frenchman! Or even with a Norman!! Astonishment at the very idea cannot be sufficiently excited.

However, they went and what is more surprising, they were received; and as the Norman affected the hospitable good fellow and pretended he

---

11. Lieutenant Thomas Reed.

was glad to see them, it is hardly matter of impeachment against their acuteness that they should have imagined themselves *welcome*: had it been otherwise, in all probability they would not have staid.

Down they sat and the dinner (in a plentiful country, with the aid of French cookery) could hardly be insufficient. A huge frowzy [seedy] fille waited at table. They all ate much alike; but their conversation was more adapted to tower of Babel times than to those even of revolutionised France. The host spoke no English; the guide *little, very* little French; O[tway] no language living or dead: but he chattered and jawed and ate and drank and laughed and *joked*!! till he rendered it imperative upon T[homas] to apologise for him: which was done (as I was informed, for I was not present) nearly in the following terms: – '*Monsieur, excusez mon ami, il est un* Jean Bull.' [Sir excuse my friend, he is a John Bull].[12] The master of the house, turning to the *fille*, addressed her thus '*Marie, sais-tu ce que c'est qu'un* Jean Bull?' [Marie, do you know what a John Bull is?] '*Non, Monsieur; mais qu'apparemment c'est une drole de bete.*' [No sir, but apparently it's a funny beast] '*Je m'en vais donc te dire. C'est, vraiment, une bete, qui jase, jase, jase incessamment, qui babille, et (si que l'on pourroit entendre ses galimatias) ne sauroit mot qu'il dit lui-meme*'. [So I am going to tell you, really a beast, which chatters, chatters, chatters incessantly, which babbles and (if one could hear his unintelligible talk) would not know a word that he said to himself]. This story would never have reached us, had not the honest man come to an inhabitant at headquarters, to ascertain what sort of people he had been honoured with, on the occasion in question.

At length few were settled at F[orge]s [les-Eaux], and if we did not find it a place of public amusement, I believe some of us fabricated a small quantity of a private nature. The little town being barely adequate to the accommodation of the headquarter *functionaries* (consisting of the Staff and a squadron), the rest were sent to neighbouring villages. G[aille] F[ontaine] held a squadron most conveniently; and it was not too far off to admit of the officers coming to dine at the mess,[13] which was established in the house of the *maire* of F[orge]s, who had moreover, become a sort of contractor.

---

12. Note by Smith – O[tway] however, happened to be an *Irishman*.
13. Note by Smith – It was here that Larry Murphy [Patrick Egan] got *well paid* for interfering with his servant's business; and by way of receipt, the man was accommodated with three hundred lashes, the second servant that had incurred the sentence of a court martial (through being on Larry's [Egan's] establishment), in the course of little more than a month; and he took care to see justice executed with his own eyes, though it

During the time we remained among these honest and peaceable people (though there were ideas both of a *Republican* and of an *Imperial* cast among them), one or two most 'untoward occurrences' took place, to which I shall make no apology for alluding.

A fair was held in the town of F[orge]s; and I should stop to say how much I was edified by a regular traveller, or bagman, on behalf of *Jose Maria Farina* (the eau de cologne man),[14] did I not believe as much in the hippocratic virtues of *Mr Farina's* water, as I do in those of the Pope's and did I not call to mind the tragic occurrences which plunged us all into sorrow and almost into disgrace.

One of our dragoons waylaid a farmer, riding home from the fair and shot him dead! An officer, stationed at G[aillefontaine], had been dining at headquarters and on his way home, found the corpse, probably his accidental arrival prevented the assassin from executing his purpose of plunder, for it was ascertained (and indeed known to the soldier) that the deceased carried a considerable sum of money about him. The officer immediately returned to F[orge]s and gave the alarm. Every soldier in the town was paraded, though past ten o'clock; every pistol and carbine examined; and a man was suspected if I recollect accurately, his pistol was found though he denied having been absent from quarters and maintained, that he had put it by clean, in its proper place. His character however, was gone. The officers offered a reward of one hundred pounds for the detection of the murderer. I was on parade when this offer was published: the man quailed and turned white in the countenance: but said nothing, He was brought to general court martial and acquitted; but for years, he lived at least a *suspected murderer*.[15]

---

would have been but decent to have asked the surgeon or myself to attend for him. After this, no soldier could be prevailed upon to live with him, until a tippling old Scotchman was talked over by his captain and agreed, *conditionally*, to accept the situation. The current story was, that upon taking up their abode together, *Jock* duly primed for the occasion, paraded Larry [Patrick] and harangued him to the following effect: – 'Maister Morphy! It's no'oot o' ony regaird or respeck for you that I'm come to bide wi' you, but purely to obleege the captain; so, you see, the first time you say the thing to me that's no circumspeck, I'll no strick ye, it wad na be dacent for anauld soger like me and a man of my character, to lay my haunds uo' the like o' *you*, but I'se tell ye the upshot, I'll just dischairge ye and gang back to my duty.'

14. Giovanni Maria Farina was an Italian-born perfumier working in Germany, who created the first eau de cologne.
15. Private William Richardson was court-martialled at Abbeville on 6 October 1815 for wilful murder of a local inhabitant but was acquitted. I must thank Zack White for this information.

Long, long afterwards, another man died in his bed and confessed the crime of which poor R[ichardson] had been unjustly accused. The real murderer and R[ichardson] had been comrades, and of course occupied the same quarters. The assassin took R[ichardson]'s pistol and with it perpetrated the bloody deed, though he reaped no advantage from it. I am shocked to add, that *a woman* who lived with the murderer, was acquainted with the whole of the affair, though she never revealed anything till her paramour was beyond the reach of human vengeance.

An evening or two after this lamentable example had been set, an attempt was made to follow it, on the part of one of the smartest soldiers in the regiment. He also took his pistol, repaired to the same place and there waited for a farmer, whom he understood to be the bearer of a large sum of money. The sturdy Norman arrived well mounted, but accompanied by his son, another bold one; and between the two, the pistol was wrenched from the fellow's grasp, furnishing tolerably strong proof as to his being the intended assassin. The farmer rode back immediately and gave information; the troops were again paraded; the pistol was found to be P[ower]'s, and he was absent, not having had time to return. Circumstantial evidence could scarcely be stronger; and the culprit was sent for trial, before a general court martial; but as the *Ellenborough Act*[16] was little known, or less understood by his judges, the animus [hostile act] seems to have been left out of their consideration and his crime viewed in a purely military light. His sentence was *a thousand lashes*.[17] A civil tribunal, furnished with the same proofs, would certainly have consigned him to the gallows; but the law of evidence before courts martial is ill defined and very imperfectly understood, unless a witness can be produced who will prove as well as swear, that he *saw* the crime committed, votes in favour of a culprit will always be given. A court martial is for these and other reasons, the most lenient of all courts. But,

---

16. The Malicious Shooting or Stabbing Act of 1803 was commonly called Lord Ellenborough's Act, who was Lord Chief Justice.
17. Private Edward Power was court-martialled for robbery at Abbeville on 2 October 1815, he was found guilty and given a sentence of 1,000 lashes. Despite Smith's comments, Power had previously been court-martialled at Fuenterrabia on 23 March 1814 for unsoldierlike behaviour and sentenced to receive 400 lashes. Although not mentioned by Smith, another soldier, Private Jonathan Forrest, was also tried on 2 October for robbery, but was acquitted. It is not clear if he was part of the same incident or a completely separate one. I must again thank Zack White for this information. Power was in the same troop as Lieutenant William Hay, who describes him as gallant, but cool and determined. He also states that Power captured three cuirassiers at Waterloo.

in the case under consideration, the punishment may be considered to have been severe. I saw it, as I have said, inflicted; and I did not think so. P[ower] bore it without a complaint; and as soon as he was taken down, he turned round and spoke as follows: 'Gentlemen, you have seen me take my punishment like a soldier; I hope you will now give me my discharge; and if you don't I will vex you all.' He was as good as his word; for the space of about two years afterwards, he lived chiefly in the guard-house, being seldom if ever out of a drunken scrape. At the end of this time, the colonel gave him a blank discharge; and since then, I have learnt that he obtained a situation as *valet de chamber*.

The case here made out against his moral character is certainly very strong: but I should entertain little fear in employing this man myself. He was, even after this ugly passage in his history, looked upon as the regimental pattern. If a new article of dress or equipment came out and a neat soldier was wanted to exhibit the same, either to the general or any authority, P[ower] was selected for the purpose; and he might then be sent *alone* to any distance. He would return sober and steady, do up his horse, put his appointments by in perfect order; and then, but not till then, get drunk and into the guardhouse, where perhaps, he would stay till again required on some similar occasion. The poor fellow had lost a wife to whom he was much attached; and from the period of her death they said, he became an altered man, took to dissipated habits and it was asserted among his comrades, that the affair for which he was punished would never have entered his head, but for the other which preceded it. There seemed to have been a sort of insanity about him.

These things by no means embroiled us with the people; they had the good sense to know that soldiers are at least, not better than citizens and they were pleased with the promptitude evinced by the officers to detect the offenders and bring them to justice. So different indeed, had our general conduct been from what they imagined inseparably connected with that of a victorious army, that we *jumped* into their good graces almost at once and as connected with the incidents now related, I may mention another, also of a bloody though less tragic nature, which amused and even gratified the whole neighbourhood.

One of our sergeants, a quiet inoffensive man, was quartered in a farmhouse, where there lived (as I shall hereafter shew to be a national habit) the old father and two or three sons. One of these had been at

Moscow, as a horse grenadier under Napoleon and was (as all the *Old Guard* were to a man) excessively insolent. The sergeant bore with his vapouring for a long time, until the fellow went so far as to accuse him of cowardice. Our friend now, in his turn, became the provocatory and challenged him to fight with their swords. *La Vieille Garde* accepted with alacrity, piquing himself, as all his countrymen do, on his dexterity in the use of that weapon. They had hardly commenced the action till the sergeant wounded him. The man of Moscow (a sort of phenomenon in France, which saw but few of that army come back) now begged his life. The sergeant granted it; and afterwards was not only permitted to live in peace, but rose high in the estimation of everybody, not excepting the family in general and his quondam [former] tormentor in particular.

The two autumnal months which were passed in F[orge]s, though perhaps monotonous, were by no means unpleasant, at least as far as I may speak for myself. The sort of life was new, though France was by this time not quite so; but those who take the manners of the Parisians as examples of French customs and character elsewhere make a vast mistake. The language was the same in the *Seine Inferieure* as we had previously been accustomed to and in some things, the economy was identical; but we were certainly among people of a different character.

It was my fortune to be quartered in the house of the apothecary, at once the most conceited and arrogant as well as the ugliest fellow I had yet come in contact with, in the latter respect he had the *advantage* even of Larry Murphy [Patrick Egan]. This son of Galen[18] had some *queer* points in his character, which it may be amusing to describe. He said he was not a Frenchman, but a subject of the Emperor of Austria, having been born somewhere in the Netherlands, while that country formed part of the Austrian dominions. However, as being born in a stable does not necessarily constitute the infant a *foal*, his having been *dropped* in Blankenbourg [Blankenberge] could hardly entitle him to be called an Austrian, the more questionably, as he had learned his craft at Rouen. I shall call him *Mephistophiles*, as by that *tour du mot* [turn of word], I preserve not only the real initial, but a sort of similarity of sound, which one of my readers at least, will recognise.

---

18. Galen of Pergamon was a Greek physician.

Monsieur Mephistophiles thought it *beaucoup d'honneur* to have the aide major under his roof: but I had not been there many days, till I was forced into a quarrel, upon the meanest of all pretences. It did not suit my finances to live at our always expensive and at that time, extravagant mess; nor was I the only Staff officer who staid away. Accordingly, the rations were of consequence, even to ourselves; while in the eyes of the natives, they appeared to be *profusion*. In the first few days, John Chiswick did his best in the cooking department; but *Meinherr* and *Meinfrau Mephistoph* threw obstacles in his way, till we could hardly get anything at all. It was then represented to me, that if we were to hand the prog over to them, they would cook it much better and by adding their own share, furnish amazing good dinners.[19] In order to save trouble, I consented and we really did find it for our advantage, their dinner hour being postponed to meet my views. We got on tolerably well now, having no trouble about domestic matters.

*Mephistophiles* however, besides his ugliness, had other very odd and some rather suspicious, peculiarities. He not only never wore a hat himself, but disapproved of other people wearing one. Probably some of my readers may be aware, that a shoemaker's knife, after long use and frequent sharpening wears to a point, the blade degenerating into a triangle. Such a knife *Mephistophiles* always carried in his pocket. With it he cut everything that came in his way and with it he carved the meat at his table. He had been a violent partisan of former governments, a furious republican first and a staunch imperialist afterwards; and he had been imprudent enough to express himself strongly against the existing order of things: in fact it got abroad that he had boasted of his ability to poison all the English soldiers and I was absolutely cautioned not to eat anything produced by him. All that the man had really said, I believe was, that he had poison enough in his shop for such a purpose; and I can only say that, during my abode under his roof, I saw nothing about him worse than vanity. But upon one occasion, he took me into an adjacent wood for a walk and pulling out the knife, said he could stick it into any tree, at thirty yards distance with unerring aim. He did so; and I could hardly

---

19. Note by Smith – It will be shewn more particularly hereafter that the allowance granted to British troops was considered, by the French, more than adequate, though our men had, when left to their own management, at all times enough to do to make the ends meet.

help imagining that there might be some sinister intention on his part, by drawing me into a situation where it would have been a very simple thing to have missed a tree and hit myself.

In the meantime, my friend J B [James Castley] had been leading a similar sort of life in the house of the physician of the Norman Cheltenham [Spa]. This was however, a princely fellow, who kept an excellent table and for a French doctor, a respectable establishment in which there was absolutely an approach to *comfort*. I had no occasion to envy Joe [James] however, for the house was almost as open to me as to himself; nor had the worthy doctor a dinner party to which his *confrere* [colleague] was not invited. He was wealthy and had some landed property I believe, in right of his wife. This lady was good natured, Joe [James] said she was rather *too much* so and even troublesome, through the kindness of her disposition. The doctor gave her, her own way and would have been all the more civil to my friend had the wife not complained of his shyness: as it was, the *mari* [husband] wondered in silence; but upon a subject of this nature, much cannot be said. Joe [James] *erred* (in their eyes) through native delicacy and manly British principle, which had taught him, as I hope it had most of us, not to violate the confidence of the man who treats us with hospitality. 'They manage these things (differently, at least, if not) better in France.'

In the vicinity of this little town were two families of some celebrity: one of the ancient, the other of the modern *noblesse*, that is the head of the latter, had received a title from Bonaparte and had been a high officer in his household. I believe he had pretensions of a more antique nature; but he had permitted all to be swallowed up by his recent ephemeral distinction. The most remarkable thing connected with this gentleman was, that one of his daughters had been married to the younger C[aulaincourt][20] (who perished in the Russian expedition) at the moment of his departure and was now a maiden widow.[21] There was a son, who had been a colonel in

---

20. General Auguste Comte de Caulaincourt was killed at Borodino in 1812. His father was General Gabriel de Caulaincourt and brother of Armand de Caulaincourt, a close advisor of Napoleon's.
21. Auguste Caulaincourt married Henriette d'Aubusson, daughter of the Marquis de Castelnouvel, on 12 July 1812. The marquis was prominent in Napoleon's government and a Count of the Empire, but retired to his estates after the Hundred Days. Pierre Raymond d'Aubusson, Marquis de Castelnouvel, was Mayor of Le Thile-Riberpre, not far from Gaillefontaine. His son was Augustine d'Abusson de la Feuillade.

the same service; but he was imprudent enough to exhibit his vindictive feelings in so outrageous a manner, that the circumstance reached the ears of government, through the medium of some of the inhabitants, who knew that our officers had treated him with unrequired and unmerited hospitality. Had he been a soldier of fortune, raised from the ranks, much else would not have been looked for and probably no such opportunities would have been afforded. He was obliged to keep himself *au secret* and the father was thrown into a state of considerable uneasiness about him. The other family was loyal *a l'outrance* [excessively] and nothing was good enough for us in their opinion.[22] They had suffered much by the changes which had taken place, but appeared now to be quite happy. They too had a son, quite a gentleman, who had been partially educated in England and spoke the language well. I believe there were no other people of similar rank near us: the town being occupied by shopkeepers, persons in or retired from business, little lawyers, publicans and sinners of various descriptions; but it was singular in an exemption which does not attach to all watering-places: what wickedness prevailed in it was chiefly, if not entirely, confined to the male sex; and this characteristic we found to be general throughout the country. The young women are in France, virtuous to an almost inconceivable and as some of our rakes complained, to a very inconvenient degree.

At F[orges] I received an invitation to visit my friend, of the Quarter Master General's department, with whom I rode into Paris, on a former occasion. He described the gaieties of this singular place in such colours and so depicted the pleasures and comforts of his own residence in a village a few miles out of town, that I could not resist. At the same time, I may add, that his lady required 'a cast of my office.' I hastened to *St Denis* and from thence to *Dugny*,[23] where I was hardly sorry to find that the necessity for my appearance had been superseded. Nature, like time and tide, would not wait for my arrival; and another pill had been done the needful. However, as few had projected some amusement during *straw time*, we did revisit the metropolis; and I was even more amused than I had been on the former occasion. By this time the Russians, Austrians

---

22. The other family would appear to be the Roys family who owned the Chateau of Gaillefontaine after Etienne des Roys had married Jenny Hoche, only daughter of Marshal Hoche, in 1814.
23. Now in north Paris near Le Bourget airport.

and all the hordes, had found their way to the banks of the Seine and a motley assemblage indeed was *there*. The British infantry were still in their camps and doing the same sort of duty, in the discharge of which we had left them. But to describe the Palais Royal would be to contend with overpowering beggary. The animosity between the Parisians and Prussians had risen to a vast height; and had been *exacerbated* by the circumstance of the latter having been newly clothed at the expense of the former.

I was sitting with another English officer one evening in the well-known rotunda,[24] when a great uproar was raised in the garden. An attempt was instantly made to shut us in and all the gates were closed in a twinkling; so that those who happened to be within them could not get out and those who were exclusives could not find their way in. I saw no propriety for my own part, in being thus caged, as I and all present had in no way been concerned in the quarrel; and among the party were several Prussian officers. One of them, a stout burly fellow, planted himself in the gateway and in spite of every attempt to close it by that ingenious piece of armour called a *key*, he kept the iron barrier open, inviting those who pleased to enter and exhorting those who wished it to depart. Being in uniform, I chose to remain where I was and took my friend (who wore *mufti* on that occasion) under my protection, resolved to see the fun. The object was to drive the brawlers into a corner of the garden at the point of the bayonet, then and there to select such and so many as might seem meet to the authorities. The forces on this occasion consisted of a subaltern's guard, composed of English, *Prusses* and French citizens (de la Garde National) commanded by an officer of the last. This poor man had to parade his heterogeneous troops, tell them off and give the word in three different languages. As far as his mother tongue went, I believe he acquitted himself to the satisfaction of his *customers*: but if I may judge of his *German* tact from his *English*, a more perfect club of conglomeration, upon a slender scale, was never seen. He faced them in a wrong direction, then scolded, then begged pardon and then tried it again, amid roars of *laughter* (of all sounds the most awful and impressive to the ears of a Frenchman), with no better success. My friend Mathews hists him off to the life in his exhibition of the Yankee volunteers, on a drill day. The

---

24. This stood at the end of the Palais Royale.

grocer or tailor, or haberdasher or saddler or whatever he was, had no doubt a book in his pocket, but he was probably ashamed to use it. How the disturbance ended I had no curiosity to inquire; for it was only one of twenty similar brawls which took place in the Palais Royal every day.

Going away we had rather an *adventure*, though not a very reputable one. I was to pass the night at my companion's quarters, at *St Denis*. Beyond the *porte* of that name we found a cab and took our seats within it. The driver delayed so long in a neighbouring wine house, that we started without him. Finding, however that there would be considerable difficulty in exploring the road in the dark, we had no better choice than to return. The fellow, after some time took his place, as yet only *grumbling*. Near the barrier another cut-throat looking rascal mounted by his side, who he said, was his brother. We jogged on till we got into the open space which stretched towards St Denis, from the foot of *Montmartre*, when our *cocher* demanded, in a tone of the most intolerable insolence, why we had dared to drive away with his carriage. We assigned our reasons; but they were by no means satisfactory. The scamp wanted a quarrel and had drunk himself up to a fight. He now stopped and began to exclaim, that he belonged to the *Garde Imperiale*, with a huge volume of nonsense to the same exploded purpose, which I cannot pretend to recollect. We desired him to forget his military character and to attend to his perambulatory business; we knew him only as a cab-man and what was of more consequence, we knew the number of his cab. He did not care a *sacre* for all that; he had been a *brave soldat* and would cry, while he had breath sufficient, '*Vive l'Empereur!*' It now became intolerable, for the *soi-disant* brother joined in the abuse. We then resolved to give them a good licking. For my own part I am but a short man, about five feet six inches with arms in proportion; but my friend measured more than six feet, with a pair of arms tremendously long and fists consistently bony. He gave the blackguards a gentle reminder in the chops (the faces of the ragamuffins being turned towards us while they continued to fill the cab with their abuse). This was returned by an attempt to brandish the whip: but French *whips* are unwieldy weapons and *Frenchmen* are not the most dexterous in the world at using them. By this act they both came within point-blank reach of our four bunches and they certainly got an undesired keepsake. We were driven then to St Denis in peace, saving and excepting a little growling and grumbling, (always allowable on the part of a defeated foe) and were rewarded for our valour, by evading the payment of our fare. Just as we left the cab, a piquet of the town guard lighted by flambeaux, passed by and we hailed them with information that this cabriolet-man had been behaving in the most insolent manner and was a *Bonapartist* into the bargain. The latter circumstance might perhaps, have been better suppressed, for the fellow was excited by wine and probably felt an attachment for his old master, which it was ungenerous, if not impossible to eradicate. The guard would have captured him *sur le champ* [on the field], had he not shewn a very commendable dexterity in driving away, laughing at them but still shouting '*Vive l'Empereur!*' We did not give his number, which the *Garde National* was desirous to obtain; but going to Paris next day, we met him driving his cab with a very enlarged nose and a pair of black eyes, worthy of Tom Cribb[25] himself.[26] I had known at the moment that my friend's fists had not been wielded in vain; for the sound was *proof* and the falling of the ex-Imperial Guardsman upon the back of his horse amounted to *conviction*.

My trip on this occasion was anything but satisfactory. To have enjoyed Paris, I ought to have lived in it; but the gentleman whose guest I was, resided two or three leagues off. I saw Louis XVIII once more on the day of opening the Chambers and I saw what was a far more interesting sight, about ten thousand *citizens* (National Guards) attending him. The equipment of these men, all at their own expense, rather astonished me. I had never *played* at soldiers myself; and had always, from the time I held a commission, been employed in the *serious* business of medico-military life, so far as a medical officer can be supposed to be: but I must acknowledge that the aspect of the *army* which marched over the *Pont des Tuilleries* surprised me. I am confident that they would have met the same number of regular troops, upon almost equal terms.

Bonaparte, it is unquestionable, had made the French (I am not called upon to say by what means) a *military nation*. Even the disbanded and unprovided for officers of his army, those who were not obnoxious to the Bourbons and who were permitted to retire to their homes, but who had every reason to find fault with the turn that affairs had taken, as regarded their own fortunes at least, wore out their uniforms, with an

---

25. Tom Cribb was a world champion English bareknuckle boxer.
26. Note by Smith – Whether I had killed *the brother* or not, I never heard; but I visited *la Morgue* for several days, without seeing his corpse.

affectionate regard to pride and economy, which Englishmen would hardly understand.

It is a matter of astonishment to every continental foreigner who visits London, that he sees few if any *soldiers*. 'Where are your troops?' is the common query. 'How can you keep order, preserve public property, or exhibit a procession without soldiers?' Upon my word I do not know what reply should be made. Soldiers, in time of peace, are the prettiest of all toys and the best adapted of all ornaments for the purposes alluded to, but John Bull would not stand them. He likes a watchman, or a constable in a blue coat and yellow buttons, with whom he can have a tussle for his incarceration, though incarceration is the inevitable result of his misdeeds, notwithstanding the *civil* character of the police. At length the thing has been viewed in a proper light, sure I am that it must have long been felt to be an absurdity. We have now, in a part of this enormously populated metropolis, a force well organised, and well adapted to the exigencies of the inhabitants; but these will not yet believe it, because they hear of *sergeants* &c a vague term, which in the *army*, applies to a very humble, but in the *law* to very exalted rank.

I ought in strict order, to have observed that a troop of the regiment had been sent from F[orge]s to a pleasant and retired village, about a league from headquarters,[27] to which I was to repair on my return from Paris, at the end of ten days.[28] I had heard much in praise of my new station, where I reckoned upon being snug all the winter; but the sequel will shew that he only is blessed *who expecteth nothing*. My new landlord had been over to F[orges] to call upon me and learning that I bore a fair character, both *en garcon* and *en medecin*, sketched out such plans of rural felicity, that Paris had no charms for me and I would on no account apply for a prolongation of leave. Aware of the comfortable quarters to which I was to return, I invited my friend with whom I was staying at Dugny,[29] to spend a few weeks with me in *Argueil*, (such being the name of my future station.) He agreed to visit *Argyll* [Argueil] as soon as arrangements could be mutually made and as a pledge of sincerity, allowed me to carry off one of his sons, whom at a stated time, he was to come and redeem. The redemption

---

27. Argueil.
28. Note by Smith – These and three days which I had spent at Brussels, before we took the field, form the sum total of my absence from the regiment during four entire years.
29. Near Le Bourguet in northern Paris.

however did not take place till nearly six months afterwards, owing to circumstances over which neither father nor protector had any control; and during the whole of this period, I was *acting papa*. The circumstance (and I speak it to the credit of the rugged ears of soldiers and the suspected inclination of their wives) gave me great importance in all eyes. Little *James* was a universal favourite with both French and English, sensible beyond conception, even at his then tender age;[30] nor had I any difficulty either in finding proper persons to take care of him when from home, or conveyance for him on a march. Everyone who sported a *wheel*, became a candidate for him as a passenger; but as the quartermaster-sergeant's wife and daughter were upon the whole the most eligible, I uniformly handed him over to their charge, when obliged to mount for a march. The chap quickly learnt to speak French like a book;[31] and among other incredible things related of Chiswick, Jem [James] afterwards told his father, that C[hiswick] had taught him to say his prayers![32]

My little companion travelled cheerfully by the diligence as far as Gisors, the delight of the coachman, for (for we sat in the front) and that place we reached in a regular manner. Clumsy as are to the present day the Norman coaches, ponderous as are the loads they carry and numerous the passengers, (amounting to twenty or thirty here and there) they got along at a great rate. Upon this occasion we were dragged by four punchy roans which trotted and galloped along the chaussee to my astonishment. The driver *sat on the left* of his passengers which is the usage in France,[33]

---

30. Note by Smith – He was barely nine, and yet he learnt all the movements of the chessboard, merely by looking on while J B [James Castley] and I were doing as well as we could to play.
31. Note by Smith – Many of the soldiers' children, born in France, or brought up there during several years of their infancy, could speak no *lingo* but the *patois* they learnt among their native playfellows and associates. The *mother tongue* went for nothing whatever. Some of them on coming home, did not know a word of English.
32. Note by Smith – I should be paying J[ames]'s mother a sorry compliment; did I suppose that C[hiswick] was his original instructor in these important matters: probably C[hiswick] taught him some *new* prayers, or made a point of hearing him repeat his orisons with more regularity than it was in my own power to have attended to.
33. Note by Smith – In France they do everything in a manner diametrically opposite to English usage; perhaps I may quote a few examples without impertinence. A French horseman, or charioteer, always passes another on the *right* side of the road: a Frenchman rides with stirrup leathers so long that his toes only and they scarcely, can touch the stirrup: he is never to be seen with a snaffle, always with a severe *bit* in his horse's mouth (in fact, I believe the snaffle is altogether an invention of *English* judgement and mercy: *mouths* go for nothing elsewhere, power only being consulted.

with the reins hooked under the breastwork, or flap of the cabriolet, only taking them in his hand when the animals flagged and wanted a little rousing and then merely for the purpose of shaking their mouths, and *blowing them up* with his own. At *Pontoise* we were accommodated with a postilion, who rode the near wheeler; and the coachman from that moment had nothing to do but chat with his companions.[34] I found him

---

French horse cutlery is commonly rusty, if iron (we say nothing of steel) but those who are particular as to *propriete* use *plated* things of this nature, which are easily cleaned. There is commonly some abominable and useless appendage to the saddle, in the shape of a *shabrac* [shabraque] (generally shabby to a laughable degree), a tremendous imitation of an Arabian headstall, only loading the unfortunate animal and helping to sweat and swelter him. The first thing done to a horse when bought out for a journey, is to give him as much water as he will swallow; he thus has the advantage of appearing *round in the barrel*, as we would say. When mounted, he is ridden at a moderate pace along the road but pushed as hard as he can go when passing through a town. The Frenchman rides to attract notice to himself, never to shew his horse to advantage and where there is no one to admire, he flags. The pace is an amble, a scrambling motion, unknown to English horses or riders. Trotting, galloping, nay even *walking*, they consequently cannot endure. Many a cast trooper, which knew no paces but these three, on being purchased by *Messieurs*, was broken in or rather broken *down*, to this execrable, though easy method of progression, easy to the rider perhaps, but wearing and tearing for the animal. And so, in numerous other things, the nations differ. In horsemanship I give it decidedly *against* them; how it may be in the following matters, I shall not judge, *chacun a non gout* [no one has taste]. The French are in many things, sensible, shrewd and reasonable, where I have thought my own countrymen inconsistent and absurd. They eat their eggs for instance without a spoon; their spoons and forks are all curled in the opposite direction to ours; their windows open like folding doors, while ours *used* to slide up and down; the last dish at a French table is fish; the ladies never leave the gentlemen; they call certain things, for which we have no terms in polite English, by their vulgar, if we must not say their *proper* names; and certain operations which in England are concealed with as much care as if one were committing a disgraceful and voluntary act, are matters of notoriety to all the members of the family at least, if not to all their acquaintances. The physician called into see a sick *demoiselle*, has no occasion to beat about the bush with mothers and aunts and nurses; whatever be the complaint, the *brother*, or the *man servant* will inform him with the utmost alacrity and overdone eagerness, as to the actual or recent state of the case.

34. Note by Smith – On a subsequent visit to France, I travelled by the diligence to Rouen, in company with my sister, and a North American physician, who seemed to be almost heart-broken at quitting the country in which he had been educated. We occupied the *coupe* and no gentleman's carriage could be more easy. But what will the *Jehus* [reckless coachmen] of England say, when I assure them, *upon my honour as an officer and a gentleman*, that the postilion (for we had no *cocher* [coachman]) who sat on the near wheeler, as already described, drove seven in hand!! My Lord Mayor, and even the King's body coachman for state occasions, may not credit me, but it is fact: and he performed it in form and manner following: – *Three wheelers abreast*, himself mounted on the near one, dressed in a white cotton night-cap and sky-blue smock frock; then two leaders (3+2=5), two *attaches* on the offside, with strings instead of reins, which he also

(as for my own part I have always found such people) civil and obliging. Intelligence I do not look for in such a station, but even with that I not unfrequently meet, the more readily perhaps because I abstain from topics of conversation, or matters of inquiry beyond their scope or province.

From *Gisors* we obtained some conveyance or other to *Gournay* [en-Bray]; and there, to my utter perplexity, I learned that the regiment was on the move. I had resolved to stop all night at this town; but the report which now reached me was under present circumstances, perfectly alarming. Had I been alone I could have disregarded inconvenience, hired a guide for a franc or two and stumped off to *Argyll* [Argueil]: but charged with the care of a friend's right eye, there could be no proceeding in any such manner; and of course, either leaving him behind or losing sight of him was out of the question; and the travelling resources of Gournay [en-Bray] were exceedingly limited.

I was short too of money, a campaign however brief in Paris, is of all others the best adapted to lighten burdens of this nature and mine I confess, had not been very heavy. At length I found an honest fellow who accommodated me with a chaise, pair of horses and driver, to convey us to Argueil, careless about hire or anything else. The post-master took my *promise to pay* and the postilion was profuse in his gratitude when presented with a five-franc piece.

Late in the evening, jolted to death over a miserable cart road and uncertain of our fate, we reached the highland territory and I had every reason to deplore the change of that was about to take place. The kindness of my host and family was beyond description; and I believe they honestly regretted the measure about to be carried into execution. The truth might be that they anticipated a grievous change

---

had in hand: these beasts might be called *on-lookers*, for as to any duty they performed, it was quite optional, a smack of the *cart whip* now and then however, put them to their mettle. Then we had two others in front of the aforesaid leaders, making nine in all!!! But these two had a special rider or postilion. This was altogether *absurd* and acknowledged to be *unnecessary*; for on reaching the barriers of Rouen, all the horses were cast off, excepting the legitimate five. Through the town, therefore, we went, with the four auxiliaries tied behind the *dil[igence]*; and as there is a very steep hill *within* the city, on the way to Dieppe, no advantage could be taken (even where it was most imperatively wanted) of our extra force. The horses still remained behind; nor was it till we had cleared the liberties and perhaps hardly required their aid, that they were appointed to their proper stations. If a reason were to be required for such an apparently preposterous regulation, I dare say the French would be ready with a *smart* one.

for the worse. The removal of our brigade was directed for the purpose of leaving the country open to a column of the Prussian army, which was on its march homewards; and what *we* had left undone in the way of insulting and tormenting the people, they promptly and efficiently supplied. But more of this *anon*.

The troop was to move from Argueil to F[orges] on the following morning. I retained the chaise [*sic*] till we reached the latter place and then handed Jem [James] over to Mrs S[idley][35] and her fair daughter. The authorities of F[orges] were standing in the streets, quite au *desespoir* [in despair] at the loss of their acquaintances and declaring that we were regarded among the people *comme les enfans du pays* [children of the country]. Tears were shed, not so copiously from the eyes of the *younger* beauties as perhaps from those of the shopkeepers, who were about to lose many good customers and receive *task-masters* and tormentors in their place. But there was no remedy. The main consolation on either side seemed to be, that the separation would only be temporary and that we should resume our old quarters as soon as the road should be cleared of the vindictive people who were about to occupy them.

The same day we reached a miserable little market town, about ten miles from Dieppe, situated upon no line of communication whatever it may be detected in a map of the department *La Seine Inferieure*, by the name of B[acqueville en Caux].[36]

B[acqueville en Caux], thou abominable hole! Siberian exile itself can hardly be worse than was the life I for one was doomed to lead, through sundry dreary weeks, within they dull and detestable limits. How cordially do I abhor they very name and how fervently do I purpose never to see thee again. Thou art the only spot upon which my tent has ever been pitched, or my tabernacle erected, which I have not so much as a *morbid* curiosity to pass through once more. I did at a subsequent period, travel within a brief league of thee; but I turned my face in the opposite direction.

B[acqueville en Caux] is more than thirty miles from F[orges] and admits of no comparison with any recognised place of human congregation. There was not a good house in it and in the middle of the *place*, or square

---

35. The Quartermaster was Richard Sidley.
36. When at Bacqueville, two troops were detached at Avremesnil.

(where by the way, there was rather a plentiful market twice a week) stood several rows of booths, constructed of *mud* and now in a state of ruin. Our friends of the Emerald Isle denominated them *Irish-town*, saying that they closely resembled the suburbs of some of the Hibernian cities. But a little scene took place on my arrival, which this may be the proper occasion to describe.

The regiment had got into B[acqueville en Caux] before me,[37] and the out-quarter troops had gone to their respective cantonments. On my arrival I found the surgeon, the vet, the Adjutant and Larry Murphy [Patrick Egan] in deep, but rather crusty consultation as far at least, as *Larry* [Patrick] was concerned: the question under consideration being his procedure to an outpost with a detachment, of which Jock L's[38] troop formed no part. I may, perhaps observe here, that when one detachment only is formed, the duty of the senior Assistant Surgeon is to accompany it; if there be two, the junior goes with another; but much depends upon the Surgeon, who in our regiment took a fancy to have me at headquarters whenever he could. Larry [Patrick] had no personal objection to obey the order for detachment duty; but Jock had run mutinous on his hands and declared (for I believe he never *swore*) that he would not go from his troop lest he should lose his *saddle*! Had Jock thought during seven years for an excuse, he could not have found one more frivolous, had he said

---

37. Note by Smith – One feature of my character will strike the reader, no doubt. I generally appear to have *followed* and seldom to have *accompanied* the regiment. The truth is (since I must now reveal it) that, in quiet and peaceable times, I preferred setting out an hour or two after the troops, for the following reasons. (Murphy [Egan] had others; but the annexed are mine). I rose as early as the trumpeters, commonly took an hour or two of writing, looked out of the window, or went to the spot to see the starting. The commanding officer indulged my fancies, because he knew I should not be later in arriving at quarters than those who set out earlier. I liked to ride smart, it is better for an *officer's* horse than walking; and what was equivalent to all other reasons, Joe B [James Castley] (also one of the privileged), was my constant companion. Larry [Patrick], when present, generally rode *before* the squadrons, although the regulations of the service enjoin the surgeon to be a *follower*. For a fancy of this kind, he was once brought to a General Court Martial: had he been in the rear (to administer assistance to weary and sick men), this would not have happened to him; but the affair took place before he employed the *rapariga* to carry his *portmantle* to his new station.
The band
Among the performers were three blacks, one of whom was consumptive and died in the hospital, which at the time, was established in the house occupied by the *Soeurs de la Charite*.
38. As the Returns for the regiment for 1815 are not extant, it is impossible to identify his servant.

that he would not go to an out-quarter lest the ants should eat him, it would have been equally to the point. While the difficulty in question was under discussion, I espied Jock standing aloof and made a signal for him to come behind one of the booths. I asked him how he could be so ridiculous as to refuse to go with Mr Murphy [Egan] to an excellent out-quarter, where both he and his master had every chance of living in clover? I represented, that by compelling *me* to go, he would be inflicting a real punishment and I could *put a spoke in his wheel* for doing it, that he would in the country have his master all to himself and could do with him as he liked, whereas at headquarters, he would be watched by everybody in general and the Adjutant in particular, who was no friend to him. These and other arguments, not necessary to be recapitulated, wrought upon Jock and he relented.

I then returned to the group already described and after listening in silence to a variety of considerations pressed upon Murphy [Egan] in vain, without saying that I had talked Jock over, I agreed to a proposal made by Joe [James], which was that in his opinion, the *uglier* of the two ought to go out. 'Done!' said I, 'done, Larry [Patrick] & I will toss up which *is* the ugly one.' Larry [Egan] who would not risk the interposition of providence upon an occasion so important, turned away and went off to the house of a ruined nobleman, whose land steward had become the proprietor of the *seignieurial* mansion and estates during the *assignat* system; and the Comte de [Martel] lodged Murphy [Egan] in a humble though neat cottage, adjacent to the chateau, now inhabited by the rascal in question.[39]

This affair being settled to general satisfaction, I turned my attention to my future abode and found it unpromising enough. The very name of the lady (for I was to be quartered in the house of a widow) sounded ominous: *Madame Boue* [mud]! a dirty prospect! Mrs or rather *Mother Mud*. One small back room, stinking, and hardly habitable, on account of filth and vermin and Mrs. Mud, the greatest woman (in her own opinion)

---

39. Note by Smith – There were many incidents of this nature which came to our knowledge; but there were others which it is gratifying to allude to. Sometimes it is true, an unprincipled servant took advantage of the general convulsion to seize his employer's property; but in other cases, the property was saved by means of the honesty and dexterity of dependents. Where they could not remit proceeds to their exiled masters, they held possession, under an affected adherence to the new system; and when the Peace of Amiens and even that of 1814 were brought about, they faithfully accounted for their stewardship and made a nominal *re-sale*.

throughout the town and neighbourhood. She kept a cloth shop and not only a shop in the house, but a stall in the square. Notwithstanding this, which in our *boutiquier* country, would be looked upon as an invincible barrier to celebrity, she was a great personage. Mother Mud had been at vast pains to denounce all the adherents to the recently exploded system, of whom she had either knowledge or suspicion and was consequently detested as a firebrand among her neighbours.

The most distinguished of these had been the talented Felix Lepeletier,[40] whose estate was in the immediate vicinity of B[acqueville en Caux]. The old jade had taken all the pains in her power to bring ruin upon the mistaken partisan, (whose political bias I have not the least inclination to defend) while perhaps her *duty* would have been to lie *perdue* at least. The government was active enough and Lepeletier was among those who felt its *minor* vengeance as a *deporte*. While we remained in B[acqueville en Caux], Lepeletier was sold up and as I believe, he had been of the Egyptian expedition,[41] there were a few Arabian horses (now to be sure rather aged) to be knocked down with the rest of the stock. In this overthrow, Mother Mud absolutely exulted and exhorted me by all means to purchase one of the Arabians (for they would go for next to nothing) and she should be most happy to send an agent to the sale and even to pay the money for me, I declined and she wondered.

We were now in the very heart of *Pays de Caux*, celebrated by the Reverend T[homas] F[rognall] Dibdin, on account of the stupendous, tremendous, awful and incomprehensible head-dresses worn by the women.[42] Whoever will take the trouble to look into his 'Bibliographical

---

40. Despite fighting for the king during the early days of the Revolution, Lepeletier remained in Paris with his brother Louis-Michel until his murder in 1793 (the first 'martyr' to enter the Pantheon). He then joined the Jacobin Club and entered politics and financed a number of newspapers. When Napoleon took power he was one of the Jacobins deported to Cayenne, but returned to France in 1803. He took advantage of an amnesty offered on Napoleon's coronation in 1804 but refused the proffered Legion of Honour. Ordered to remove himself further away than Versailles, he was to reside at Bacqueville-en-Caux where he became mayor and president of the canton. Lepeletier refused the oath of loyalty to King Louis XVIII in 1814 and rallied to Napoleon's cause in 1815. On the return of Louis he was arrested and gaoled. He remained in exile in Belgium for three years but then returned to France and supported Louis Philippe's reign initially before returning to his republican roots.
41. I cannot find any evidence that Lepeletier went on the Egyptian Expedition.
42. This refers to Dibdin's *Bibliographical, Antiquarian and Picturesque Tour in France and Germany published in 1821.*

Tour' &c will see the effigies of a *fille de chamber* at Dieppe and I can bear testimony to the fidelity of the representation. Every Sunday, Mother Mud dressed herself in this *absurdity* and came stalking into our apartment, with the coffee, more like a turkey (for I will not degrade the beautiful Argus [a large tailed pheasant native to SE Asia] by such a comparison) than a rational being. 'Look at my cap, Messieurs; behold (*voila*) the streamers of fine lawn, down to my very *fesses* [buttocks] and the *sommet* [peak] of my headdress, so high that I was obliged to stoop to get in at the door. Do you not admire me? There are now only two of us in this town, who preserve the costume du pays, Madamoiselle Mabille is one and *moi, je suis l'autre, regardexz bien, je marche tout a mon aise*. [me, I am the other, take a good look, I am comfortable walking]'.

I shall only observe, that the aforesaid Mabille was the acknowledged *belle* of the neighbourhood, that she was *very* handsome, perhaps *affected*, said by the old Muddy woman to have been too intimate with Lepeletier, who was now the demon, as formerly he had been the *deity* of the neighbourhood, but I never believed a single word of Madame Boue's scandal.

The ugly harridan had one redeeming quality: she made excellent coffee and taught John Chiswick to do the same;[43] but it happened, almost every Sunday, when we uniformly had the pleasure of Mrs Boue's company, to bring in the coffee, that she wanted to introduce some of her Protestant friends.

Considerable numbers of these were in the neighbourhood; and they were Napoleonists to a man: indeed they had every reason to be so, but it would have been prudent not to have brought them into our society. Madame Mud did not take these things into consideration; and at last did thrust one of her friends upon us, *as a Protestant*. We received the fellow as well as we could (one Sunday evening), and pressed him to drink with us. We proposed a toast; he filled; 'Louis XVIII' said we, 'and Bonaparte' added he. We turned him out as a matter of course, for his impertinence, though neither he nor myself cared a pinch of snuff about

---

43. Note by Smith – Madame Boue's method of making coffee was distinguished (as Chiswick told me) by the introduction of a little flannel bag, containing the powder, into the boiling water; which bag she never entirely emptied; rejecting part only of its contents and retaining a certain portion of what had already been boiled, when new coffee was introduced.

king or emperor. Madame Mud was terribly mortified at the ill success of her kind offices, in bringing men of the same religion together. I doubt not she went away saying to *herself*, as Paul Pry[44] does to the audience, that she would never do another kind action.

Near B[acqueville en Caux] there were some old families, still possessed of their hereditary property, and well entitled to shew themselves in their appropriate elegance and superiority. Ladies, handsome and accomplished, elderly and young, but all *amiable* and many of them lovely, no longer secluded themselves from the gaze of military eyes; for those to which they were now exposed were not the glances of libertines of low derivation. Our officers found a ready welcome, wherever they sought acquaintance.

An accidental circumstance introduced me to the interior of *one* of these families, which, as being rather of a *military* nature, it may be more appropriate to quote than might be pardonable with respect to others. One of our non-commissioned officers, on a *relay* party, contrived either through drunkenness or carelessness, the former being the more probable cause, to be attacked and disfigured, if not wounded, on Louis the Eighteenth's highway. His case excited attention and he was conveyed to the nearest chateau, belonging to a gentleman, a *noble*, (as the case might be), where 'oil and wine' were not wanting for his consolation. He was not much respected in the regiment: nevertheless, on the following day an elegant young gentleman rode into B[acqueville en Caux], and applied to the commanding officer for assistance on behalf of this man, who was then lying grievously wounded, in his father's house. The Adjutant and I rode off with the youth; and were quite surprised at finding Corporal P[enniston][45] lying in state, *not* (for it would be an ungentlemanly reflection on the tact and taste of the family to represent it otherwise) in one of the best bedrooms of the house, but in the very best servants' room. We examined and cross-examined him, puzzled and perplexed him, as to the cause of his injuries; but we could get nothing satisfactory out of him. Wounds or bruises he certainly had: and I did the best I could to dress them. They were even so severe that I did not like removing him that day. We proposed therefore to bring the hospital waggon over on

---

44. The play *Paul Pry*, a farce in three acts by John Poole, was premiered in 1825.
45. Probably Corporal John Penniston, as he was the only corporal with this initial.

the following: and this proposal on our part was succeeded on theirs by a cordial invitation to dine at the chateau upon the occasion. In this family I observed, what has been a subject of frequent notice in France, that the children were few in number. In many others we had seen the same thing, a *son* and a *daughter* composing the whole; and the deviations (whatever may be the cause) from this were apparently exceptions to the general fact. One of the dishes at this dinner consisted of *red herrings*; and one of the liqueurs, introduced after coffee, was *rum*. Horseradish (to eaters of roast-beef so essential a necessary) we were long indeed in finding. It was never to be obtained from the *marchands de legumes* [vegetable vendors]; and we were on the point of giving up the *ros–bif* in despair, when someone (J B [James Castley] I believe) immortalised himself by the discovery, that horseradish was cultivated by the apothecaries and to be had from them only.

While upon *culinaries*, I shall give some account of a *bifteck* [beef steak] with which I was treated at a gentleman's house (not in Normandy however) and which was not professed to be 'a la [Fiorentina[46]]' I had received sundry hints to keep a corner for the national dish; and less of course I could not do. I took very little *bouillon* and no *bouilli* at all, expecting my own little ration and confident as to its pre-eminent elegance. I was still very hungry when it did arrive: but then, what was it? A *bifteck* literally not worth a d[amn]! A slice of the *bouilli*, of the beef previously boiled senseless in the soup, cut thin, and dried up in the frying-pan! This, O members of the *Lyceum* Club,[47] was a beefsteak, *a la*, I shall not say what!

Cautions had reached us, that we were not quite safe among our Norman neighbours; and orders had been issued never to part with our arms, night or day. About four o'clock one morning an alarm was raised of 'fire' which I dare say, every man construed into the signal for an attack upon his throat and brain-box. I remember, all prill [tipsy] as I was, jumping up, buckling on my sabre and sallying to the door with immense precaution. It was however, a real fire at the auberge; and our dragoons shewed a dexterity in extinguishing it and thereby saving the whole town, paralleled only by the crew of Admiral Anson, upon a similar occasion

---

46. A traditional steak of veal or heifer char-grilled.
47. The Lyceum Club in the 1820s was a 'beefsteak' club, it should not be confused with the Lyceum Club founded in 1904.

at Canton.⁴⁸ Every one of our fellows, however, turned out with his sabre and carbine.

About this time, I was ordered to the little Norman town of *Neufchatel* [en-Bray], where a board of medical men was to examine the claims of wounded officers, who applied for the *year's pay*. The reader may consider it impertinent perhaps, to introduce the word *Norman*; but I lost a letter directed to me at the same place, upon a subsequent occasion, in consequence of its travelling into Switzerland. It found me at last with the following note upon it, written by the postmaster of *Neufchatel* [Neuchatel, Switzerland]: – '*Pas pour las Suisse; voir Seine Inferieure.*' [Not for Switzerland, see Seine Inferior]. Nor did I get it till long after the event had taken place about which its purport was to instruct me.

The 'year's pay' was an act of liberality, characteristic of our present most gracious and benevolent Sovereign's reign, though he as yet bore the title of Prince Regent. The pensions, on a scale of munificence utterly unprecedented (and so extensive that government considered it impossible to continue them upon their original footing)⁴⁹ were altogether distinct. The year's pay was granted for the purpose of covering the expenses of an officer during his cure. Now on active service, there can be no expense, though there may be suffering an inconvenience; consequently the thing was a royal gift. It had been first announced in 1814. I sat upon several boards at Lisbon and in no instance was our recommendation disregarded. The officer presenting himself might be perfectly well at the time; or his injury had in several instances, been so trifling as to have almost escaped his own recollection. All that we required was a voucher from some medical officer, that the gentleman had been seen wounded at, or soon after, the time at which he received it and then we certified accordingly, 'recommending him the year's pay granted for the cure of wounds.'

---

48. During Admiral Anson's circumnavigation, they arrived at Canton in 1743. Whilst here, the crew helped to extinguish a fire which threatened the city.
49. Note by Smith – Pensions for the loss of limbs, or for wounds equivalent to such privations, were at first to be augmented, upon a scale of such a nature that, if the officer rose in rank, his pension was augmented accordingly. Subsequently, the pension was fixed for life at the sum to which the officer happened to be entitled when he sustained the injury; thus if he lost an arm or an eye, as a subaltern and subsequently rose to the rank of colonel, the pension remained at the degree of its original grant. It was a jocular observation in the army, that the way to make a fortune was, to lose *one eye*, both legs and an arm, equivalent for a lieutenant to nearly £300 a year, besides half-pay &c &c.

The officers who presented themselves on this occasion were all cavalrymen and chiefly belonging to the German Legion. They dined together and were polite enough to invite us (three in number); but for reasons not requisite to specify, we preferred to dine by ourselves.

We had left one of our officer's sick, upon our removal from *Cheltenham* [Forges-les-Eaux] and being now within eight miles of him, I resolved to beat up his quarters, my messmate Joe B [James Castley] having promised to take a day there also and ride home with me. A most uproarious visit this turned out. Our sick friend [Otway], of whom I have already had occasion to make mention, was not the most tranquil character; he was rich and to the last degree hospitable. Two such blades coming to enliven his solitude, would have been quite enough, had there been no more of it; but we found him with a rattling scamp of Oxford or Cambridge, who was up to every sort of mischief; and the night before Joe [James] and I took leave, the fellow played a trick upon me, which might in a country where the police was so well regulated, have cost him dear, had it been detected.

Dieppe is (among other parallel circumstances) comparable to our Brighton, because it is the nearest point to the metropolis upon the coast, in the most respects it is far superior, as regards natural situation. There is neither a palace, nor a place like the Steyne;[50] but there is a venerable old castle, and the neighbourhood is classical, for near it Henri IV performed some of his exploits.[51] There is a considerable fishery here, in which respect it also takes precedence of Brighton and the supply of Paris depends chiefly on this resource. All persons versed in the history of Louis XIV are acquainted with the tragic event of a fish disappointment, as connected with *Vatel*,[52] his Majesty's maître d'hôtel, which the court was on a visit at Chantilly. Whether it arises from this or from some other circumstance, there exists a sort of sumptuary law at Paris, by which the fish-carts of Dieppe are regulated like the English mail coaches. If

---

50. The Steyne was a stony area of ground just to the west of 'Old Brighton'.
51. Note by Smith – I doubt whether it is so generally known as it ought to be, that the *Arques [la-Bataille]*, celebrated in the wars of the illustrious Henri Quatre, is close to Dieppe. There is another *Arques*, a considerable town, near St Omer and as we shall see in the matter of *Azincourt*, sometimes mistaken for the classical one.
52. François Vatel was responsible for an extravagant banquet for 2,000 people in honour of Louis XIV at the Chateau de Chantilly in 1671. According to surviving letters from witnesses, Vatel was so distraught over a late seafood delivery that he killed himself by running himself through with his sword. His corpse was discovered by a servant bringing news of the arrival of the fish delivery.

they arrive after the time prescribed, the conductor is fined heavily for every minute's delay. These carts are long, uncouth and to appearance, ill adapted for the purpose. The fish is thrown into them among straw and there are regular relays of horses; nothing interferes with their progress and the quickest method of transportation to Paris is to jump into a steamer at Brighton, into a fish cart at Dieppe and stand erect all the way by Forges, Gournay, Clermont &c to town. Seats and accommodation of every description, are quite out of the question; but there is speed.[53] The trick alluded to was simply the abstraction of a linchpin, from one of these carts, as we were going home from a game at billiards. Our Oxonian contrived to perform this feat and to transfer his plunder to my *sabretache* and I did not discover the affair till I had nearly got home next day.

I took up my abode at the house of Mephistophiles, which had been my former quarters [at Forges-les-Eaux]. His ugliness himself was at *Ruin*[54] but madame was an hospitable representative. My sick friend had his quarters in the house of the *juge de paix* [Justice of the Peace], who was one of the most pragmatical fellows I ever met with.

We heard sad accounts of Prussian insolence. For about six weeks our exasperated allies had been passing through, or in occupation of the place. The contrast between their temper, habits &c and our own, had rendered them quite intolerable to the people. The mayor having notice that a detachment of this army was expected, prepared a dinner for as many as might find their way to his house; but unfortunately, in serving the soup, the cook forgot or declined to separate the vegetables. This gave mortal offence; his worship was ordered in and the cabbage dashed in his face, with the following censure: – '*Cochon Francais, comment ose-tu server les legumes dans la soupe?*' [French pig, how dare you serve the vegetables in the soup.]

The day of our return to B[acqueville en Caux] came at last and we were to commence operations with a *dejeune a la fourchette* [breakfast with a fork], at the house of the *cidevant* maire, already spoken of. We sat down at ten and rose at two: after which the ex-magistrate, Joe [James] and myself, rode thirty-five miles at scores; in the course of which journey, I

---

53. The journey amounts to about 80 miles.
54. Note by Smith – Rouen was about twenty-five miles from our headquarters; and possessed numerous attractions. *Growler* [Otway] was (for a reason that may appear in the sequel) constantly going backwards and forwards, on his way to Paris; and invariably said, that he had either just come from, or was going to *Ruin*.

found out that I was loaded with the linchpin. A few humorous incidents occurred in the course of this ride, which probably were chargeable upon a certain quantum of prime champagne we had encargoed; but by the time Joe [James] and I reached our muddy quarters at B[acqueville en Caux], we felt an inordinate craving for dinner and discussed a proper quantity (of quality there may be little to say), as soon as the *Chiswick* department of the family could arrange for us.

Dieppe was about ten miles off and once or twice I paid it a visit. I think it (and I have been there since) rather a pleasant place. All the world knows it to be celebrated for ivory manufactures: among other articles, for chessmen. Joe B [James Castley] and myself were heartily tired of our own resources and cards offered but little variety to two people, (who by the way, could amuse themselves infinitely better); so I agreed to teach him chess, if he would buy a set of men. This my friend did and in a very short time learnt to beat me.

Living so much in the country, I ought perhaps, to have inspected the agricultural economy of the Normans. Many reasons might be assigned for my not having done so. It is a rich district; nothing is more common than the sight of two or three hundred turkeys in a stubble field; and the country is *inclosed* (an unusual thing in France) by hedges, these again studded with timber, as we are accustomed to see in England. The Normans have the reputation of being the *Yorkshire* of our friends over the water. Perhaps they are acute; but I met with no instance of roguery among them, for my own part, nor did I hear of any. It is to be borne in mind that during the time of our residence among them, there was a doubt as to the length they might venture with their armed visitors, about which our friends of Picardy and the Boulonnois might, at a future period, have less scruple. Be this as it may, I have a most favourable impression concerning the inhabitants of Normandy and hope, ere I die, to find myself among them again.

# Chapter 12

# Neufchatel-en-Bray

One frosty morning we were routed out of this abominable den, and proceeded to Neufchatel, a more civilized place, by ten thousand degrees, where for some weeks, we really enjoyed *ourselves*. This Neufchatel [-en-Bray] is the *chef lieu* [chief town] of an arrondissement, the seat of a *tribunal de la premiere instance*, famous for little cylindrical cheeses and a town of great consequence, when compared with those of which, for some time we had been occupants.

For my own part I found an asylum in the house of the judge, or president; and certainly I never was better lodged while a *militaire*; but owing to an impression that the first advances should proceed from the established parties and not from the stranger (as we are accustomed to at home), I did not reap all the advantages that were intended for me by my kind entertainers; nor was it until towards the period of our departure that I was properly instructed in the etiquette of proceeding. The first duty of a French military man, in taking possession of his *billet de logement*, is to make himself presentable; his next to render his *homage* to the master of the house; who then as a matter of course, requests his company to dinner. So it is in civil life; the stranger on his arrival in a new place of abode, calls upon all whose acquaintance he seeks and such as approve of his pretensions and desire his society, return the visit. It is quite the reverse in our country; and I give the preference to our national usage; for although to be overlooked and neglected cannot be palatable to a stranger, this is seldom if ever done without reason: and to *pay* visits which remain unreturned would be more galling still.

I owed great part of my education in these and similar matters to a lady, who had been *dame d'honneur* to the Empress Josephine.[1] She

---

1. Adelaide de la Rochefoucauld was appointed *dame d'honneur* (Mistress of the Robes) from 1804–10.

was a relation of an old deaf Baroness de Rabbit,[2] in whose house Joe B [James Castley] had his quarters and in which, he, myself, little James, and Larry [Patrick] (when we could not avoid it, or required diversion of a peculiar kind) messed. At this time, the officers were scattered about in twos and threes, living as they could and *where* they found convenience. Joe [James] and I must have led rather a hard life at this time, had it not been for the chessboard; for one or two of our friends, knowing that we could create neither disturbance nor disorder in the *baronne's* house owing to the infirmity alluded to, were fond of dropping in during the long evenings. Let it be recollected that we were now in the midst of winter and that claret and cognac were excessively cheap. Cigars we had more difficulty in finding, of the right sort; but through the assistance of our sutler, who was an accomplished smuggler, we did even at this time, contrive to obtain them.

Our accommodation in Joe's [James'] quarters was rendered the more comfortable, as there was another female relative of old Madame De Lapin resident there, who took the strangest fancy I ever met with on the part of a woman. She was assuredly *insane* and this plea can be the only one sufficient to account for her conduct. She was young, but not handsome, at the same time her manners were of the gentle and attractive description, so characteristic of French females, even in the lower ranks of life. Larry Murphy [Patrick Egan] took up the cause of Cupid; but I believe, without success. Our occasional visitor however, resorted to a method of procedure which was so absurd and ludicrous as to drive the poor girl to make certain disclosures, which were too amusing to be disregarded.

Murphy [Egan] piqued himself upon his gallantry and Gallic accomplishments, along with other qualifications, to which he had about as much pretension as to bear as to become a professor of dancing, or an elephant to chop logic. He *thought* he spoke French in purity and perfection; but it always seemed to me likely that the *Duc de Feltre*[3] had humanely sent him out of the country, on a former occasion, lest he

---

2. Note by Smith – Madame la Baronne de Lapin. Joe [James] lived in her house for many weeks and she hardly knew it. She was one of those good old souls, that acquire many kind friends towards the arrival of their last breath. The Baroness of Rabbit was very rich.
3. Henry Clarke Duc d'Feltre, Minister of War, released Patrick Egan from being a prisoner of war.

should commit himself on the score of seditious speeches. Of his person I say nothing, though of that he was vain beyond measure.

Notwithstanding sundry other advantages which nature, education and travelling *ought to have* bestowed upon the person who had been indebted to these for the perfection of character and accomplishments, Murphy [Egan] disdained to proceed by a straight-forward course to his purpose. He poked about the house till an opportunity occurred of speaking to the silly creature clandestinely. He then told her he wanted a laundress, that if she knew one, he would be obliged if she would recommend her and be the medium of intercourse. His object in making this odd proposal, was to have opportunities of slipping *billets-doux* into the bag. This sort of traffic, all I believe, upon his side, went on for some time, without our knowledge; but at length, the stupid thing who was the prize at which Larry [Patrick] aimed, quarrelled with him, laid the whole circumstances before us and handed over his *morceaux*; and choicer specimens I have seldom seen, whether their bad French, Irish blarney, fusty sentiment or barefaced impudence, or the whole together be taken into account. Upon a subsequent occasion and in another part of the country, these *billets tendres* were produced to the author's face, after he had denied the fact of having written anything of the kind.

Near N[eufchatel-en-Bray] there was a village, in which some of our regiment were quartered; the *seigneur* took his name from the place and with his son affected the society of the English officers. I dare say they cared as much about us in their hearts as they did about the Prussians; but their deportment was courteous and their behaviour even hospitable. They were staunch friends of the Bourbons; but in their immediate neighbourhood a *parvenu* had started into wealth and therefore into no small degree of consequence, by means to say the least of them questionable. He was a vulgar fellow; but having an officer in his house, he crept into an acquaintance among us and on one occasion I met our aristocratic friends at his table. We had a great quarrel about Bonaparte, our host maintaining it was not true that he had been carried to St Helena, that we (the English) had him somewhere hid, ready to be let loose upon the unfortunate French, the first time they did anything to displease us, so that by exciting another war and ruining the country, we should have a pretext to partition the territory, a measure, by the by that not a few sensible people had already laid their account with. Calais and Boulogne were to have fallen to the share of England, as a matter of course: and I rather think that the people of Calais themselves would have exhibited no very decided reluctance to the arrangement.

 Still the life we led here, owing in a considerable measure, to the dreary season of the year and our slight intercourse with the people of the place and neighbourhood, was dull to a proverb. Almost my sole amusement was furnished by Murphy [Egan] and his man Jock. Jock was by no means a bad fellow; but he was stricter in his religious *notions* than in his *practice*; and the poor man was a very inconsistent professor when *schnapps* were accessible. He was a hard-baked Presbyterian and as he and I had once entered upon a religious discussion, Jock frequently came to me, when in trouble of a conscientious cast. Upon one occasion, I met him reeling drunk in the streets, after Murphy [Egan] had been complaining that he could not find him or hear of him anywhere. 'Larry [Patrick] said I, 'Mr Murphy [Egan] is looking all over the town for you.' 'Maister Morphy [Egan]! what's he to me, I should like to know, the bigoted body! What need I go to him on a Friday? He'll no eat a bit o'my wife's cookery; but he's gaun to hae a grand denner the next Lord's Day, a crying sin and shame on the part of an officer.' It was too true about the profanation of the Sabbath: and I am sorry to confess that I was an eye-witness of the transaction. The dinner was intended to be in the French fashion; but as upon all notable occasions Larry [Patrick] made a jumble, so did he upon that in question. A priest, one of the family where he resided, was invited; and I believe the banquet had been got up in honour of him; but he did not arrive till towards the end of the business. A dish of roast beef had been removed, but they had forgotten or omitted to carry off the horseradish with it. This article accordingly remained until the priest and a pair of boiled fowls entered the apartment. The reverend gentleman spread it all about the town next day that he had dined with one of the English surgeons, but never saw such a thing at a table before as boiled fowls and horseradish. The French are not generally speaking, famous for inquiring into the real meaning of things: they see, they flatter themselves that they perfectly comprehend all and jump rashly to conclusions.

 I must not however, allow it to be supposed that our friend Jock was '*like master like man.*' Far from it, Jock L was one of the best characters in the regiment: the worst thing they could say against him was that he rather sought occasions of being 'inspired;' and the next to that was his being 'a swaddler.'[4] Now in some regiments, this latter would have passed as a very venial transgression, if one at all; but with us such were few in number. Jock, it must be confessed was but an unfavourable sample, though his professions were rather high. Being by birth a Scotchman, he had as a matter of course in his tender years, learned his bible nearly by rote and like many of his countrymen, could not divest himself of these early impressions, when placed in scenes of trial and temptation, though they served to influence his conduct. Jock was rather on the wane at the time under review and had a wife and a family, all the members of which were singularly well conducted; and he himself never failed in respect or deference to any officer, excepting to his *domestic*, Larry Murphy [Patrick Egan], who was after all, rather his tyrant by repute and appearance, than in reality; for Jock was his match at all points and kept him in wonderful good order. Murphy made a sad example of himself on one occasion, which occurred at this time. He had gone out to dine with a detached squadron and after dinner a handicap was instituted; in the course of which, his sporting cost him his best horse, the one, to wit upon which he had ridden to the place and was to have returned home. Larry [Patrick] no sooner found out the extent of his misfortune, than he began to make a poor mouth, saying he was ruined and all that. There was a celebrated horse in the regiment at that time (which afterwards, by the by, came into my own possession) called '*The Doctor*.' The fellow had been in every one of the peninsular battles, was a Waterloo *beast* and a first-rate hunter: but he had a curious trick of refusing the bit. Excepting Chiswick, I seldom met with anyone who could cleverly bridle him; and when I rode him myself, I was extremely circumspect not to let any stranger attempt to get him ready for me.[5] Upon the occasion in question, Murphy [Egan] was

---

4. An old offensive name for an Irish Protestant.
5. Note by Smith – This requires elucidation. The *Doctor* was an animal who would submit to be bridled only in one way. At one of the grand reviews, I put him up for a feed, while myself and another officer were taking *café au lait*. I desired the French ostler by no means to attempt to bridle my horse, but to let me do it myself. While my friend and I were at breakfast (after a very long ride), the cry came into the house that the Duke of Wellington was gone past. Up I started, desiring to pay the reckoning, while I went to bridle the *Doctor*. I ran to the stable and found as I had feared, that the ostler with his sky-blue smock frock and white nightcap, had already given the *Doctor* a dunch [a blow] in the teeth with the bit; this was conclusive. I scolded; and declared that all the 40,000 men round the corner of the auberge could not bridle that horse *now*. Those who are acquainted with the *gear* of a cavalry man's horse, that part of it for instance, called the

offered the *Doctor* as a gift, if he could bridle him. 'Och' says he, 'I'll do that in a twinkling.' The *Doctor* however, knew his powers too well and fought a stout battle with Larry [Patrick], which ended in the biped's defeat. Bridling was out of the question, and poor Murphy [Egan], was for the nonce [time being], reduced to his ten toes. Next morning however, they returned his nag with a caution not to be so eager to put him in danger upon a similar occasion.

While we were in these quarters, the depot troops, accompanied by the band of the regiment, joined us. Everything in the shape of man, woman or child, found its way to Neufchatel and what we might have wanted in looks was amply made up in numbers. I believe the arrangements for the stay of the army within the French territory were by this time completed; and we had scarcely got familiarised to these comfortable appendages when another removal overtook us.

Before however, desiring the reader to follow our line of march, (not by any means the least interesting of those we ourselves had tracked), I must apprise the medical profession that I got into a few consultations with the Norman faculty. Upon one particular occasion, I was both amused and provoked with their *modus medendi* [therapeutic method]. The nature of the case requires not to be told; but so it was, that all the *medici* pretended to wait for my decision. Upon seeing the patient (a young lady by the by, whose heart was more concerned in the malady than her system), I was convinced that there existed deception and strenuously advised the administration of an active remedy. The particular article of the *materia medica* [medical materials] need not be quoted; but it was one which Frenchmen are not bold enough to employ. These gentlemen however, could not refuse their consent: although they stipulated for delay, promising most faithfully that as soon as the paroxysm should be over,

---

*head-stall* will (but no others can) understand me when I relate the sequel. I called for a piece of bread; this was brought. The *Doctor* seized it greedily and while his mouth was open, I slipped the snaffle into it and hooked it to the head-stall. I had him now safe enough for all useful purposes; for his mouth was a remarkably fine one and required no bit. Still however, he was not fit *to be seen* at a grand review; and I expected to carry the regimental bridle in my hand, the horse now looking like a man without a hat, a Turk without a turban, or an old woman without a cap. While contemplating this doleful prospect, a smart English groom, who had been observing our proceedings, came to me and said, 'I know your horse's trick, Sir and will bridle him in a moment.' Hardly sooner said than done; and the *Doctor* was immediately fixed, with the heavy bosses on his nob [head], wherewith we made a fair enough appearance.

they would put my prescription in force. It was in vain that I endeavoured to impress upon their minds that the object was to cut the paroxysm short *by* the medicine. '*Bien, Monsieur, bien: on suivra vos conseils aussitot que l'occasion se passera.*' [Good sir, we will follow your advice as soon as the opportunity arises] No, no; but calomel, to the amount of four or five grains, was no more to be administered than as much corrosive sublimate. During one of these visits, I encountered the apothecary, in full military uniform,[6] blustering like Hector,[7] because the physician was rather late and had spoken disrespectfully of him in the exercise of his calling. The man of pills talked of challenging and I know not what.

Living in the house of the judge, it might be supposed that I formed some acquaintance with the jurisprudence of France: but I never more than once entered his court; and upon that occasion he was not present. The good old gentleman was on his last, I must not say *legs*, for judges in France sit, as well as those in England very much, as Sterne says 'at their ease'. However, he partook of the hospitable propensities of his neighbours and upon some occasions gave a dinner to his *bar*. Such an event occurred a day or two before our departure: and as I had presented myself by this time, a point was made of sending me an invitation, which a prior engagement I exceedingly lament to say, deprived me of the pleasure of accepting. I should have liked much, at least I should like much *now*, to have seen the *Cicero*[8] of Neufchatel in private life; but fate ordained otherwise.

Our friend Growler [Otway] has for some time been overlooked; but I must recall him to recollection. With all his pride, the man had no small share of good-nature; but was of a disposition which amounted to a puzzle. Sometimes he would be civil and obliging, but at others he would shew his teeth, in a way that many did not like. For my own part, I wished to have no dealings with him that could be avoided and I took the very earliest opportunity of drawing my pay from the regimental agents. It is not however for the purpose of venting any spleen, or quoting any old grudge (which I am doubtful about the existence of), that I recur to him now. While we were at the place called *Cheltenham* [Forges-les-Eaux], he married the beautiful daughter of a celebrated character, then residing in

---

6. Note by Smith – He belonged to the National Guard.
7. Hector, son of the Trojan king Priam appears in the *Iliad*, where he is portrayed as a good father and loving husband
8. Marcus Cicero, a Roman stateman and lawyer.

Paris;[9] and the pursuit of this scheme cost him many journeys, *via Ruin [Rouen]* , as we have said elsewhere.

He always asked for a '*Clane pleet*' [Clean plate] at table; and after a tour in Holland, he observed, that 'the Heague [Hague] was a mighty clane pleece.' He deplored the arrival of an accomplished officer as there would now be no more *pace*, Mr [Barrington] knowing his value as a subject. The style in which he replied to Joe [James] and myself, when we wished him joy of his marriage, will not bear to be written; the man who could use it must have little deserved the prize he had secured.

*Ruin a la Gr* [Rouen Grand Mare] I never visited till years afterwards, when I passed some time in France as a civilian. But for many months, we were within easy reach of it. At that time it must have been a place of considerable and even of unusual importance, for it was the *chef lieu* [chief town] of British cavalry quarters. Normandy, the *lower* I mean, for we had nothing to do with the *upper*, of which the capital is Caen, abounded with illustrations of an almost classical nature, illustrations of the most important kind, viz, the *objects* themselves spoken of in the page of history. Here and there we encountered chateaux, celebrated in the wars of Henri IV;[10] and castles or churches, or some other indications of still more ancient days, when the Normans looked upon England as their own and the English in their turn, laid claim to Normandy.

At length we marched out of this little *metropolis*, for the ostensible purpose of taking up our *alignment* in the Army of Occupation. Previous to this, an abridgement of the allied forces had taken place and 150,000 troops only were to remain, forming an arc, which was to extend from the sea on the western coast, to the Alps on the eastern boundary of the kingdom. The British were quartered near their own country; to them were joined several subsidiary corps;[11] beyond which were the Russians

---

9. Paymaster William Loftus Otway married Sibelia Barrington in 1815, the daughter of Sir Jonah Barrington, an Irish judge and politician, most noted for his amusing memoirs.
10. Note by Smith – The Chateau de Menieres was within a league of N[euchatel en Bray] and had been a place of retreat for *La belle Gabrielle*. Some of our officers were quartered there and had a little difficulty, on the day of their arrival, about dining. The maitre protested that nothing could be got ready after Mons Le Baron de M[esniere]'s dinner. 'O, then' said our friends, 'we will dine with the baron, send our compliments and say so.' 'Messieurs' was the rejoinder, 'c'est un peu trop fort' [It's a little too strong].
11. Note by Smith – There were about five thousand Danes; about the same number of Saxons, &c; which assembled at the grand reviews along with the British contingent, partly composed of the Hanoverians or Kings' German Legion.

and Prussians; the Austrian contingent forming the other wing and touching upon their territories, behind Switzerland.

Under this arrangement our immediate destination was Picardy, or rather that part of the ancient province which had for nearly a quarter of a century been designated the Department of the North. We passed through the celebrated city of Abbeville; and had occasion to halt there for three days, while arrangements were completing for our permanent accommodation. Abbeville is a town of great resources, as well as importance; but as it is by this time well enough known to British travellers, to make any allusion to its lions would be only so much impertinence. Distant as it is from the field of Waterloo,[12] the cannonade was heard distinctly upon the ramparts, owing partly no doubt, to the vibration of the connecting ground, but in a great measure to the direction of the wind.

Before we reached Abbeville, we had an amusing scene with Murphy [Egan]. At one of the intermediate halting places, Larry [Patrick] himself arrived with the troops; but *Jock* being dismounted, followed upon a baggage-waggon, among the women and *childer*. It so happened that Joe B.'s [James Castley's] horse, my own and Murphy's [Egan's], were all put into the same stable. Joe's [James'] man and mine having performed their preliminary duties, were *non inventi* [not to be found] when Jock arrived with his convoy. There was no getting into the stable, Chiswick had gone away with the key. Though Larry's [Patrick's] horse had been fed, Jock was blamed for delay. Chiswick still more so, for his insolence in locking up the stable. We knew not where to find the men at the moment, though we were perfectly aware, that at a reasonably early hour they would be with their animals, to which little or nothing could be done, beyond giving them corn, during the time the servants had been making good their quarters and getting their own dinner. Murphy's [Egan's] wrath mounted high; but for that we cared less than for the starving state of the kind beast which had carried him. Feeling for the poor animal's situation, we did our best to find the men (who were not upon this occasion quartered in the same houses with ourselves); and as we went along, Murphy [Egan] exhaled so many complaints and uttered so many threats against our people, (against my man in particular, who was always most to be depended upon in such *emergencies*), that we were obliged to take him to task, J.B. [James Castley] by saying, in his good-humoured way, that he would lay any bet Chiswick

---

12. Nearly 100 miles.

would have the best of the interview, for he would assign a sufficient reasons for having locked the stable and I by declaring that I would not be the subject of the pangs Larry [Patrick] was then enduring through his rage for a stable-full of horses. This was but adding fuel to fire and death by sentence of a court martial was the least poor Chiswick had to expect. At length we found the men and Murphy [Egan] became as calm as a cup of tea, when confronted with servants who *had lived long* with their masters. He simply demanded the key of the stable where his horse stood, (being *senior* officer) and the reply he got from Chiswick was the following, 'Oh, you want the key, do you? Here it is, I shall keep it safe enough: I fed your horse as soon as we came in and if L[arry]'s [Patrick's] is come, he must give me my corn again.' Larry [Patrick] neither obtained the key (for Chiswick knew better than to trust him with it), nor had the grace to thank him for feeding his charger. *Impotent rage* is one of the most ludicrous exhibitions that can be made to bystanders, while it must be one of the most mortifying sensations to him who is the subject of it.

Abbeville lies upon the Somme, and here we smelt peat reek. '*La Tourbe de Picardie*' [Picardy Peat] about which volumes have been written, was now to be *seen*. There are mosses on the banks of the river, which copiously supply that species of fuel. There will hereafter be occasion to mention the coal mines of France, though the staple for the chimney-corner there is wood. On the River Canche we found the little fortified town of Hesdin, a dull and miserable place, of no strength and commanded like many stronger towns which we had seen, by neighbouring heights. It might however, check the advance of an army for a few hours and thereby give time to arrange an orderly retreat. At the time of our transit we saw no troops, although it commonly contained and at a subsequent period did contain a regular garrison. It was here that I saw for the first time, men walking upon pattens [protective overshoes – often raised] and for this sensible practice we afterwards discovered valid reasons. They walk upon pattens in the north of France for the same cause that they stride upon stilts in the south, because they would otherwise sink in the mire.[13] Sometimes

---

13. Note by Smith – So deep is the soil, so bottomless the abyss of clay or mud in these parts, that there is a story current of a farmer, who, going to a christening or some other jollification, took up his wife behind the saddle. In the course of the journey, Bucephalus dipped his hind legs too low in the earth's crust; but recovering himself, after a desperate plunge, the master arrived safe at his friend's door. Welcomes were given; but these were hardly pronounced when inquiry was made concerning Madame's

on subsequent occasions, I was fain when quartered in a boggy hamlet, to go out to dine mounted on a pair of these conveniences and propped by a stout long staff. Besides this, a lantern was an indispensable article of equipage. As the government however, could not or would not mend the by-ways, the state of the lanes about the habitations of the agriculturists was in winter, such as to render them impassable, either on horse shoes or any other. Indeed, the infantry which occupied some of these communes were not unfrequently conveyed to their parades in carts. The pattens are different from those used by the females of England, being much broader in the rings and more steadfast.

At length we took up our permanent station, as we had every reason to suppose for several years, but such a station! We had our headquarters in a little bourg on the high road from Abbeville to Saint Omer,[14] in which there was but one habitation either clean, or clear of vermin. The inhabitants were little jobbers in wool and dye-stuffs and of course, *all* their hands and most of their faces were dirty. Our first impressions were the more unfavourable, on account of the state of the weather and the temper of some of the people. We came among them in a shower of sleet and we missed the cordiality which had so frequently graced our former reception. This was partly owing perhaps, to their low grade in society; but it was partly ascribable no doubt, to their unpleasant anticipations: not that they looked for ill treatment at our hands, but these quiet and insignificant *folk* had been unused to the domination of military occupiers. We had not been long among them however, till they felt the benefit of our *custom*; and some of them became very sycophantish, most of them obliging.

In the first instance I got into this town by mistake, as I was to be detached to a neighbouring village with an out-quarter squadron. Where this village lay, nobody knew; all that I could learn was, that it lay off the road from Hesdin and that I had come twice as far as would have been necessary: but I could never be far wrong if at headquarters; and as all my principal friends were there, I resolved to dry myself at Joe B's [James Castley]'s fireside; but such a side of a fire I have seldom seen. The moment the *fille* attempted to light it, volumes of *sharp-eye* smoke

---

    absence. 'My wife! What, is she not here? I saw her mount the horse, but when, where, or how she contrived to get down again, I cannot tell.' The poor woman arrived in two or three hours, begrimed to the eyes.
14. Headquarters were at Fruges.

came pouring upon us, so that nothing but a retreat was conceivable. The old dame consoled us by saying that all the houses in the town were subjected to the same curse. We asked if she had no other apartment; as lodging where she had placed my friend was impossible, at least kindling a fire was out of the question. The reply was that she had an apartment, which she had never been able to make use of for the same reason; that in fact it was worse than the other; but we might judge for ourselves. To judgement we accordingly proceeded; but our judgement was quickly satisfied, on perceiving that cataracts of smoke were pouring down the chimney, derived from the adjoining houses. This was conclusive, if not consolatory and I wished my friend joy of his prospects, go where I might I could hardly be worse off, even if *turned out*.[15]

I next day proceeded to my station and found myself in a very different sort of place,[16] though being last comer, I was worst served in point of quarters, notwithstanding my right of choosing was comparatively high. It was a rule among us, never *to turn out* after occupation.[17] The retired village in which our squadron was now deposited, possessed several charms, though the season of the year was unfavourable to their display. There were five good houses in it; but unfortunately we were six officers in number, so that one was comparatively ill off. The society of the commune was, as in all other parts of the kingdom, in a divided state. The restoration of the Bourbons was at least a temporary misfortune, for it roused feelings which had been long dormant and excited certain ideas of interest and advantage in many quarters where they had been long unknown. The royal family had been blotted out of memory and came to the throne and kingdom of their ancestors as nearly strangers as persons could be who had once been seen by any of the existing generation. In our secluded quarters, there were two or

---

15. Note by Smith – There have been more disputes perhaps, in active military life, about the insignificant matters of smoky apartments, barns, conservatories, ice-houses and pleasure grounds, chateaux and palaces, trees, banks, ditches, posts, straw, faggots, pails of water, doors, window-shutters, cow-houses, stables, pigsties, space of all sorts for blankets and oil-decks, chairs and benches, ropes and similar comforts and conveniences for a night's lodging, than about all the important operations of a campaign put together.
16. This is likely to be Ruisseauville where William Hay was also quartered (he writes Brugesville).
17. Accomodation was allocated initially, but any senior officers arriving later had the right to demand a billet, even if already occupied, turning their juniors out. Here the regiment had agreed not to 'turn out' juniors.

three red hot *Bonapartists*, but they were held in equilibrio by as many *Ultras*. There was at one time, an idea that it was better for us to be quartered on the B[onapartist]s than among the U[ltra]s and the theory may appear to be sound. It was natural to look for civility on the part of those whose tables had been overturned, while it must be confessed, that some glaring instances occurred of insolent presumption among the men 'of the ascendant.' Individually we cared little about our landlord's politics at any time; but I confess that I preferred living under an Ultra's roof: for my experience told greatly in their favour. They were upon the whole, more agreeable in their manners, less quarrelsome in their dispositions, gratified rather than mortified at recent occurrences and when *right minded*, ready to behave towards us as *friends*. They were, if not *individually* of the old school, generally influenced by its principles and polished by its courtesies. They were *the French* of whom in our youth we had *read*; whereas the *Republican Imperialists* were quite another race, new to Europe, the reputed scourge of everything which those educated in habits of order and moderation had been accustomed to respect and the terror of all that domestic life held sacred. I do not say that we found them *hyaenas in their own dens*, for perhaps there is no country in which the social and familiar duties are better performed than in France; but when dragged from the bosoms of their families and *compelled* to carry arms into foreign territories, they either forgot or disregarded all the ties of humane consideration; and something of this sort they brought from the sands of Egypt, from the sierras of the Peninsula, from the marshes of Poland and *a few*, even from the ice and snows of Russia.

It was my misfortune, as *turning out* was not encouraged in the regiment, to get into a house still in course of construction. My landlord was not only *hospitable* in his way, but had obtained no small consequence among his neighbours, from the circumstance of his house being an officer's quarter. Had we been fewer in number, a sergeant would have probably taken up his abode with him; but *the authorities* had entered his style of accommodation upon the higher list, and it was impossible, in the first instance, for us to ascertain what would have been more suitable. C\*\* was a retired agriculturist, who having realised some property, had set about building himself a mansion, in which to spend the evening of his days as quietly and his wealth, as frugally as possible; but the noise of carpenters was incessant and disturbed me very much. He did not mind it; six was his hour of rising, for he had been accustomed to labour all his life: notwithstanding this, he possessed certain aspiring ideas which were by no means to his discredit. One day he gave a dinner, I believe on my own account and gave me *carte blanche* for the rest of the officers. One came (and it was good-natured enough of him to do so) but we dined at twelve o'clock: and the dame of the establishment did not presume to sit down with her husband's guests. She served. This sort of attention ran a course among the Ultras and Royalists. I was invited to several other *grand dinners*, all at or about twelve o'clock. Nevertheless, it was an object with me to penetrate into the recesses of the *Picards*, who had a general reputation for hoarding wealth, though from their appearance, they might have been judged worth nothing. '*Ils sont apparamment en misere, mais ils ont des ecus*,' [They are apparently in misery, but they have ecus] was the universal proverb concerning them.

We were now among people distinguished for simple manners and kind dispositions. It would be wrong to say that their simplicity arose from the contracted list of their wants, for they appeared to live in considerable comfort, I might without impropriety say even in luxury. The *necessaries* of life, as the middling classes are accustomed to style them in England, were here matters of very subordinate contemplation. *Bread* was the chief object of domestic care; a pound of butcher's meat went for a long way among them; while *game* (I shall not say much of fish) and claret were seen and seen profusely in all directions. Still there were drawbacks, of which the good people themselves were insensible. A knife, even at the table of a substantial person, was never placed, although a four-pronged silver fork was upon all occasions to be found. If a knife was asked for (and it never was demanded but by an Englishman) we either were accommodated with an instrument barely capable of cutting hot butter, or (what was equally frequent) some polite guest pulled a huge clasper from his unmentionable pocket and giving the blade a few rubs upon his arm (as a barber does a razor on his strop) handed it to the stranger. This would spoil many a person's dinner. I was once at Apothecary's Hall when a gentleman was purchasing medicine; but he would not take it, because the man who had made it up had *bitten* the cork before putting it into the phial. Such a fastidious associate could not live among French people. Fortunately for the truly delicate, here the operations of cooking are not carried on in the straight-forward, honest manner of certain houses, in which the *bif* is grilled before one's eyes and makes the *chops* ready before the *steaks* are.

In private houses like those in question, there was nothing *bad*; the manners of our entertainers differed no doubt from those to which we had been accustomed: but hospitality and kindness made ample amends. For my own part, I was not rich enough to be fastidious and where there was no degradation, it became me to investigate men and manners in all ranks. The medical man is called to assist alike the poor and the wealthy, the humble and the elevated. I never had a dislike to the company of the latter, a society of which I have seen almost as much as *can* be seen; but I always considered myself rather at the command of the humbler performers on a painful scene, when there might be a choice of preference. This may account for my having mixed more among the *roturiers* [commoners] than I should have done had I been otherwise circumstanced; but their thanks and attentions were gratifying.

A vacancy having occurred, I was lodged in the house of an eminent royalist, an aged gentleman, whose family consisted of two elderly spinster daughters (one of whom took a villainous quantity of snuff) and whose hospitality knew almost no bounds. Upon one of the occasions when I had been pressed to dine with them, the priest was invited. It was not the first time I had been in his company, he was an intelligent old man, whose period of exile had been passed in Westphalia and he was a great partisan of the restored dynasty. Indeed, the clergy were so without exception; but one circumstance, not very remarkable in itself (inasmuch as it can be easily accounted for) presented a strange aspect. There were no priests to be met with, or at least but a few, who were between an advanced and a very young period of life. There seemed to have been a stagnation in the state of the clerical market for twenty years at least and so it was. The intermediates had been removed; the sufferers in the cause of royalty had been restored; and their assistants were lads, who took things gladly as they found them.

I have some knowledge of the English clergy, of the Scottish and of the Portuguese, as well as of the French. Of the first I have nothing to say, excepting that they are all learned enough; but while some are too rich, a great proportion too is scandalously poor. As to our *Caledonian* friends, there is not a man among them who neglects or dares to neglect his duty and the general provision for their support is upon so equitable and well distributed a scale, that while no one can honourably make a fortune, no one suffers privations; and as for *learning*, it is more equally distributed than in the sister kingdom. The *Portuguese* clergy were (with few exceptions) ignorant of their duties, immoral in their lives, disreputable in society and bigoted to a system which cannot last long. Of the *French* I am bound to speak in terms of very high commendation. They devote themselves to their people; are quiet and unobtrusive; always as far as I have seen, ready to encourage and join in benevolent action; not very learned, but intelligent and disposed to be careful *pastors* rather than accomplished and attractive *preachers*.[18]

Nevertheless, they hardly appeared to have a character in common with their parishioners, not being scions of the highest stock in the kingdom (resembling perhaps in this respect, the parallel state of those in Scotland). They were barely *gentry*, though still above the rank and level of the bulk of their neighbours and they were *unambitious*. Their peculiar costume at all times and in all places, distinguished them so much and so remarkably that it was dangerous to pass a *priest*, if one happened to be riding a shy-horse. The general aspect of the black, portly, clerical animal, was of itself enough to cause a start; but when with a politeness altogether peculiar to *the Sorbonne*, he took off his huge *triangular* hat, which he conceived to be the *sine qua non* of good manners, he often received a curse in return, instead of *a compliment*. Our horsemanship was put so much to the test by them, that Joe B [James Castley] and I considered the accidental sight of a priest as *malominous* [foreboding] as that of a magpie; and of this bird, unless encountered in couples, we both *affected* to entertain an enormous dread. If we lamed a horse, missed the person we went to call upon, got no lunch where we had calculated upon it, lost our way (a very common occurrence), had a bad day's shooting, or found the dinner spoilt, or any other untoward event had happened, we recalled to mind that we had either met a single priest, or seen nothing but single magpies, just as the gossips, upon finding a new-born child with a peculiar mark upon it, cast back their recollection and quote some grand event that must, through the medium of the maternal imagination, have left its indelibles upon the infant, which could have had no more

---

18. Note by Smith – Of one worthy *cure* his people used to say, *qu'il ne savait pas precher* [that he did not know how to preach]; nor did he ever make the attempt.

concern with the *fancies* of the mother, than with the *cap* or *wig* which she might have worn upon her head.

To be consistent however, I must go on with *events*, reserving general remarks for future occasions.

In this miry village was found an unoccupied house, where the mess was established. The walls were bare of every decoration excepting *whitewash*; but we had a humorous artist among us who knew all the events of Murphy's [Egan's] history; and upon these walls he was accustomed to amuse us, as well as himself, by drawing striking likenesses of our surgical hero with rods charred in the fire. He also decorated his own apartment with descriptive illustrations, to the great amusement of all who were admitted to 'a view.' One of these scenes was truly humorous. When Larry [Patrick] was proceeding to join the regiment in the peninsula, he hired a young man and his wife as servants; and having got within a day's march tolerably well (by means that need not be explained), he was thrown upon his own resources and made his first appearance as a pedestrian, his portmanteau being carried on the head of the female, the husband at the same time bearing the provender. This was admirably sketched, the principal figure being a striking resemblance of features and general aspect, as well as of peculiar manners. There were other allusions, which would not be understood, unless through the medium of a tedious and tiresome explanation.

The grand curiosity of the kind however, was a full-length portrait, on the wall of the messroom; round which were several quotations from the foul-clothes-bag, formerly mentioned. The original knew nothing of this till he found himself seated opposite to it one day when he came to dine. The quotations were more staggering than the drawing, which was by no means a caricature.

In such ways we contrived to pass long evenings at a dreary time of year and a period of existence which was particularly uninteresting. My own stay in the village was much shortened, for I was ordered to headquarters [Fruges], which at this time were established in the smoky place to which I had been introduced a few weeks previously. Being the seat of government for the canton, it was a more considerable station than the one I had left; though the inhabitants were either small shop-keepers, manufacturers of various coarse articles, or persons of a corresponding class. It had the advantage, however of being on one of the high roads to Paris, though not that most frequented and our regimental drill ground was the celebrated field of *Azincourt*! Society there was none, but what we furnished one another with and there was as little here possibly it might be said, there was even less of an amusing nature, than we had seen at B[acqueville-en-Caux], in the Pay de Caux. Still there was an interesting occupation for the curious, in surveying the scene and recalling the particulars of Henry the Fifth's great victory, since the achievement of which a period of more than four centuries had elapsed. The battle was fought upon the 25th day of October 1415; but even at this distance of time, there was great facility in forming an accurate idea of the peculiarities of the ground, to which in *some* measure the good fortune of the English was owing.

There is no position, in the military acceptation of the term; but the open space upon which the shock of the two armies took place, was covered on either flank by a wood. That into which Henry threw a body of archers, belongs not to the village or commune of *Azincourt*, but to the neighbouring one of *Tramecourt*; and we were assured that some of the identical trees were still standing. The space is very narrow and afforded facilities for a small force to present as extended a front as a large one: but to describe the battle would be to repeat an oft-told tale and one which would be inappropriate here. Perhaps it may be considered a remarkable coincidence, that a portion of another victorious English army should have been accustomed to hold their assemblies here: and still more so, that the decorations awarded on account of their victory should have been delivered on this spot. It was on the field of Azincourt that we received our Waterloo medals; but although it is hardly conceivable that this circumstance could have been entirely of an accidental nature, there was not that advantage taken of the event which would have been the case among a body of the *native* troops, similarly circumstanced. The neighbours said we filled our snuff-boxes with the soil. Perhaps we ought to have done so.

The village of Azincourt, an exceedingly mean and paltry one, possessing the common character of dirty lanes, obscure hovels and utter want of comfort, familiar to all who have visited the north of France, is situated near the high road from St Omer to Abbeville and not more than fifteen or sixteen miles from the former city.

While we were still in these quarters, a very interesting occurrence, of a domestic nature took place, which may be here described with consistency and I trust without wounding the feelings of anyone concerned. In fact, there is nothing to state but what is every way honourable to human nature; but it might not be agreeable to be too circumstantial. I shall therefore, not only avoid mentioning names, but so disguise allusions that few if any, but the parties will recognise the circumstances: these, however I shall take not liberty with, but condense them into as close a form as may be consistent with veracity and authenticity.

I have had more than one occasion to record, with sentiments of gratitude, the kindness which was intended to myself in particular, by a fine young officer who fell at Waterloo. But he was not kind to me only. During his short military career (and it was a *very* short one, for he died a cornet [John Lockhart]), he was eminently successful in winning the good will of everybody. Perhaps there had seldom been seen in a regiment so universal a favourite: the kindness of his disposition, his generous propensities, his gentlemanly deportment and his knowledge of his duty, contributed to adorn a character, which must have led to great eminence in his profession, had providence thought proper to spare his life long enough. It was however, ordained otherwise.

It had been shewn that he was the greatest benefactor the regiment had met with for some time, down to within a few minutes of his own death. He was killed in the charge;[19] and buried where he lay on the following morning, by the surviving officers, the Major [James Bridger] reading the service of the church and every eye moistened. The same melancholy respects were paid to the remains of his brother subaltern [Lieutenant Lindsey Bertie], whose corpse was found not far from that of the cornet: and two finer youths perished not (if perish be an allowable word) upon that day of carnage.

---

19. Note by Smith – Perhaps it may be considered an improper occasion to introduce a very humble, though faithful follower of the regiment to notice; but his claims have been strongly forced upon that of the writer. A dog, of no particular breed and by no means attractive in his appearance, had voluntarily enlisted at Lisbon and (as was regular) attached himself to the troop, in which the officer above-mentioned did duty. The animal accompanied the regiment through all the Peninsular campaigns and arrived with it in England. He acknowledged no particular master, but always travelled with this troop; and in Flanders, where the horses were frequently groomed in the open air, he was always on duty, keeping off the idle boys, in fact he seemed to have an instinctive dislike for the race so called. He was at his post in the early part of the 18th of June, but was seen no more after the charge. It was supposed that he had gone into the melee with the horses and had been trampled to death. [It does not appear that the dog was ever named as William Hay also mentions its death along with his own dog 'Dash' during the charge.]

In the course of the spring, while (as I have said) we were still in the neighbourhood of Azincourt, the father of the first mentioned gentleman arrived at the regiment[20] accompanied by a friend, who I believe, has published one of the most interesting accounts of the campaign of 1815.[21] The object was (now that time had fortified the paternal mind for such an undertaking, though it had not yet extinguished his grief) to obtain accurate information concerning the site of his son's grave. The commanding officer recommended to his attention another who had received a commission for his excellent general conduct and who had been present at the finding and interment of the body. They went into the Netherlands, and visited the spot. When [John Carruthers] returned, he told me that the journey had been a most interesting and affecting one. The parent felt deeply the revival of recollections that bore him back to the years of protection, years which had linked his heart with that of his son: he described him not only as the heir and hope of the family, but as his own personal friend, as one in whom he already placed deep confidence and to whom he looked for future happiness. Everything however of this nature, was now wrecked; but the manly heart of the sire, was prepared to encounter whatever affecting memorials of his loss might present themselves.

The party visited the fatal spot. The plough had been lately tracing its furrows over the last resting place of the brave defenders, whose remains now formed far too precious a manure for the soil of Belgium; but the grave of our friend still remained as his companions in arms had left it, with such alterations only as the footsteps of curiosity and the vicissitudes of a winter season, might have affected. The labours of the agriculturist had not yet reached the narrow abode of our favourite. His visitors had the satisfaction therefore, of believing that all which *natural* events had left of him was entire and that no mutilation but that of the hostile rencontre had been inflicted. The parent knelt near the bones of his beloved son, wept and gave a period to the claims of feeling, but he declined the proposal of removing the sacred deposit: 'No, we can find no grave for him so honourable! Let him remain where he is!'

---

20. Lockhart was the eldest son of William Elliott of Borthwickbrae, MP for Selkirk, who had assumed the additional surname of Lockhart on marriage.
21. This was Sir Walter Scott, a close friend of William Elliott Lockhart.

The officer who performed the duty of conductor on this melancholy occasion, gave such satisfaction, that the result was a comfortable retreat for the rest of his life. I allude to this, because I am confident the perusal of the story would be gratifying to those most intimately concerned. Our friend was desirous to retire if he could do without making too great a sacrifice. Mr [Elliott] was colonel of a corps of yeomanry;[22] the Adjutancy of which at or soon after this period, became vacant. A fitter person for the appointment could hardly have been found; and in a short time we lost our gallant comrade, who went to a distant part of the kingdom, where he is still to be found, in happiness and prosperity.

About the beginning of summer we moved from this neighbourhood to the vicinity of the coast; and soon afterwards the cavalry division was reduced to six regiments, forming three brigades, of two each and a troop of artillery. It was a fine handy little force, the attention of which was now given to the maintenance of their efficiency and the improvement of their dexterity in military exercises. During the summer, each brigade assembled for field practice within its own cantonments, an arrangement which was far from being to us the least *interesting*, or would perhaps by the reader be considered the least *amusing* part of our system: but we did not commence these assemblies with regularity, until settled in those quarters which we occupied for years; and in which some of us at least, considered ourselves at home. Our domestic economy fell into usage and received but little interruption till a short time before the breaking up of the army and their evacuation of the French territory. It will be more in order however, to sketch the progress towards these and corresponding and connected matters. So let us now leave Picardy, for the country near Boulogne, a place whose name is as familiar to English ears as that of Margate.

The distance between our old and new headquarters[23] was not more than a dozen miles; and some of our out-post communes even bordered upon one or two of those we had now removed from. I presume that, when dispersed through the new *country*, our regiment could not occupy a square surface of less than from thirty to forty miles. The brigade consisted of another, which probably [covered] not quite as great an

---

22. He was colonel of the Roxburgh Yeomanry Cavalry.
23. The regiment were ordered to Desvres and the nearby villages of Longfosse and Courset on 27 May 1816.

extent; the artillery were snugly gathered into, or close to one little town on the high road to Paris; but as we had a chaplain,[24] to whom the whole spiritual consolation of this flock was confided, I am sure, excepting in the Highlands of Scotland, there is no clergyman whose duties can lie wider than did those of my reverend friend. He contrived to preach his *parish* though about once in three weeks, when the weather was favourable; and as the hospitals required regular extra and (through the misdeeds perhaps of us of the faculty) occasional duty, I am obliged to confess that his *priestship* wrought hard enough for his rank, pay and allowances. He was and I am happy to be able to say is, a man of easy temper and one of the best *tete-a-tete* companions I ever knew. He was much liked and respected in our regiment, to the officers of which I had the pleasure of introducing him; he did his duty conscientiously, kindly and ably. The worst thing I knew of him was his *drum-head sermons*, which were *too short* to be satisfactory to one who had studied divinity in a university. But he had a redeeming practice: he shortened the tiresome liturgy, which if those who profess the intention of bringing it out of the confusion into which it was thrown (something after the manner of our corps at Canterbury) in the good days of King Edward VI do not consider necessary, I presume, for one to hope that they will at least correct its 'vain repetitions.' On the blank Sundays, that is when we could not have the chaplain to preach, prayers were read in quarters by the commanding officer.

I think we changed for the better as to headquarters, by this movement: but I am not sure that either men or horses found the chalky soil of the Boulonnois preferable to the plains of Picardy. The country was rather more interesting to the eye; but under foot there was less substance. Rye we found to be the staple product; but our vicinity to the coast and the neighbourhood of a seaport, rendered all considerations of that nature immaterial to us. When we removed into D[esvres], a place the farthest possible removed from all pretensions either to dignity or celebrity (except from its being in the route, and even on the road by which Caesar marched to embark for Britain) we found the little folk bustling about, like bees in a hive, when some suspicious object approaches. We were not the first specimen of the English army they had seen; for the year preceding, a

---

24. Note by Smith – My Peninsular and Nivelles friend had, by this time, been appointed to the brigade. This was Chaplain Robert Tunney.

division had passed through on its way to Calais. This consisted among others, of some highland regiments; and at the sight of the Scottish savages, one young woman told me she fainted away. However the Gael[25] staid long enough in the place, to impart very different feelings and to verify in his own case, the homely proverb of his country, respecting the *singed cat*.[26]

D[esvres] is not more than ten miles from Boulogne, to which we had easy access, by a well-kept road, rather hilly but in some parts pleasant enough, especially in summer; for it ran through two forests, one of which contained more than 20,000 acres of timber and the other about 10,000. Between them, or rather on the skirt of the larger, the river [La] Lianne pursues its course, forming at its embouchure, the celebrated harbour of Boulogne, celebrated less on a commercial than on a military account. It was here, while the army of Austerlitz (certainly misnamed of England) held their revels on the heights above, that Boney constructed and prepared his bateaux, or renowned, if not by some considered *fabulous* flat-bottomed boats, second only to the mysterious and *truly* fabulous rafts. They perished in their very cradle; not a splinter of one of them was to be found when we took up our abode in this neighbourhood; and the people seemed to deride the very idea of an armament finding its way to England, which dared never even venture to sea. That Napoleon at this time seriously intended the invasion of England is more than questionable; but it is also more than probable that he considered himself in a state to take advantage of a favourable opportunity of trying the experiment, or at least of creating confusion and doing mischief. None such occurred; and he marched off to Vienna. While these threats were coming from Boulogne, the English cruisers were occasionally treating it to a bombardment and throwing their cannonballs into the streets and houses. The place, no doubt enjoyed some degree of prosperity, while a force of about 200,000 was encamped above its chimnies [*sic*] and *L'Empereur* held his court within a league of its market; but this was not unmixed with alarm.

Behind our little town of D[esvres] runs a chain of hills, not of much height but of curious form. They extend from one of their extremities,

---

25. A Scottish Highlander.
26. The Old Scottish Proverb 'He's like a singed cat, better than he's likely' – meaning that he's better than he looks or seems.

which dips upon the coast between Boulogne and Etaples, by a semi-circular sweep, round the ancient *Moria*, thus cutting off one district of the Boulonnois from another, back to the sea again near Calais, forming a sort of natural boundary to a lower region which is not unfurnished with objects of interest. In this chain there is one remarkable eminence, a browsing place for sheep, the mutton of which is celebrated for its excellence and is of the same sort as that which is so much esteemed in England under the name of *Southdown*. In fact, the hill is covered with nothing but grass, thyme and other wild flowers and juniper bushes. It is a mark for sailors when approaching the port of Boulogne; and is towards the sea, a very conspicuous object. Had the invasion of our country been actually attempted, a fire was to have been made upon its summit by certain persons in the neighbourhood, who were ill affected towards the Emperor and had, through many privations, maintained their attachments to the Bourbons. This hill must be distinct from the heights on the opposite coast; for in favourable weather, the chalky cliffs of England are clearly visible to the naked eye. One gentleman, whom I forbear to point out more particularly, had been hid in a chateau under the hill for ten years; and he was in the secret of this undertaking, if not even actually engaged in it.

The forest scenery I used greatly to admire. In summer, the alleys green and velvet swards, the glancing shades, the variegated flowers, together with the nodding foliage, not to talk of feathered choristers, the hum of insects, or the sound of the woodman's axe, seduced me frequently to retirement. Here accompanied by my spaniel and furnished with a book, I used to pass many a quiet hour seldom intruded on, unless by those who trod their way to labour of one appropriate sort or other. These simple people might have wondered at the sight of an idle gentleman in such a situation; but by way of a blind, or for the satisfaction of curiosity, I commonly carried my gun, though not always powder and shot. In winter we had tolerable amusement after woodcocks and snipes in the marshy bottoms; but in summer rabbits were all we could expect to meet with. The neighbourhood abounds singularly in the first mentioned article and the forests formed one of their favourite tracks in their transitory flights, for thousands were netted every winter.

Shortly after our settlement in our new and I may say, our final quarters, Lord Combermere,[27] the commander of the cavalry, turned out a captain of our regiment, in order to establish himself in the chateau, which had been the imperial residence during the theory of invading England.[28] There appeared to me to be better looking houses in the neighbourhood; but probably the internal accommodation was unrivalled; and while it was near Boulogne, it had also the advantage of lying by the side of the great road. After his lordship's departure for Barbados, Sir H[enry] Fane[29] took up his abode in the same house. These were noble uses to which to put the habitation of a usurper who crowned himself; but there was rather a reverse of fortune in this instance as well as in that of Renaix.

The term *reverse of fortune*, calls to my recollection many instances of an illustrative nature, which occurred among the people we were lodged with. In one place a butcher's shop was kept by a man who, in the Imperial army had commanded a squadron. I have seen one of the same rank conducting a dung cart: he farmed a few acres and dressed himself, *a la militaire* on Sunday (as long only, I suppose as the uniform lasted) and was vain of his sabre, which hung throughout the week upon the kitchen wall. Him have I seen in a blue smock-frock and nightcap, which had once been white, driving his team a-field, full many a time.

The character of the French, for gaiety of manner, if not genuine resignation amid reverses of fortune, was exemplified upon a very large scale, under the eye of every nation in Europe; but more particularly that of our own, in the instance of the royal partisans, who followed the exiled court. It is but due to the adherents of the dynasty of usurpation (if *dynasty* it be not absurd to style it), to give them credit for corresponding equanimity, that is generally speaking. Among the *emigres*, there were probably few who had not been torn from possessions which had been long in their families; and there were probably not many who had expectations of future elevation disappointed. To *keep and maintain* were the ideas with which these had been born and educated: whereas the *military* men of Bonaparte were, for the most part soldiers of fortune and *rising* at the

---

27. Lieutenant General Stapleton Cotton, 1st Viscount Combermere, took command of the cavalry after the Earl of Uxbridge was severely wounded at Waterloo.
28. This was the Chateau d'Pont de Briques at Saint Leonard, Napoleon's headquarters from 1803–05.
29. Major General Henry Fane.

time to what the others had fallen from, to what they had not the least experience of; and consequently, it might be a fair inference, that their chagrin at losing would be less acute at first and sooner blunted. Few also had to leave their homes in consequence of political conduct: the amnesty being wide and their claim to a considerable extent acknowledged. The facts just quoted of 'beating their swords into plough-shares,' and their spears into slaughter-knives for sheep and oxen, may serve to shew that they had resources at *hand*, to which the *pauvre ancienne noblesse* could not resort, at least in their circumstances and probably would not have resorted to, under others of a more promising nature. I remember the wife of a banker, who for many years had been pointed at in the place as a *noblewoman*, who had done the most extraordinary thing arising out of the revolution, in sharing the loaf of the bread-maker.

As from this time there was little change in the locality of our position and still less in the features of the life we led down to the period of our return to England, a more particular account of our situation and mode of procedure may not be unacceptable. For my own part I was two years in the little town of Desvres, in the course of which, chiefly from my professional pursuits and the ready exercise of my office among the poorer people, I obtained considerable knowledge of their character and became tolerably acquainted with their private history. This I am sure of, that a great deal of news (alias gossip) was brought to me, which the other gentlemen could not well learn. I had a great ally in the town surgeon, but a still greater in the priest, a character of whom I can never think but with the highest veneration. He was aged, but tall, upright and polished as highly in his manners, as we should expect to be the case with a perfect French gentleman of the older school; but, what was better, I knew him to be benevolent and liberal:[30] and I never doubted that in his religious

---

30. Note by Smith – One instance of this, as occurring in Catholic clergymen, I beg to relate. An officer (whose wife was a native of the place, and therefore one of this gentleman's flock) had a child to baptise, and our own chaplain [Tunney], being on the spot for another purpose, the two priests met. The *cure* was asked by the mother to perform the ceremony; but believing the form of the English church to be substantially the same as that of his own, he merely requested to know if it was so; and upon being assured that the infant would be baptised in the name, &c, he said, 'it is equally valid and I cannot think of interfering with my English brother's duty unnecessarily,' politely taking leave. He would have staid to see the ceremony, but he alleged as a reason, the fear of giving umbrage to ignorant persons, whom it was his care not to offend where he could help it. Had this man been a bishop, I am sure he would have been one of the Fenelon sort.

profession he was sincere. All our dead were interred in the churchyard[31] and our own chaplain read the protestant funeral service there, as would be done in any English burying-ground.

The mode of quartering the regiment, under the circumstances now alluded to, was the following; and the description given of our own state and condition, may be applicable to the majority of this extraordinary army. The Army of Occupation formed, as has been related, a cordon extending from the sea coast to the borders of Switzerland; and it may not be impertinent at this distance of time, to refresh our recollection by remarking that it consisted of four great contingents of English, Prussians, Russians, and Austrians, amounting at first to one hundred and fifty thousand and afterwards diminished to a hundred and twenty thousand, in the whole. The English contingent was on the right of this cordon (supposing the front to be towards Paris), the Austrians, I believe upon the left. A certain number of fortified places was given up to the allies; among those which fell to our share, were Cambrai, Valenciennes and Bouchain, the headquarters of the Duke of Wellington being established in the first-named city. In these *enviable* situations, the troops (consisting of course of infantry) did regular garrison duty and in point of economy found perhaps, but slight difference between their *actual* and what would in corresponding circumstances, be their *English* manner of life.

The brigade of which we formed a part, belonged to the right wing of the British contingent and threw out one of its flanks to the very *beach*. The most convenient villages were selected for regimental headquarters, there being a necessity for concentrating regimental resources upon one spot: such as the hospital; the Adjutant's office; the quartermaster's stores; the riding house,[32] armourers', sadlers', tailors' shops, &c &c, with the persons in charge of these establishments, not the least important of which perhaps, was *the school*.[33] Besides, there commonly was a troop

---

31. This would be the churchyard of St Saveur at Desvres.
32. Note by Smith – Riding schools are not *necessaries* of military life: a good master can do without them, however convenient where they are to be had. While we were in these quarters, the drills went on very well in the open air; and a whole regiment was altered from dragoons to lancers and highly accomplished, not only in the new exercise for the men, but also in the new method of managing the horses; a circumstance highly to the credit of their riding department. [The regiment became lancers on 28 September 1816.]
33. Note by Smith – The teacher of our men was a very decent person, of the genuine Dominie Sampson case [a character in Scott's *Guy Mannering* – 'a poor humble scholar'];

and sometimes a squadron either in the town, or quartered in the nearest hamlets, who were considered as belonging to headquarters. These were every few months, changed by which arrangement all had their turn of convenience and superintendence. The commanding officer either lived in a chateau close by, or in the best house the town afforded; while the rest of us took quarters as well as we could, but in places of this sort there was no great choice. In the course of our movements, I had the luck to be sometimes in the house of a gentleman (*nobleman* always in France) and sometimes in the filthy and inconvenient cottage[34] of a farmer.

The soldiers were dispersed all around and some of them to considerable distances. It was not the matter of *distance* however, which formed the characteristic of their situation. Had they been regularly detached in *bodies*, to any distance whatever, they might still have had little or no merit in their good behaviour, either under the roof of a barrack or the continual observation of officers. But it was far otherwise, every little habitation, where the poverty of the inmates did not preclude the possibility of admitting another, had its dragoon and his horse; some two; but few had more; and nothing can speak more forcibly in praise of the non-commissioned officers who were distributed among them, or of the men themselves, than the very sparing list of complaints which was presented against those, who, if they had not in point of fact more money at their disposal than the people they were among, were more disposed to make an inconsiderate use of what they had. The article of the rations however, was a great card on both sides; and one which was tolerably well played. The single men readily handed these over to the family, who gladly undertook to cook and add vegetables to the daily pound of meat and pound and a half of bread received by the soldier;[35] who on his part,

---

and his characteristics were all the more remarkable on account of the contrast of his situation. He was much respected however and gave great satisfaction. But what will be said when I reveal the fact, that he always took his charge to divine service and led the sacred concert, he himself being a Roman Catholic!

34. Note by Smith – A cottage, as here alluded to (or small farmhouse), will present a very different aspect from that which is so called in England. Clumsiness, make-shifts and inconvenience of every description are abundant; nor is its very plenty of the comfortable sort.

35. Note by Smith – The daily ration issued to the English soldier on service, for which he pays I believe, four-pence per diem, is as above stated, with a portion of fire-wood. The liquor, commonly of spirits sometimes of wine, is a gift from government and forms no just ground of complaint when not forthcoming. It is often withheld from

was left master of more time by this arrangement than he could have been, had the culinary duties been added to those which he had elsewhere to perform. The rations were drawn every third day; and that day was commonly one of fatigue and trouble unusual to the parties employed. It will be recollected, that for a detachment of thirty men and horses (all getting their supplies at the same time), besides a formidable pile of loaves and lumps of beef, there were several cwt. of hay and corn to be conveyed, I think the farmers furnished straw for the litter, in consideration of their receiving the manure. But the bustle these operations always caused in a little town, gave it the appearance of a market; with this singularity that all the purchasers were in military costume. Of course, it was the practice to bring waggons for the purpose of conveyance. Our own horses had enough to do in attending the field-days; and the men to keep them up for military purposes, without performing this sort of service, which would have lowered their condition to an almost painful degree. In each cantonment there was a place of rendezvous, or parade, for squads, troops, &c and one general *point d'assemblee* for the whole regiment when required.

In summer our intercourse was constant; but when winter came on, we thought of roads, but looked for them in vain. Among the communities, or groups of houses, in which all the inhabitants of one parish were gathered

---

ill conducted soldiers, at the discretion of the commanding officer. The ration of the French soldier is much below the English scale. His staple is bread; and with a trifling quantity of meat and a little time to grub in the fields, he will cook a superb mess soup. It is a proverb in France, 'C'est la soupe qui fait le soldat' [It's the soup that makes the soldier]. Where an Englishman would see nothing but useless or noxious weeds and be sure of poisoning himself, the Frenchman selects a bunch of fragrant and wholesome vegetables for his broth. We once taught our soldiers to apply tourniquets in cases of emergency; why not teach them to swim and give them lessons in herborizing, as well as in many corresponding matters of the greatest utility on active service? The Adjutant or sergeant-major, marches them out to bathe; why not let them accompany the Surgeon, or the Assistant-Surgeon on *foraging* parties of this nature? Everything we trample under foot is not a weed, though that is a term of such general application. I do not pretend that in such articles much direct nourishment would be found; but they might make disagreeable food plateable; and even correct perhaps, certain noxious qualities of what is now and then unavoidably resorted to. The ration of the French *officer* is in proportion to his rank: after putting *us* for a short time upon this allowance in kind, we received a compensation in money. This to the field officers and captains, was a gain; to the subalterns about an equivalent. There is no difference in the ration of the English officer and that of the soldier. It is so much *per man*. Regimental officers pay about the half of the men's rate for their provisions; Staff officers nothing. I lost nearly a shilling a day by promotion.

round the church or near a chateau, but always among trees (which if they sheltered from the wind, excluded the sun) the lanes or *rues*, became impracticable. Ponds of water, bogs and the usual phenomena of *green lanes* in *wet* weather, taught us the necessity of disregarding boundaries and clearing obstacles in all directions, for crossing the country. It was bad enough for the cavalry, but in most situations we *could* contrive to get on; our friends however of the infantry, who were in similar situations, had to be conveyed to their musters, drills &c in waggons. The inhabitants moved upon the pattens already spoken of, which had very large rings, the wooden work being supported upon high clumps of iron and to steady the beginner, a long pole was found serviceable. We found out the prudence of resorting to the custom of 'Rome,' in this respect; and when lodged among these sloughs, I have been glad to borrow such a carriage, to go to dinner. Clogs, goloshes and all that sort of finery, would have been as inconvenient to the full, as silk stockings and *arraphostic* shoes.[36]

In consequence of these inconveniences, our quarters in winter were not locally the same. There were villages with which we could communicate very well in fine weather, occupied by troops for the convenience of the field-days; but when the season called for a discontinuance of this kind of work, it became necessary to place them upon something like a road, as more frequent inspections in quarters were then necessary, than during the period of regular assembling in one field under the eye of the general.

At this time Murphy [Egan] was on detached duty with one squadron or other; and now and then some laughable story of his proceedings reached us. My station was headquarters, from which I was not removed for years; but there were several detachments to which I was obliged to have an eye, making the periodical inspections required by the regulations of the service and dividing with the surgeon (at his own desire) the annoyance of going to casualties. These were sometimes disagreeable occurrences enough in the *day* time, as (according to the well-known rule of human perversity) the summons generally came when, all the morning's work being over, one was going to shoot, to pay a visit or to dinner; but this was a trifling matter, compared to what it was when, in the dead silence of the *night*, a ride of ten or a dozen miles was to be taken, occasionally after all,

---

36. Arraphostic shoes were first advertised in the early 1820s. Being made from a single piece of leather without any seams, they were claimed to be virtually waterproof.

upon a false alarm. I know not how often I had to act for Murphy [Egan], who was characteristically fond of the pleasures of the nearest *town* and when a *job* occurred, they either could not or would not take the pains to, or were glad of the pretext not to find him. After a brief and perhaps a *sham* search, a messenger was sent to headquarters.

It has been repeatedly remarked, that horses have a peculiar faculty of finding their way back (*home* to their stable, I suppose) by the track they have already gone over. These rides by night afforded me several illustrations on this curious point. That a horse should ever *recollect* the features, turnings and crossings of *roads*, is almost more than we should be inclined to believe; but under the circumstances alluded to, when the track was among the mazes of a forest, across ploughed fields, through gaps in hedges, with (now and then) a stile to leap or a brook in the way and only one practicable place in the shape of a ford, or one approximation of the banks, that an animal whose nose is supposed to be of little use but to breathe through, should most accurately and (as I have found it) inevitably follow all this maze in a dark night would be *surprising* in a solitary instance. On these occasions, I always had a conductor *out*, but I never brought him *back*, the animal I rode being then perfectly acquainted with the quartermaster-general-ship required on such occasions. Nor do I recollect an instance of a mistake, excepting sometimes on my own part, when perhaps, I had for a time no idea of the course the quadruped was taking, till at some recognised point, I became convinced that he was right and that if I had set my *reason* in opposition to his instinct, we should have both gone wrong. For a long time I had an experienced old gentleman to carry me at night: and he not only knew where Chiswick lived, (in the stable, when *possible*) but where to walk cautiously and when to trot out, requiring neither hints nor instructions on these dreary occasions. By daylight he was more reserved and commonly expected orders; but I found it the case with horses in general: and when a horseman loses himself, the wisest thing that he can do, is to let the animal take his own way.

A very striking feature in our economy and pursuits, not of a military nature, is to be found in the matter of *field sports*. In everything of this nature we eclipsed the natives. We had better guns and (though the article was severely prohibited) better powder. That which is used for these purposes in France is of a very coarse description and such as men accustomed to percussion locks and Dartford manufacture,[37] can hardly use with safety, there being not unfrequently a distinct interval, first between pulling the trigger and the ignition of the priming and then between this and the discharge: so that it is possible the last may not take place till the gun is removed from the shoulder.

There was a pack of fox-hounds kept by the officers of the brigade and the sport was commonly fair enough; but it was an indulgence in which for several reasons, (the chief one being that of duty) I was obliged to be very sparing. A hunting surgeon, even in civil life, is next thing to ridiculous; and had I taken to this sort of occupation in the army, I should have rendered myself perfectly so. I have seen some medical Nimrods,[38] and have occasionally heard remarks, of which I should not have liked to be the subject. However, *chacun a son gout* [everyone to their own taste]; and if these gentlemen amused themselves, they did it not at my expense. My fancy was to be thoroughly acquainted with the hospital and state of the regiment's health and to amuse myself when my work was over. Nor were resources wanting of a nature analogous to the one in question. The less expensive diversion (both as to money and time) of coursing, we could command in great perfection, owing to the fields being without enclosures. If a hare was started upon one of these plains, the only chance for its escape was getting into a wood. This we commonly prevented by running her down before she could reach one; and sometimes we had what is termed a *burst* of two miles or even more. The French were greatly obliged to the *fox-hunters* for ridding the country of these destructive animals (though I believe, they were so scarce as to require importation from England and cubs I know were at a premium); but the *greyhounds* were an abomination, there was to the best of my belief and recollection, some law or usage of the chase in France, by which no one could employ *levriers* [greyhounds] unless one of their legs was *hamstrung*, the hare then having *fair play* for it! Greyhounds hamstrung!! And yet some allowance ought to be made for the different nature of the country, as English dogs could hardly fail to take, there being nothing but straight-forward running for it.

---

37. In 1812, John Hall founded a factory at Dartford for making gunpowder, calling it 'Dartford Gunpowder'. The percussion cap was introduced in the early 1820s, being a single-use percussion device allowing muzzle-loaded firearms to fire reliably in any weather conditions.
38. Mighty hunters.

Nevertheless, no sight was more common in the fields than that of a ploughman keeping a sharp look-out for a squat [lair]. Wherever he discovered this, certain death was the consequence. When he went forth to his work, he commonly carried a musquet (if he had been a soldier, which was the ordinary case in France), and made use of it in the un-sportsman like manner described. Puss had no warning, no law, but was made sure of as she sat, she was then taken to market and thence to the pot.

Since the convulsions of the revolution, the game-laws of France, which under the old regime had been more oppressive than our own, had undergone a fundamental alteration. In fact, there was at this time hardly any law upon the subject. Property had changed hands, not only in so general but in so minute a manner, that game belonged to everybody; for in the space of an acre of ground there might be a dozen of freeholds, '*Morceau-ci et morceau-la*' [piece of this and piece of that], as a farmer once told me, run-riggs as the Scotch formerly had, so that if the proprietor of a strip of oats chose to be tenacious of his rights, his neighbour who cultivated half a dozen pecks of rye or barley, would repay his presumption in such a way that like the Kilkenny cats,[39] nothing would be left of either but the *souvenance* [remembrance]. So it became necessarily an affair of *give and take*; and whoever had a gun and could command time enough, might shoot all over the country without molestation,[40] provided he had

---

39. Note by Smith – If two of these ferocious animals be shut up all night together, they quarrel, fight and even devour *each other*; so that no vestige of either is, for the most part to be found in the morning, excepting now and then a *tail*. When they amount to ten or twelve, which is frequently the case the danger is diminished, as there would be a difficulty in disposing of so many *bones* within one victorious combatant. [Kilkenny cats were fabled cats which fought to the death.]
40. Note by Smith – An exception is, perhaps to be made to the ground immediately attached to a gentleman's residence. There something is occasionally found in the shape of a preserve; and a sort of keeper, called *garde champetre* [rural guard], has the charge. This functionary may demand a sight of the *porte d'armes*. The person of this description with whom we became best acquainted, was like Liston in the Burgomaster of Saardam [an Italian opera first performed in 1827], 'Read it, easily said, read it, read it yourself!' We handed him anything we chose and he used to express himself perfectly satisfied. For my own part, I once presented him with a map of the department, which I had about me, but his politeness would not permit him to look at it. The fact was as officers, we required no *porte d'armes* whatever; all we had to do was to avoid private trespass; and to give the people justice, they never interfered with us in the least, but were on the contrary, universally disposed to promote our arrangements. [This would appear to refer to the huntsman mentioned by William Hay, who he says was known to all as 'John Major'.]

a *porte d'armes*. This, which is equivalent to our game certificate and required no qualification, as far as I am aware, might be had for a very few francs these were considered money well laid out; a fact which it only required a fall of snow to prove. Upon one such occasion, our little market-place exhibited several scores of hares for sale at two francs each; and partridges, woodcocks in particular, snipes, quails and rabbits, might be had proportionately cheap.

A more serious kind of sport sometimes occurred in the shape of a *wolf hunt*. This was a rare occurrence and excited general attention. It was conducted in something like the following manner. First of all, it was necessary to scare these ravenous animals into some corner, or more frequently, into a forest. The ranger thereof, generally a nobleman, or person of superior rank, then summoned the posse to repair to a certain place at a certain hour, properly armed and prepared for chasse aux loups [a wolf hunt], all the country roused as a matter of course, but not entirely of choice; and as a curious scene was exhibited on such occasions, we (the English officers) were generally eager enough to go.

The beast or beasts, as the case might be, being shut up in their retreat, as large a circle was formed round the forest as the number of the forces would permit. Then began the noise of hallooing, screeching and horning, which increased as the circle contracted. The woods being entered at all points, the alarmed objects of the hunt retreated towards the centre, where in course of time, their lair was discovered, dogs of course, being among the *poursuivants* [pursuers]. Then came the tug, guns going off, now a *dog* shot, here a *wolf* and there a *man*!

I do not think the French care much about *angling*. There was no want of trout-streams and scarcity of trout; but these they either took with their hands or netted. Angling was a sport left to ourselves and such as were fond of it got their tackle from home. In the course of a ride one day, through a dreary part of the country now spoken of, I overtook a middle-aged man in the undress of a naval officer, (that is, he had the anchor on his buttons), with a rod in his hand. He gave me to understand that he had been resident in the neighbourhood since the peace of 1814 and that he had remained without the slightest annoyance or molestation during the Hundred Days. He spoke highly in praise of the people, who were unobtrusive and even kind; where he lived I did not inquire, it would have been impertinent, for he was one who evidently did not wish to throw himself in the way of his countrymen, and his retirement was entitled to respect. I never saw him upon any other occasion, nor could I learn that any other of us had done so. We proceeded together till we reached the stream in which he was about to pursue his simple pastime, upon the success of which perhaps, his dinner mainly depended, and when I say this, I mean no unkindness.

Fresh-water fish attracted the less notice, as Boulogne had an excellent market for the plunder of the sea. It is to be supposed that every article of provision was at this time screwed up to the highest possible pitch, as the officers of the army were not there for any purposes of thrift and messmen in particular were celebrated for extravagance. Our man, who was not the best of managers, once wanted a turbot, (the ordinary price being two or three francs); the *poissarde* [fishwoman] demanded ten; and being refused, she told him that it was the only good one in the market and he might go home without fish if he liked; but if he did, he would hear what the officers would say to him. There was a vast difference between making our own purchases of *everything* and employing an honest agent of the place for the purpose.

The headquarter mess (for every detachment had its little club where practicable) was established in a large house belonging to the justice of the canton. This gentleman did not, pro-tem, reside in it, having a chateau about a mile off; where he shut himself up and with him we had no intercourse. He was a smoke-dried old fellow, who wore powder and a pigtail and led a very recluse life. There was no officer in his chateau, a burden he evaded, either in virtue of his office, or in consideration of his accommodating the mess.

In this house, operations, both legal and culinary, were carried regularly on. The courts of the district were held by his worship, on market-days on one side and we dined daily on the other.[41]

How this functionary managed matters I know not; but, on a subsequent occasion, in a *chef lieu* not far off, I stumbled upon the *juge de la paix* giving *audience* in his kitchen to one man, with a bottle of beer on a table between them; and the magistrate informed me that his duty

---

41. Noted by Smith – But in this house (and in the mess room) all our regimental courts-martial were held. There came an order to appoint regimental deputy-judge-advocates. I expected the appointment, in consequence of an application to know if I would take it; but it was given to an officer who had been originally intended for the bar.

was of a peculiarly perplexing nature, as the seat of justice was on the border of four ancient provinces, to one or other of which some part of the canton belonged; so that he had the common law, or usages, of each of these to apply, as well as the national or Napoleon code, according to the exigencies of the case.

Perhaps however, there may be some to whom the term *canton* does not, without explanation clearly convey its meaning. Every parish, or in modern French language, *commune*, has its magistrate, or *maire*,[42] (mayor certainly being the English word for it, though head-borough might come nearer the mark) and this person has an assistant denominated the *adjoint*, acting for, and representing him in his absence. Sometimes, and very frequently the *seigneur* is the *maire*; but he is often little better than a peasant in his aspect and no better in his speech or scholarship.[43] I do not know what is the legal qualification to fill the office, which is one of no emolument, though respectable and influential. His duty is to superintend the police, to execute the orders of government and *perform the marriage ceremony*! I believe that in certain cases, he communicates with that great man, the *sous-prefet*. A certain number of circumjacent communes form a canton, in the centre of which the justice holds his court and his powers are more extensive than, though distinct from, those of the *marie*; he settles litigations upon a small scale, and, if I am not misinformed, is subordinate to the *tribunal de la premiere instance*. So many cantons form an *arrondissement*, or great division of the department or shire. In each of these and in one of the principal towns, resides the *sous-prefet*, or chief civil authority, acting under the *prefet* of the department, so very great an officer, that I never saw one. The *prefet* reports to the minister of the interior; receives and communicates his instructions; and as nothing required of government can be done without passing through this channel, a system better contrived for gaining time could hardly be devised. This may be either an advantage or a disadvantage; of the latter I met with an example in attempting to establish an hospital for a troop of artillery. First I had a host of difficulties thrown in my way by the mayor of the place, a shrewd and intriguing attorney; then I had his excuses to receive for delays on the part of the *sous-prefet*, who had to represent to the

---

42. The Maire of Desvres changed in 1816 from Furcy Legrix to Jean-Marie Harelle.
43. Note by Smith – The *marie* of the village near Bavay, was an example of this genus.

*prefet* who had to report to the minister, then wait his excellency's leisure to receive an answer, which when it came, consisted of queries, these had to be sent back from Arras to the *sous-prefet* at Boulogne; thence to be remitted to Mons le Marie, by him to be put to mem[o] my answers having to travel in this round-about way to Paris and back and up and down again: so that three weeks were spent upon a plain matter of duty, which almost as few sentences would have effectually accomplished.

Talking of marrying, the following story may serve to illustrate how they then managed these things in France. An officer of the Staff, who had been long attached to the regiment and with whom I was upon terms of particular intimacy, was ordered to Cambray [Cambrai]. Before his departure, he informed me that he was in a scrape with a young lady in the place and that there was a necessity for carrying her off; the parents having refused their consent to a marriage. I declared I would have nothing to do in any job of the sort, unless he would pledge himself that his object was an honourable one. This he assured me was the case; and moreover, that the consequence of leaving the girl behind, would be more dreadful to her than eloping, a measure which would infallibly reduce her father and mother to the necessity of doing what they at present turned up their noses at. The parties were too respectable to make this a matter of levity on my part; and there was too strong a mutual attachment to admit of its being a trifle in my friend's estimation. I knew the family and was on good terms with them. Mademoiselle had sanctioned his confidence in me; knowing as both of them did, that if I could not assist, I would not reveal. We talked matters seriously over and the result was my engagement in the affair. R*** had many friends, each of whom would have gladly lent a hand in such a business; but he paid me the compliment of preference, for various reasons; among others, he thought me dexterous and prudent, as well as likely to take the trouble of afterwards healing the breach about to be made.

The only thing to be done then, was to devise the most feasible plan of operation. First, it was essential to be furnished with a double passport; this R[44] obtained without difficulty at Boulogne, *pour lui-meme, et pour 'Madame son epouse'* [For himself and for his wife]. So far, so good. The

---

44. Both Ron McGuigan and I have been unable to identify the Staff officer R who had married, it is quite possible that Smith has given a false initial as he did with many other names.

second step in the process was, making and handing over the lady's *pacquet*, which there was a necessity for consigning to the care of the lover, a day or two before the route, in order that it might be incorporated among his own baggage. This was accomplished by throwing the articles to him out of a window and so far all went right.[45] Thirdly, we had to decide upon *time* of flight, *place* of meeting and *circumstances* of every description. We thought otherwise. In a day or two there was to be a great fair in the town, and her father's house, like all others in the place, would be filled with *cousins* from the country. There would be a general concentration of attention upon the great and important event of dinner, in all quarters, about the middle of the day, during which the *country* would be deserted; and no opportunity so likely to prove free from observation or interruption could possibly occur. It was agreed therefore, that the elopement should take place as soon after twelve as possible, on the day of the fair; when the town would contain at least a thousand people, more than at other times: but all their eyes would be turned upon one another, and our little tricks would escape scrutiny, for the moment.

Secondly, Mr R, who was to take formal leave of everyone overnight, was to mount his horse at seven in the morning and march off, no one to know in what direction, to halt at the nearest town, hire a chaise and have it in waiting at a particular spot, about five miles off.

Thirdly, J J[46] was to dress in mufti, (a costume in which he had never been seen in those parts)[47] wait for the lady in an obscure lane and *walk* with her, (riding under these circumstances, might have drawn attention and our English chargers would have spoiled the whole with a little French demoiselle on their back, who knew infinitely more of the *menage* [housework] than she did of the *manege* [ride]) by by-roads, well known to himself. Should any question, *par hazard*, be put by a *gens-d'arme*, a thing not impossible, though, under the circumstances, unlikely, (these

---

45. Note by Smith – If the story be considered worth understanding, I ought to observe that the window of my friend's apartment 'gave upon' that of the heroine; so that conferences between them were very easily managed and through this channel the arrangements were made. R was at the time quartered in the house of Mademoiselle's aunt, a rich old dame, with whom she was a favourite and of whom I believe, she was looked upon as the heir.
46. Again, it has proven impossible to identify this officer, there being no one with the initials J J.
47. Note by Smith – His wardrobe is described in another place: at this time he had his regimentals and a shooting dress only, and had never been seen in any other.

*gentry* being at dinner, as well as their *concitoyens* [fellow citizens]) J J was considered a very fit person to bamboozle with his answers.

So far as I have given the *programme*, the plot succeeded *a la merveille* [perfectly]. I put on a black coat and round hat, sneaked out of the town and after a long time, was joined by my fair companion, who confessed that her flight had been greatly facilitated, though grievously delayed, by her only brother (a big unlucky boy, come from school for the holidays) having over-eaten himself and taken fit in consequence. While all the party was busily engaged in the work of resuscitation, Mademoiselle, with a keen eye upon her dearer engagements, slipped away. Finding from her account, that we had a clear start of three or four hours before they could possibly miss her, I walked her more leisurely and with greater insouciance [recklessness], than would otherwise have been the case, to the spot where we found the chaise, R and (one of our officers) the son of a noble lord,[48] who was also in the secret.

Handing over my precious charge to R, I said, 'I have played *my* part, take care you do not now put your own foot in it.' I believe I have escaped to this hour without suspicion of having been at all concerned in the abduction. The blame and the execrations fell upon our noble associate, who had no more to do with it than a cloud can have with the moon, that is to say, he merely made a screen for us. He had gone with R to the place whence they brought the carriage and had been *seen* with him: but, if the *girl* was not invisible, I was.

After all, it is a funny little history; and I shall take the liberty of writing it out. As soon as we had consigned the fugitives to the chaise, they drove off. There was a way round the town whence the chaise was hired, by which they might have got clear away and neither father nor mother, sister nor brother, would have been able to track them. But it most unluckily happened that the postilion rebelled. He had, through the untoward circumstances, on the lady's part, at the projected time of starting, been kept so long waiting, that it was more than his place was worth to proceed without fresh horses. The laws of travelling in France are such as leave no discretionary exercise in the power of *any* travelling party. To contend appeared to be the worse of two evils and so there was no help but to return and conceal *Madame* (we shall now call her) as well as possible.

---

48. Almost certainly the Honourable Augustus Stanhope.

Passing through this town, situated in the high road from Calais to the metropolis and the residence of my worthy but *uninitiated* friend the pastor, his reverence espied R in the carriage; and having had some transaction with him about a saddle, he stopped the driver in order to make final inquiry concerning the bargain. A parley was inevitable; but the man in orders never saw, or at least took no notice of the lady. The chaise ultimately passed on; and no untoward event seemed now to impede the progress of the fugitives. But while they were bowling thus smoothly along the road to Cambray [Cambrai], a storm was brewing at home. R's trusty servant was in the secret and had been left behind, for more than one purpose, during a day or two. One part of his business was to announce to me the state of the family pulse, upon making the discovery; before I should present myself *in propria persona*. The lady was missed in the course of the elopement evening; but, at that time conjectures favourable to their wishes were conjured up. In the course of the ensuing day, the tempest rose to such a height, that I requested an audience, which was granted. The only difficult part I had to play throughout this long-protracted business, occurred *now*. Upon entering the house, I was received with French politeness; but found *pa* in despondency, and *ma* in a huge rage, not however with *me*, for they looked upon my humble servant to be as innocent as a child in the womb. It was that specious fellow St [John],[49] who had carried off their daughter. Could I tell them anything about her? Where was she gone to? 'Who could have believed it?' said Madam, 'and he spoke French so fluently!' 'No!' rejoined Monsieur, 'he did not understand French at all.' Now this was mere spite; for R*** was one of three (and there were no more than three among us) who did speak the language and understand it *thoroughly*. St [John] was the second, who the third was, I leave the reader to guess.

I then entered upon the hypocritical task of consolation and reconciliation. I gave a hint that pursuit was vain, that by this time they must be on English ground, that their measures had been well taken, and the wisest thing that could be done would be to consent to the marriage. 'No, never,' said the enraged father; 'Never! He may keep the girl; but I will prosecute him for robbing me of her clothes; she is a minor and has

---

49. Cornet William St John, 12th Light Dragoons.

nothing of her own.' This was '*un peu trop fort*; [a little too strong]' and I had enough to do to preserve my gravity.

Nothing satisfactory resulted from this interview. St [John] was loaded with reproaches, which he was not present to hear; and my advice was taken as to the propriety of seeing the chaplain, lest he should have performed the marriage ceremony. Not imagining what had occurred, after delivering over my charge and believing that his reverence was as much as in the dark as the Bishop of London, I highly approved of the suggestion, which to the dismay of those most concerned, was acted upon the following morning.

At an early hour the good folk started for clerical headquarters and obtained an interview with the *minister*. They were thereby instructed which way to go; for upon asking him if he knew anything of Mr. R, he *naively* informed them, that he had seen him pass through to Cambray [Cambrai] the day before yesterday, though he knew nothing about any *lady* being with him. This was enough. Pursuit was forthwith made; and a day or two after their settlement in Cambray [Cambrai], my friend with '*Madame son epouse*,' [Madam his wife] was caught taking a walk on the ramparts and the fair fugitive brought back in triumph, to the humbler place of her nativity. Thus, for a time, all loured upon their prospects; but the enterprise had the anticipated result of mollifying and reducing to reason the *obdurate* parents.

As soon as she got back, I was summoned to a council and could hardly help admiring the nonchalance with which she bore the event. Probably she was living in hope; and knew of course, with whom she had to deal, better than I did. In a short time, R obtained a few days leave and came down for the purpose of fulfilling his engagements: but although *M le Cure* had the complaisance to marry them in the church, according to the Roman Catholic form, it went for nothing in the eye of the law: for the *marie* would not act without the consent of R's mother, who was yet alive.

To English ears, of all the absurdities which can be sounded, that of seeking the consent of a parent after one is of age, much less after coming to years of advanced maturity, is perhaps, among the greatest: but so it is. In this matter, the French law appears to recognise no achievement of *personal* discretion; for so long as a parent, a grandparent, or a collateral, (such as an uncle or aunt) exists, a reference is necessary. In case of refusal, I believe there is some tedious or troublesome remedy; but these have a control, which they are called upon to exercise, in one way or other. So was it with poor R. His mother resided near London, but decidedly objected to her son marrying a *papist*. Many letters passed to and fro, between England and Cambray [Cambrai]; but it was long ere we got anything like a glimpse of satisfaction. At length R's sister wrote to say, that the old lady had consented; and this letter was sent down to me, as a floorer for the mayor. The bride's father and mother were more anxiously interested in the result now than they had been before in preventing it; and we imagined that our troubles were at an end. However, the mayor all but laughed at the *consent*, conveyed in this shape: he required a formal act on the part of Mrs R, countersigned and sealed in the chancery of the French embassy at London!! I now lost my temper; and declared that there was no woman in France worth so much trouble as they were putting us to, that I would never *have* a French wife, as long as this law continued in force and that, I do not know, in short, what I said; but I had no great confidence in the opinion of this cabbage merchant and therefore took that of his predecessor, a *gentleman* as well as a man of sense and experience. He assured me, that the thing was as had been represented and that there was no remedy but the one pointed out. I represented the vast absurdity of enjoining such a measure on the part of an obscure old woman, such as Mr R's mother; who, *as it happened*, lived near London and therefore the thing might be practicable, but that if her abode had been in the North of Scotland, in Wales, or a remote region of Ireland, such an arrangement would be hopeless, and a great deal of misery, if not even of disgrace, entailed upon innocent parties. Reason was of no use (even though admitted to be to the purpose) where it had to quarrel with law; and so for a time, we were *bogged*.

At last Mrs R went through the requisite formalities, (though by this time a little grandchild had opened its eyes to the light). The mayor no longer hesitated; he and the town-clerk performed their mummery; then came the English priest (we had had the French one long before) and then the christening, all in one day. I had the honour of *standing* interpreter to the bride and godfather to the daughter, without sitting down. It was upon this occasion that the venerable cure declined to perform. Thus ended this stage of a tedious business. The sequel of the story I know but imperfectly. My friend R is no more; and I have been told that Madame got married again, in the scene of these adventures.

Among the other trifles I have to record, as forming an era in this history, was our success in clearing the mess-house of *rats*. I relate our exploits in this sort of sport, because I think the revelation of it may be generally useful. Many plans have been devised for the same purpose: such as smoking with sulphur, poisoning (a method that often recoils upon the sportsman), drowning or entrapping for that purpose, not to mention steel snappers and various other contrivances of a corresponding nature. The most effectual method however yet known, is to unprop the tenement, as all the rats *to a man*, will desert before it falls. Hence old rickety houses contain none. We might have tried the plan of a celebrated Scottish lawyer,[50] but should have found, (as he did) our remonstrances unheeded; we resolved therefore to bring the first one we could apprehend, before a court-martial. It was not long ere a rascal was caught in the fact of reconnoitring the *sideboard*, late one evening, when only two or three of us had remained and were very quiet. A trap had been prepared, of such a fashion as did not mutilate him; and he had a fair trial without handcuffs or fetters. The sentence was that his ears, tail and whiskers should all and each of them be clipped close off with a pair of scissors and that he should then be allowed to find his own way to 'the place from whence he came.' We had no more rats during *our* stay.

Our host, the justice, to whom this house and these rats, of right appertained, had as I have already signified, a chateau about a mile off. From this he and his family (consisting of a wife, one son and one daughter), *a la mode du pays* [country style], were in the habit of migrating every winter to Boulogne. This be it observed, is a practice among the gentry of the French provinces, which were it observed in England, would tend much to diffuse wealth and prosperity throughout the country, I mean, if the landed proprietors, instead of ruining themselves, in too many instances by resorting to the metropolis, would encourage a little metropolis of their own in the nearest country town. But no! London or nothing! It is not so in France. Paris is of itself a nation, composed of inhabitants differing almost as much from the

---

50. Note by Smith – One of the Scottish judges, when newly called to the bar, came home one evening from a dinner party, and found a congregation of *felines* making a great disturbance on the pantiles adjoining his apartment. He first loaded his gun, then took out a copy of the riot act, which he formally and deliberately read over; but, finding this to have no effect in dispersing the mob, he was at *length* driven to the painful though necessary duty of firing among them.

people of the provinces as they do from those of any other country; and to Paris but a few ambitious or dissipated seigneurs think of looking, as an habitual place of residence.

One winter our commanding officer's wife formed the project of hiring the chateau, during the absence of the justiciaries: but a more profound insult could not have been conveyed to a *Chevalier de St. Louis*. Hire his house! What could these people take him for? A sordid wretch who would stoop to make money by such means? They ought to be ashamed of themselves. He could never respect an Englishman again, He had no idea of the benefit a house derives from being inhabited: and though, year after year, the chateaux of France are advancing in dilapidation (repairs forming no part of their system), the sight of his house crumbling before his eyes was insufficient to mould him to the purpose.

And yet this *gentleman* (had an officer been billeted there) would have *sold* him a bottle of wine out of his cellar, or a billet of wood from his stack, or an egg from his hen-house, at a profit of fifty per cent, not only without scruple, but upon no other terms. It was as common as ordering wine at a tavern, to call the servant of *any man's* establishment where we happened to be quartered and demand an account of the cellar, as well as the price of the wine we selected!

In the summer of [1816] it rained incessantly; and we had a most uncomfortable time of it: we censured, with little ceremony, the place of our abode, much to the vexation of the inhabitants, who endeavoured in vain to assure us that, if the weather were as it ought to be, we should have been much pleased with our quarters.

While we were here Freemasonry became all the fashion. There was a lodge in the regiment to which the officers went almost in a body, to be initiated; and the mysteries were in very high repute and splendour at Boulogne. The master of the regimental lodge was a singular character. He was at once the father and the chronicler of the corps; being an old non-commissioned officer, who was past all duty, who never wore regimentals, unless at half-yearly inspections (and seldom even then) who was allowed to follow us about from place to place and do as he liked. His appearance was exceedingly venerable, his deportment respectful, almost to excess towards the officers and his influence in the ranks unbounded. I suppose there was not one among the *older* soldiers, who would not rather have offended the colonel himself than old Billy

Barlow,[51] as *we* styled him; Mr Barlow always among the commons. From respect to his age and character, the mess had presented him with a handsome silver vase, capable of holding nearly half a gallon; and on public days, William Barlow was frequently requested to come with his cup to the mess-room, whence he never retired without bearing it off full of claret.

The last duty he had performed was that of hospital sergeant, so that the doctor had a particular share of his respect. His ruddy countenance accorded particularly well with his thin white hairs, (he adhered to the old military fashion of wearing a queue); But he had a few curious fancies: one of which was a moral *hydrophobia*. The old gentleman had for many years avoided washing his face; and yet it was not only the cleanest but the clearest complexion among us. He managed without 'the element,' by rubbing hard with a soft towel; but towels are not *abstergents*. Old Billy wanted little in addition to the celebrity he already enjoyed and all that was considered essential to the comfort of his evening was peace, with freedom from interference. Towards the close of his history however, Masonry involved him in notoriety, which flattered him to a great degree. I suppose he made a dozen officers competent to work their way into any lodge in Europe; and the rage which pervaded us in this matter re-juveniled the old boy so much, that having taken a trip to Dublin, (under the Grand Lodge of which the regimental one held its authority), he found that the lodge, which had gone by the number of the regiment, had become vacant; and he returned in triumph with a new warrant, removing us from among the hundreds, to a station not very far from number one and identifying 'for ever' the number of the [12th] Dragoons, with that of the forfeiture.

From the summer of 1816 till that of 1818, we remained in these quarters. Hunting and shooting, coursing and fishing, billiards, which and other collateral amusements, formed the amount of the general catalogue. I do not recollect that a single act of mischief was perpetrated during the whole of this long period, notwithstanding the facilities that the dispersion of the soldiers might be supposed to have afforded. The value of non-commissioned officers was most fully proved in the course of this service. We had a very praise-worthy establishment, men

---

51. No senior NCO of the regiment with the name of Barlow has been found in the records.

of sobriety, diligence, influence and integrity. They went from house to house; their eyes were never off their charge and the common soldiers not only obeyed their orders with alacrity, but respected their personal characters sincerely. It is proverbial in the army, that the sergeants of the Guards are jewels in the colonel's hat: and so I acknowledge them to be, for more trustworthy persons I never met with (and I have often encountered them in important situations); but I cannot look back to the period under review, without pleasing recollections of the character and conduct of our own sergeants, both major and minor.

There is a regiment of the line, which played a distinguished part in the Peninsular war, the ranks of which abounded with broken-down *gentlemen*. Of course, like other corps, they had their proportions of sick and wounded: and of these a certain number became patients in the General Hospitals. It was my lot to have rather an influential charge wherever I happened to be stationed and the elegant epistles, petitions, memorials, memoranda and suggestions I used to receive from *Messrs Les Soldats* of this corps, were at once vexatious and amusing. One man in particular, a full private, a portly fine looking personage, stated himself to be the son of a general officer, describing who his father was, I had no reason to doubt his story. He wanted some change of diet, and wrote a letter fit for the First Lord of the Treasury to see and sufficient to have obtained him a seat among the commissioners of customs, at least. Another spark, not more than twenty-two years of age, was a wardmaster under me; he was already crippled with the gout from hereditary disposition. How *he* could have become a private soldier I never could comprehend, for his conduct was unexceptionable, in every respect. We obtained for him the local rank of corporal and felt great confidence and interest in him. While he was discharging the duty of the situation in which he had been placed, the colonel of another regiment came sick to the station. Corporal *[52] claimed the close relationship of *brother*; and the colonel made but an awkward defence. There was little doubt, on the part of the medical officers, that the *ral*[53] had presented 'a true bill;' but he

---
52. It has proven impossible to identify this 'corporal'.
53. Note by Smith – 'I have a letter from my son Tom, in Portugal,' said a woman to her gossip; 'he gets on famously; he has not been a soldier more than two years, and he is a *general*, already.' 'A general!' said the other, 'impossible!' 'Fact, I assure you, he is either a *general* or a *corporal*. I have lent the letter, but I am positive he has got among the Rals.' When taking over the charge of a hospital, upon one occasion, in the Peninsula, I was

wanted nothing of his relative beyond his good word and good opinion. Many of these men were recruited from London and among a crowd derived from that source, there must have been many imprudent young men, who had received a good education.

We had a few *gentlemen* however, of our own in the ranks. Four of them may be spoken of with no great impropriety.

The first a young Irishman, whose appearance was much in his favour; but his health was bad; and he had not been long with us when we had to invalid and discharge him. Before marching off, however he had the modesty to solicit the hand of an officer's fair daughter! Being as a matter of course refused, he vowed vengeance against the father and maintained that he was a better man than himself, inasmuch as he had it in his power to purchase his whole breed, seed and generation. Nothing however, came of it; the father is still alive and I hope will long continue so; and the young lady has taken the name of a very worthy officer, yet in the regiment.

Number two was of the same country; but *distinguished* from almost all his compatriots by modesty. We performed an important surgical operation upon him, for a very painful complaint, which gave him instantaneous relief. He was employed in the Adjutant's office, being an admirable clerk. How he got his discharge I do not remember; probably at the reduction in 1818, when these compliments were going in profusion: but some years afterwards, an Irish gentleman, learning that a detachment of the regiment was passing near his residence, invited the officers to dine at his house and some accepted. Everything was conducted in the best style; and after the cloth was drawn, Mr [**]'s son came in to pay his respects. This was no other than the *ci-devant scribe*.

Of the third *gentleman* I am bound by every consideration to speak in terms of high respect. He enlisted while a *minor*, under a feigned name; and so engaging were his manners and appearance, and so superior was his address, that to put him into the ranks was on all hands, considered a repugnant measure. At this time the hospital sergeant had been invalided, and there was a vacancy on the *medical staff.* Even the Adjutant proposed

---

appealed to, in very moving terms, by a patient, who described his situation as peculiarly uncomfortable, inasmuch as he had once been an officer himself. My predecessor observed, that he had no cause for complaint, as he was getting on again, being now a *corporal*.

that we should take this youth under our wing, for he was 'a great scholar.' S [Robinson] assented and we had no reason to repent. Westlake[54] turned out, not only to be intelligent and to possess the manners of a well brought up youth, but acquirements that might have put some of his superiors to the blush. He was a good Latin scholar, spoke French with perfect fluency, understood accounts, wrote a good hand and dabbled in poetry and music. Nevertheless he attended strictly to his duty; and the doctors resisted every attempt to get him away from the hospital into the Adjutant's office, where he was very soon coveted. From corporal we got him made sergeant; without having done a single day's *military* duty, or having been *instructed* in his exercise. Still he learnt it, as ingenious young people will many things, merely by seeing how others perform them. The best proof of the soundness of these remarks which can be adduced, is that the last time the writer heard of him, he was permitted to be a sergeant-major, and in the high road to a commission. W[estlake] is one with whom I should be proud to shake hands, any day; and I hope his prospects will be fully realised.

But we had another character among us of a very different stamp. This was an illiterate, *harum-scarum* private, a slovenly little vagabond, not able to write his own name, who fell heir to a property of £3,000 a year!! This was a greater blow to the regiment than Waterloo had been. Teddy O'Brien with £3,000 a year at his disposal! The equilibrium was for ever destroyed, unless he could be disposed of. But Mr O'Brien was too valuable a card, to be thrown away so easily. His agent came over from Ireland to obtain his *mark* to some deeds, among others, as we understood, to settlements on behalf of his sisters. Still there remained this *enormous* income at his disposal. It was a regimental puzzle what to do with our squire. The captain of his troop (a land-owner himself in Ireland) would have borrowed the money, but he found the amount so large that he could not think of it: so the agent, by this gentleman's advice, invested the proceeds in the funds, as fast as they became tangible; and it was decided (as Teddy O'Brien would not be turned out of the regiment) that while he remained in it, he should receive no more than £360 per annum, payable at the rate of £30 per month.

Soldiers in general, who have but a shilling per diem, nominal pay,[55] can hardly make the two ends of the month meet. When the 24th

---

54. It has proven impossible to find the real identity of this soldier.
55. Note by Smith – Something more in the cavalry; but the extra expenses are sufficient drawback.

comes round, the imprudent are in debt; and the better conducted, after paying for intermediate supplies, can have but a few shillings to receive. Therefore, such a man, if liked in a troop, was sure to have all and each of their suffrages. Affection, both of men and women, has its price; and he who has most money, provided he applies it with even a decimal of dexterity, will procure most regard.

O'Brien was of course a greater man in the ranks than he would have been, had he purchased the troop right out, or even commanded the regiment. When *thirty pound* day arrived, he was miserable till his pockets were entirely incinerated, for money to him was no better than phosphorus. He generally had little difficulty in getting leave to repair to the next town, till the explosion should be over: but Teddy seldom if ever went by himself; he commonly had a sycophant, who was anxious to accompany him; and these going together, once gave me an opportunity of witnessing a curious, though disgraceful scene. I had entered a celebrated French city, in company with another officer and had got into one of the principal streets, when we observed a crowd at the door of the governor. With this we had no business, till one from among it called to us that a man of our regiment had been killed and was now laid out in a cart for conveyance, by order of the commandant, to the hospital. I dismounted from my horse and got into the cart. There was most assuredly, a being in the shape of a man in our full-dress uniform; but so discoloured and disfigured was his countenance that though I personally knew almost every one of our seven hundred and (as it soon turned out) this hero in particular, I could not possibly identify him. Accordingly, I descended and stated to my companion that I could not make out more than that the fellow, whoever he was, seemed to be *dead drunk*. We then waited upon the commandant, who frankly told us, that he had ordered the man to be secured for his own safety and welfare and that wishing to discharge his duty to a stranger, he had ordered him to be received at the garrison hospital; but now that he had the pleasure of seeing two officers of the regiment to which the *pauvre diable* [poor devil] belonged, he would hand him over with the more readiness as one of us was a surgeon; and he hoped we would excuse him to our commanding officer, if he had been overzealous, for his apology must be found in his desire to be on good terms with the English troops. All this we most readily and cordially admitted; but (my companion not knowing a word of French) I represented, that the better plan would be to execute the original intention, that I would see the *polisson* [rascal] deposited in the hospital and take all further results upon my own shoulders.

Returning hereupon to the street, I was about to desire the people who were in charge of the cart, to proceed onwards, when *Teddy O'Brien's* phiz protruded from a neighbouring door. 'Oh, ho!' I exclaimed, 'now I understand the whole of it. This is one of your rigs, Mister O'Brien. Who is this comrade of yours? And is he really killed or not?'

'Please, Sir, favour me wid a moment's hearing and I will tell you how it all happened. You see, Sir, my pea [pay] come due yesterday; and having more money than I knew how to take care of, I got lave, and took Cannor [Connor] wid me, *thinking he was a steady man*. We had lave to stay till eight o'clock; but he got so infernally drunk by six, that I could not move him out of the town; and of coorse, happen what would, as I had brought him in I could not desart him. So, Sir, I resolved to stay all night and make the best excuse I could in the morning. Well Sir, we did very well last night; and he gat up very well this morning; but nothing would do Sir, but a glass of *eau de wie*. This of itself, I thought Sir, could not hurt him and let him have it, hoping it would clare his head; but after that he would have another; and then Sir, he swoor he would bring me a cowrt-martial if I did not trate him to a *third*. As for his bringing me to a cowrt-martial Sir, I knew that was all nansense: but I was afeard of his letting out the whole story, and getting himself flogged instead of me; and if that was to happen Sir, you know no man in the regiment would associate wid me afterwards. Whereby Sir, I was glad to kape him quiet. But as we were going along up this very street, he swore he must have some more brandy, to *putt* him to rights, before going home. Whereby Sir, I was *seduced* to give it to him; and Sir, he had not left the door of the wine-shop three paces, till he fell down a trap in the street and hort himself upon a cow's horns, that happens to live below. What do you think of his case, Sir? For I am very much alarmed about him.'

'In my opinion, he has sustained no injury beyond what *you* have inflicted upon him, by making him drunk; and the whole affair is chargeable to your door, Mr O'Brien.'

'I hope not, Sir; I did everything for the best, *upon my honour*.'

'No doubt; but your manner of *doing things for the best* is not in very high repute. I will see to the man's safety; he is going off to the garrison-hospital and I shall go with him. My advice to you is, to get home to your quarters immediately; whether you or your friend is the greater *scamp*, remains to be seen. In the meantime, I have got a duty to perform, for which I do not feel obliged to either of you, as I came here for a very different purpose.'

'Stop a moment Sir, if you please,' said O'Brien, (pulling out six or seven Napoleons), 'perhaps he may want money; pray take what you like, for my part I have no use for it.'

'O'Brien, no money will be wanted upon this occasion; and what you have left, I recommend you to hand over to your *sergeant-major*.'

He promised to do so and we parted, he to sneak home and I to accompany the convict to the place of execution. The medical officers were exceedingly polite, saw the true state of the case, asked me what they were to do; and my answer was, 'keep him till sober, then give him an *unlimited* quantity of shower-bath; by which time, a non-commissioned officer will be at hand to bring him home.'

We must now enter a little more into *military* matters. Our brigade drills have been already alluded to. They were conducted under the eye of a highly distinguished and most accomplished general. He resided in a chateau at some distance from our own headquarters; and our rendezvous was generally upon fallow ground, as near his house as could be conveniently obtained. With a slight variation according to the arrangements of the corps, we met within a few furlongs of the same spot, year after year; and the products were very acceptable to the *agriculturists*.

Our muster was however, always on the side of the great road to Paris; and the eyes of Mr Bull and his family were ever on the stretch when they saw a large body of cavalry galloping over the fields which bordered the chaussee. Occasionally they would stop the postilions; and if there appeared to be young ladies among them, some of us idlers, would make a patrol to reconnoitre. On one of these occasions, a bacon-faced fellow poked his pig's-head out of the window and hailed me thus: 'Mounseer! Quells regiments? Guards royals ou Imperials?' My reply (in plain English) flabbergasted him and set five girls laughing at poor *pa*. I may as well give it: 'Sir, there is nothing Imperial hereabout which I can see, but the thing on the top of your coach. As for the regiments, they are all English and we live in this neighbourhood.' 'Good God! Who would have thought it? That we should have seen our own *paid* soldiers riding about in this here France.'

Many such rencontres (though not always of this vulgar description) occurred. I shall relate another.

One day I happened to be standing in the place of the upper town of Boulogne, when an elderly and a younger man, both well dressed and courteous in their manners, came behind me; and after scrutinizing the buttons on the back of my pelisse, politely asked what regiment I belonged to. I told them. 'Are you in this neighbourhood?' 'We are.' 'How do you like France?' 'Very well, but give me leave to ask, in return, how *you* like it?' 'Not at all; we are going home, but it is a great comfort to see one's countrymen, *in foreign lands*.' The same day, I went to dine at one of the hotels, where another officer of the regiment was waiting for me. We there found a fat cockney, who told us he had been 'as far as *Amens* on a *wisit* to a friend, and he had *stud* it for a fortnight; but he had got within sight of *ould* England *agin* and was going to *sale* home that *wery ewening*.'

It was about this time that the English economists began to cram the towns of France. Even before *we* had done with it, Boulogne had several, I cannot venture to say how many thousand English inhabitants. When I call them *economists*, I believe it but justice to add that they were not of the same description as those who, after the removal of the Army of Occupation, took up their abode in that neighbourhood. We had much pleasant society in Boulogne at the time of our own residence; many respectable families settled in and about the spot, because there were sons or brothers, or other relatives among the troops. In fact, Boulogne became an English colony, in point of moral influence though subjected to French laws.

Provisions are cheap: we could buy a huge turbot at Boulogne for thirty or forty sous: but though bread is at a lower price than in England, butcher's provender is not much less; all sorts of game may be described as *literally* accessible to the lower orders; for game in France, is not the exclusive food or enjoyment of the nobility and the gentry. Liquors are hardly worth mentioning. Malt is unknown, certainly as a product of France; but they make a very pleasant beverage from liquorice, horse-legs, and isinglass,[56] which they sell at two-pence or three-pence a bottle in the

---

56. A form of collagen obtained from dried fish bladders used in the clarification of alcoholic drinks, especially beer.

taverns. Bordeaux wine costs those who bottle it themselves (even after sea-carriage to Boulogne) not more than ten-pence per bottle. In addition to this, there is no appearance or state to be kept up: house-rent is perhaps, not much at variance with the standard in England; taxes however, are far below it; and the man would be ridiculous who thought of wearing fine clothes and consequently raising a tailor's bill. For my own part, I never saw my private wardrobe during three years,[57] having left it in the stores at Canterbury, when we embarked, but excepting at the mess, or on a field-day, occasions upon which I was necessarily obliged to wear uniform, I went about in a shooting-dress. This is the mark of a *gentleman* in France and might be a hint for half-pay officers.

We thought we had sprung a valuable mine (which turned out however, to be a mare's nest) soon after coming into this neighbourhood. One of the Boulogne wine-merchants intimated, that he had in his cellar an immense quantity of genuine *old port*, which had in point of fact belonged to his Majesty George IV of England!! How was this? Thus it was. A vessel had been freighted at Oporto, with a cargo of bottled port for HRH the Prince Regent; but was captured, on her way to England, by a French privateer and carried into Boulogne. A merchant purchased the whole cargo as a good speculation; but for five years, it had lain in his vaults unsought-for and I believe, unknown. Frenchmen would not touch the fiery liquid; and English bred stomachs there were none. At length the uncontemplated event of our arrival recalled the wine merchant's speculation to mind; and a few dozen found their way to D[esvres], at a very moderate price. However, a second batch was not to be had upon the same terms. There was a *Peg Nicholson Knight*,[58] in Boulogne, who brought up the remainder of this cargo and sold it again at a profit of, nobody could tell how much per cent.

---

57. Note by Smith – The fact is, though I left a very good one in England, I never saw it again. When my trunks came out to D[esvres], after three years separation, I had neither coat, waistcoat, pantaloons, nor any other article of the sort or purpose left. I thanked God that my books and papers had not been made free with. Clothes I could replace, but the other *essentials* I could not. I was not the only officer who had been served in a similar manner. We had better have had our duds at Waterloo: for then, if they had been lost, we should have been compensated.
58. The only Peg Nicholson I can discover, was a dead mare in a poem by Robert Burns. Early mentions seem to indicate it might refer to new or young nobility, but I have been unable to confirm this.

Alluding to this worthy character, leads me again to Larry Murphy [Patrick Egan], whom I beg now to congratulate, in having been transferred from the most Siberian of all our out-quarters, to the most enviable, where he 'carried on the war' with great force and effect. Being stationed near Boulogne, he contrived to get spoken of in all directions. An English physician, who was settled there in private practice and who was celebrated for great powers of wit and descriptive humour (the author of some dramatic pieces, which long kept their place upon the English stage), often asked me what sort of a man this Murphy [Egan] was. I had uniformly evaded giving direct answers, because it was not a very gracious job to blacken a brother officer and because the querist was himself an army man, of rank and standing, with whom I was by no means sure that I might not be doing Larry [Patrick] a mischief, if I said candidly what I thought. However, in a short time, he found an opportunity of judging for himself.

It was the practice of the officers at this time, to have a monthly dinner at a celebrated restaurateur's in Boulogne. He was *famous*, equal at least to *Very*, the *Freres Provencaux* [Provencal brothers], or the *Beauvilliers* of Paris itself. His very sign was an invitation, *'The Woodcock Pie.'*[59] Who that has passed three days in Boulogne is not therewith acquainted? Yet let it be received as a proof of the artlessness with which the matter of these pages has been arranged, that notwithstanding the much good cheer I had in his house, I have forgotten his name and forgetfulness is not one of my failings. The night after one of these family meetings, an officer was taken ill; and Murphy [Egan] being upon more intimate terms than I happened to be at the moment, was called in and prescribed. The case, however, assumed something of an alarming aspect and other advice was sought for. Dr V** was, therefore, required to give his attendance. I had changed my uniform for the shooting-dress and had resolved to walk to D[esvres] with my gun, for the double purpose of exercising myself on a fine winter day and killing perhaps a woodcock, or a hare as I went along. I was also partial to walking (as I purpose to prove in proper time and place). Passing up the Rue St. Nicolai, I saw V** in close conversation with the consul, whom I did not personally know; so I gave the doctor a nod and was going on, when he roared out, 'Stop, J[ohn], stop, I want to

---

59. 'La tarte à la bécasse'.

speak to you most particularly.' Accordingly, I halted and ordered arms. He got rid of his majesty's representative, apparently with little ceremony and running to me, seized me by the collar, exclaiming, 'I say, what a rum one that Murphy [Egan] of yours is! What do you think? We have just had a consultation and he has ordered three drops of digitalis[60] for a man in a pleurisy.[61] Ha! Ha! Ha! My eyes! Good morning to you! Ha! Ha! Ha!' 'Three drops of digitalis for pneumonia, ha! ha! ha! I shan't be able to hit anything all the way home. What did you order?' 'Mum!' 'O, very well, I dare say it will do him more good than the digitalis.'

This same gentleman (who exercised considerable hospitality in B[oulogne]) had been an old peninsular acquaintance of mine and had had the distinguished honour of being in the regiment with that most eminent and lamented of all Irish characters, Maurice Quill[62] (another of my familiars). He, or rather his lady, gave a fancy ball, to which I was invited, as also was Murphy [Egan]. Murphy [Egan] gave me my dinner on the occasion, as his place of abode was near B[oulogne]; and we thence proceeded to dress in a house not far from the scene of amusement. Murphy [Egan] was to be decorated in Spanish and went in the character of a don of high rank; looped hat and feather, white coat, red slashed unmentionables, yellow shoes, knee-buckles, &c &c. I chose some John Bull sort of disguise, which while it conferred upon me a *character*, did not make me conspicuous. All the world and his wife had got there before us; and, among others, the parson, who was in *propria persona*, ie without any disguise or fancy dress, standing among a group of ladies, at the time we were squeezing in. He no sooner saw Don Laurentio, than he bawled out, 'That's Murphy [Egan], of the [12]th.' Murphy [Egan] turned to me, in great wrath and proved the accuracy of the clerical conjecture, by exclaiming, 'What for did you blow me?' I protested that I had not so much as opened my mouth, or even got so far into the room as himself; but that anyone who had ever seen him before, must know him in that dress, as it shewed *his figure* too accurately to deceive, notwithstanding the mask. Upon this, he returned to the wardrobe-keepers and assumed another, though as it turned out, not a more effectual disguise. In the

---

60. A drug produced from foxgloves used to lower the heartbeat and strengthening the heartbeat.
61. A lung infection.
62. Maurice Quill was the Assistant Surgeon of the 31st Foot in the Peninsula.

course of a quadrille, in which my metamorphosed friend was shewing off, the surrounding crowd pushed a person against him, who was in the character of an old clothesman. Murphy [Egan] took fire immediately and demanded what was meant? (It was just at the time that the Staff uniform had been changed and our shoulders deprived of ornaments, which have since been restored) 'Vat you shay? replied the sham Jew. You vant me buy your epauletsh; how mosh? Vill ui chow zem?' Here was a second detection, of which it was impossible to impeach *me*; and a third visit to the wardrobe became, in consequence, indispensable.

One more story about Larry [Patrick] and we shall pass to something else. About this time, he gave a grand dinner to the officers in his vicinity; but Jock and all the rank and file, had long 'discharged' him; so that he was entirely dependent upon the good humour of a young Englishman, whose character was at least questionable and his reasons for being *abroad* not less than suspicious. However, they did tolerably well together for some time and the cause of their parting may turn up in its due order. Some of the guests seeing Murphy [Egan] in a great *stew* and that things were likely to be managed curiously, amused themselves with a kind of practical jocularity that would hardly have been allowable elsewhere. The *slave* had been told to let a tongue fall and to excuse himself by saying it was a *lapsus linguce* [slip of the tongue]: for Mr Murphy [Egan] was too good a scholar not to forgive him if he made a Latin excuse. The tongue fell sure enough; but the excuse was, 'Beg pardon, Sir, but it's only a *slapsus slingo*. I'll wash it, Sir,' which he accordingly did, in cold water.

An attorney, in the northern part of Great Britain, as celebrated for convivial qualities as for professional skill, paid a visit one evening at rather a late hour, to a boon companion; and in a short while, the two gentlemen became so happy in their social *converse*, that time, place, occasion and everything else, were utterly lost sight of. About midnight however, the lawyer started up, as if struck by a sudden recollection and exclaimed, 'I must be off.' 'Why so?' 'Because I forgot that my horse has been all this time standing at the door.' 'Oh, if that be all, he shall come in.' The animal was accordingly brought into the dining-room, where he was attached to the sideboard and furnished with something to *eat*, while the master and his friend amused themselves with drinking during the residue of the night. What the housemaid did with the carpet, after the departure of the iron-shod visitor, I know not; but it is natural to suppose that tea-leaves would not be of much use.

My friend B [Castley], as will be imagined, occupied, or rather arranged, one of the best stables in D[esvres]. He and I, having some right to consider ourselves fixtures, thought it worthwhile to consult our comfort in such matters. I got into a ruinous enough shed, upon my first arrival and employed a carpenter to fit up three snug stalls. This was done, *a la Francaise*; and the morning after the job was accomplished, Chiswick was driven mad, by finding every stick and stone, rack, manger, bails, stall-boards, hay, corn, straw, litter, bridlery and saddlery, scattered all over the place. My stud at this time, consisted of three, including a friend's horse, left with me for disposal, which though a very serviceable, was an extremely disagreeable charge. Among other accomplishments, he possessed that of untying the most intricate knot which we could possibly make upon his halter, letting himself loose and then doing as he liked, if no one was present. We first tried him with a leather halter; from that we had to descend to a rope; both however proving useless, we had to *invent* a chain, by which we were at length, able to fix him. This fellow (the quietest and most submissive upon earth when under control) was no sooner left without human surveillance, than he began, one would almost imagine, to *devise* mischief. It was the *lodger* who brought down the house, upon the occasion quoted; and Chiswick was all the more irascible that it had not been done by one of our own family, which alone, in his opinion, had any right to be disorderly. The immediate consideration however, was that of *repairs*; and the horses were removed into a neighbour's premises, while John went to work; and in the course of the day, with the materials the carpenter had only *pinned* together, erected barriers which set all heels at defiance.

But I have a better story to tell about Joe B [Castley]'s stable. It was in the backyard of a house belonging to one Monsieur Poste, who never having mounted a horse in his life, hardly knew what accommodation was due to one. The way to the stable was through the family sitting-room; in which, though there was no *sideboard*, there stood a ponderous wardrobe. It happened in the roster of the almanack, that papa *Poste's* wedding-day, or birthday or saint's day, or some other anniversary, came round and all his friends were assembled to partake of his hospitality; upon which occasion my messmate had ridden out to some duty, while the festival proceeded during his absence. High dinner had been discussed and the party were about to commence their coffee, when B [Castley]'s servant entered the apartment, leading his master's horse. The noise and sight of so many fine folk gave the animal a start. The alarm was mutual, for the company all rose with one accord: some of the females screamed and the poor horse, which probably would have behaved with perfect politeness, had his nerves not been thus acted upon now mended the matter by upsetting the lumbering *garde-robe* and smashing a pile of chinaware and crockery, which (in honour of the occasion) had been displayed upon its ledge. The overturn arose from the circumstance of the stirrups not having been crossed over the saddle and one of them hooking a corner of the aforesaid piece of furniture, the scared animal pulled with might and main, until the apartment was filled with dismay and desolation. It now became a *scene* indeed, some of the company got under the table and contrived to overturn it, laden as it also was with coffee, liqueurs, cream &c &c; and among these was Mons[ieur] P[oste] himself, whose back received the contents of the cream jug. One was said to have taken shelter in the chimney, but to the accuracy of this report I am unable to speak. All the belles of D[esvres] were there and the dreadful event furnished them with gossip for weeks afterwards.

J B [Castley] and I were just going to dinner, in perfect ignorance of all this, (for B [Castley] himself was not quartered in the house) when Mons[ieur] Poste brought over the awful tidings. He looked more like the man who 'Drew Priam's curtain at the dead of night',[63] than a quiet bourgeois of D[esvres]. For some time we could not comprehend him: he exhibited his back; well, that was streaked with white paint of some sort or other, but we did not profess to be connoisseurs in painting. He told us it was *cream*: we did not doubt it, it might be cream, or anything else; all we knew was, that we had not put it there; he next attempted to describe how pleasantly he and his convives had passed the day, and how much felicity would have fallen to their lot, had not the *horrible* interruption occurred. He was now more unintelligible than ever. '*Who* had interrupted them?' was our natural inquiry. If any of the soldiers had so far forgotten themselves as to be guilty of such misconduct, we pledged our word that we would state his grievance in the proper quarter, and he might depend upon having redress. In the meantime, would he take

---

63. From Shakespeare's *Henry IV Part 1*.

a glass of wine with us? French *politesse* compelled him to consent; and under these circumstances we got the truth of the matter out of him, in something like order, method, and consistency.

'Well, Mr. Poste,' said we, 'this is very unpleasant: but who is to *blame*? Was Mr B [Castley]'s servant disorderly, in conducting the horse through the usual access?' *Poste* was candid enough to say that he did not blame the man at all: in fact, he thought *nobody* was to blame; but that he had sustained a heavy loss, the more grievous, as several pieces of China were broken, which had been in his family for generations and had never been displayed, but upon occasions of the greatest importance. We asked what he thought his loss would amount to? 'Not less than a *hundred* francs, Messieurs!' Having ascertained this point, we then inquired, 'whether B [Castley]'s horse (worth fifteen or twenty times the money) 'had been injured?' This silenced him: and he retired, expressing a hope that he should be considered entitled to some recompense.

B [Castley] was then about to start with the regiment for the first grand review in Flanders; and had to go off before this crockery business was settled; leaving me (whose orders were to remain in charge of the hospital) to arrange as well as I could with Poste. I kept the old fellow on the tenterhooks of hope, at one time and despair at another, for several weeks. Whenever he called upon me (and it was always at a late hour in the day, my avocations or amusements engrossing me till dinner-time) I received him politely, offered him wine, but talked wide of the *smash* business, as not having received full powers and instructions; remarking, that my friend was absent and that *delay* would be inevitable. At length he came a little too valiant over me: hinting in pretty broad terms, that as he could make nothing of *us*, he knew where to apply for redress. 'And suppose M[onsieur] Poste, that my friend had had his horse irremediably injured; whose fault would that have been? Would it not have been considered preposterous, that the way to your stable should be through your parlour? Would you have satisfied *us* for the loss of injury of a valuable animal, which would have gone quietly and peaceably into its stable, by a proper approach, but was alarmed at the sight of a convivial party, in a place altogether incompatible with its habits?' Poste admitted the justice and propriety of these representations; but still the facts were, that the horse had *not* been injured, while all his *cups* and *saucers* were gone to pot. It was a brittle case to be sure: and after some further negotiation, it was agreed to, 'on the one part and on the other,' that Joe [James] should pay one-half of the damage, and Poste abide by the rest of the loss. I must say, for the honour of human integrity, that when I made this proposal, Poste considered us to be men of unmeasurable merit.

At length the reviews in Flanders (which have been alluded to) began. The first took place after the harvest of 1816; and all the army was collected for the occasion. Our regiment was away nearly two months; as it was necessary to assemble larger bodies together, for a few weeks previously, than had been practicable under ordinary circumstances. The first season, I was left at home; and S [Robinson] went himself. Murphy [Egan] went also; and they made this campaign together, *tant bien que mal* [as best they could]. They came back upon terms that were, at least as amusing as serious. The officer already spoken of, as having been a patient of Murphy [Egan], fell dangerously ill, at some place in Flanders, and Larry [Patrick] was called in. The unfortunate gentleman, not finding himself better, summoned S [Robinson], who desired a consultation, the case presenting a very alarming aspect. The result was a decision that the sick man should be bled. It was the duty of Murphy [Egan] to perform the operation; but he strenuously objected to the measure, giving various reasons, some bad and some worse, for opposition to this opinion. All however, was unavailable and S [Robinson] remained with him, after the consultation to superintend, or execute the sentence. Now arose a contest, which required the interposition even of martial law to quell it. Let me give it in the form of a dialogue:-

S [Robinson], 'Mr Murphy [Egan], have the goodness to take twelve ounces of blood.'

M [Egan] 'Take twelve ounces of blood! I'll do no such thing; it would be the death of him. I know his constitution; he never would stand it."

S [Robinson], 'Well, we do not doubt your knowledge of his constitution; but there is active inflammation, and our practice must be decisive.'

M [Egan] 'I entirely disapprove of blood-letting.'

S [Robinson], 'But we have had a regular and proper consultation: you surely will not fly in the face of that and run the risk of the consequences to yourself, for so doing?'

M [Egan], 'I don't care for the *consultation*, he ought not to be bled, I say.'

S [Robinson], 'Then Sir, as your superior officer (since you lay me under the disagreeable necessity of resorting to such an alternative), I order and command you to bleed Mr [blank], one of the officers of this regiment.'

M [Egan], 'I will not do that, or any other professional act, in opposition to my judgement.'

S [Robinson], 'Well Sir, this is conduct for which I shall bring you to account hereafter. In the meantime, as I am at a distance from my quarters, lend me your lancet and I will bleed him myself.'

M [Egan], 'I will do no such thing.'

S [Robinson], 'Mr Murphy [Egan]! Attend to me! I now ask you upon your honour, as an officer and a gentleman, whether you are *possessed of a lancet*?'[64]

M [Egan],'I am not obliged to answer that question.'

S [Robinson], 'Your reply is perfectly satisfactory. It is notorious that you are *not* possessed of a lancet.'

A French apothecary was called in; and the operation was performed, under S [Robinson]'s superintendence; Larry [Patrick] protesting that he would not by his presence sanction any such murderous proceedings. After this, S [Robinson] addressed an official letter to Murphy [Egan], wherein he ordered him (as under the circumstances, he had the right and indeed it was his duty to do) to provide himself with the instruments, *lancets* in particular, which according to the rules of the service, he was obliged to have, the Apothecary General's depot at Cambrai, in the vicinity of the scene of the transaction, offering a favourable opportunity for so doing, a fact which S [Robinson] very kindly pointed out to him: but to this mandate Murphy [Egan] instigated either by old Nicholas, or some mortal lover of mischief, returned an answer, to the following effect:

Sir:
I have received your letter, with the advice conveyed in which it is not my intention to comply. I want no lancets and shall not provide myself with instruments; but I will in return, advise you to take a few lessons in French before you engage in another consultation with the medical men of this country, in order to avoid making a fool of yourself again, as you did yesterday. I have the honour, &c.

---

64. Note by Smith – S [Robinson] had his own in his pocket at the moment; but thought it his duty to be sure of Murphy's [Egan's] efficiency.

This was not to be got over; and though I must do S [Robinson] the justice to declare that he was a mild and forbearing man, Murphy [Egan] had by this time, tried both his and my own patience beyond endurance. He came down to headquarters in arrest, for S [Robinson] had been obliged to report the circumstance to the authorities. Larry being *shopped*, was anything but cause of rejoicing to me, as I knew I should have all his duty to perform in addition to my own. However, as it was, at all times, my wish to screen a brother-chip from real harm and as, through a system of conduct such as this, S [Robinson] and I had long stood, (and did much longer afterwards stand) between Murphy [Egan] and the serious displeasure of the regiment, I became uneasy at the situation to which he had reduced himself and gave him all the advice and assistance, within the compass of my power.

Murphy [Egan] being now an idle gentleman, (though not *at large*) hung about headquarters and knew what to do. He talked very big about taking S [Robinson] from his bread, should he take his bread from him; but it never went the length even of smoke. One morning I received a message to attend at S [Robinson]'s quarters, for the purpose of hearing a conversation between him and Murphy [Egan]. I went and had the pleasure of listening to the following colloquy,

S [Robinson], 'Mr Murphy [Egan], I have sent for you and J[ohn] by yourselves, as we are the three parties most concerned in this most unpleasant business, to endeavour to make some arrangement that will neither be injurious to you, nor hostile to J[ohn]'s interests, who is the only one to be benefited by your departure from the regiment. The letter you wrote me is in the hands of the Adjutant General and you will have to stand a court martial, in consequence of it. I am now speaking to you with perfect freedom from animosity, but you have been too long in the service not to be aware that you have committed a great military offence.'

M [Egan], 'Sir, I offered you satisfaction, and . . .'

S [Robinson], 'Yes; you first committed yourself with the Articles of War and the Mutiny Act; and then you wanted to bring your behaviour within the pale of a personal quarrel. I also understand that you have threatened me with personal vengeance, if I proceed in the matter'

M [Egan] 'I deny it!'

S [Robinson] 'I shall say no more on that point; but I beg to state that, if the affair ends in your honourable acquittal, *I shall consider myself bound to make you reparation.* In the meantime, there can be little doubt that you will be broke, if the matter is pressed. I am unwilling to be the agent in an affair of such serious consequence to you; and you had better attend to what I have now to propose. In the event of your being brought to a court martial I must appear as prosecutor. This I will do all in my power to evade, if you will pledge yourself *to exchange out of the regiment, by the 24th of December.'*

M [Egan] 'I will!'

S [Robinson] 'You promise then, upon your honour, that by the 24th of December, or as soon after that as you can make arrangements, you will quit the regiment? If so, I shall lose no time in withdrawing my charges.'

M [Egan] 'I do.'

Thereupon M [Egan] and myself walked out. When we got into the square he looked very melancholy and observed that this was an ugly business. I had little consolation to offer him; for I thought that a medical officer who could go about vapouring as he had done, without the means of affording relief to the sufferer, while his bounden and especial duty was to do so, deserved to be removed from so responsible a situation. But the creature now threw himself upon my good offices and asked me what he should do. 'You know, J[ohn],' said he, 'that if we go to the utmost, I shall come down. I was broke by a general court martial once before; and a second job will finish me. The letter will d[am]n me; and I would never have written it if I had not been advised by \*\*\*.[65] What *will* I do?.' I replied that I was the last man upon earth to whom such a query should be addressed, for in the event of his removal, I should obtain a step of the greatest importance to myself. However, as I could not refuse him the advice he sought, I recommended him to throw himself upon the officers in general and endeavour to obtain their interference with the Surgeon. This I thought would be a powerful influence and it proved indeed, overwhelming. S [Robinson], in spite of his sense of duty, of his unconcealed dislike to Murphy [Egan] and his avowed goodwill towards me, was compelled to yield; and in a few days, Mr Murphy [Egan] went back to his duty.

I have sometimes been told that the toleration of such a man was a discredit to the corps. I should think so myself, upon recollecting how

---

65. It is impossible to know who this refers to.

differently our ideas of duty were arranged; but the [Surgeon] was remarkable for forbearance; and Murphy's [Egan's] brother-chips did all they could to cover his sins. At a future period, he stood alone; and although the skin which clothed the animal seemed to be that of a *spaniel*, the beast was discovered to be an ill-tempered *turnspit*. I have little doubt that, had we succeeded in keeping Murphy [Egan] to his word, I should have been in the [12]th still and I have little less that I should now have been riding in S [Robinson]'s saddle.

I have already made allusion to my personal dimensions and I need not repeat at this time of day, that I belonged to a regiment of horse. The gentlemen, with whom I was accustomed to associate, knew enough about riding; but not one of them had the slightest notion of what could be done by a *pad-nagger* [walker]. From an early period of life, I had habituated myself to the use of my feet.

About this time an extraordinary character came among us,[66] of who I had heard a good deal, but had seen little; and one day the conversation turned upon the distance between D[esvres] and Boulogne. The road (I have elsewhere said) was hilly; in fact there were fourteen rises between the two places, and one of them was so formidable as to have received the titular designation of *mountain*. No one of the party could tell exactly how far the places lay asunder; some thought they were ten miles, others more others less.[67] I happened to say that I was sure I could *walk* it within three hours. 'Walk it in three hours! Why, that is as much as a horse can do.' 'Well, but I can walk faster than most horses.' 'You walk faster than a horse! A little fellow like you!' The extraordinary alluded to (whom I must not venture to identify) now addressed me, with the observation, that it was more than any man *could* do, to walk to Boulogne in three hours. I asked him what he would bet that I would not accomplish it in two and a half? 'Two and a half! Why, I will bet nothing, for I should be taking you in.' 'Well, Sir, if I am taken in it will be my own doing; but I will bet ten *Nap[oleon]s*?[68] with you and the same sum with any other gentleman present, that before this day fortnight, I walk into the gateway

---

66. It is likely that this character (who is also referred to as *Old Dignity*) was Major Overington Blunden who would have come out with the depot squadron when the regiment became lancers. Major Blunden was actually a colonel in the army and an MP.
67. The distance from Desvres to Boulogne is about 18km or 11 miles, requiring Smith to walk at the rate of 4.4 miles per hour, which is quite possible.
68. A Napoleon was a 20-franc coin.

of the upper town of Boulogne within two hours and a half from leaving this square.' 'Done,' exclaimed J B [Castley]; 'and some,' said the other. The bets were made; and part of the intermediate time employed, on my side, in ascertaining whether I was *really* to win or lose the money, for when I made the proposal I did not know. Our old extraordinary pitied 'the young man,' and was afraid he would do himself a serious injury. J B [Castley] however, soon found that there was an ugly prospect about his *Nap[oleon]s*; in fact, in the warmth of confidential friendship, I one day revealed to him that I had ascertained it all and knew that I could do the match within *two hours and twenty* minutes. The thing being a mere joke upon our man of rank and after all, little better than a convivial quiz, I should not have been sorry to have forfeited my bets (though I could ill afford the sacrifice); but I found that so many interests had been involved and entangled in the matter, that the sport was inevitably to go on. Joe [James], however, contrived to make a hedge with the dignitary, to the amount of his bet with me; so that what he lost by Paul, he was paid by Peter. The day of performance was a celebrated one. I had my choice of several and selected a fine morning. Off we went at ten, myself afoot and about a dozen of them on horseback; among whom was *old dignity*, uneasy if I got for a single moment out of his sight. At starting, something in the shape of duty detained him for a moment and a mischievous spectator informed him that I was running down the first hill (which led out of the town) as fast as I could split. The fear of foul play, for he really believed it impossible that any man could win by *fair* means, induced him to cut the cause of detention very short and to gallop after me, at the risk of his horse's knees, if not of his own neck. After this he never left my heels; but as we journeyed on, J B [Castley] and others played upon his feelings by alternately raising his hopes and exciting his fears. At one time it was, 'see how he labours, he is almost done. J[ohn], you had better give in; we will take half forfeit, you have gone far enough;' then, as we approached within a league or so of the goal, it was, 'the Bank of England to a potato: as good as won.' The old gentleman began to think I was not so great a fool as he had taken me for; and as if it had been in his power to hasten the march of *time*, he left us about half a mile from the town and rode quickly on. When we came up (in triumph) we found him under the gateway, with his watch in his hand; and holding it out to me, he very handsomely observed, 'that I had eight minutes and a quarter to spare, that I had astonished him, that I deserved my winnings, but that he feared I was greatly distressed.' As the astonishment of this Solomon was the principal object and was likely to afford the mess some future merriment, I coolly replied, 'that, so far from being distressed, I had thoughts of *walking* back again;' upon which he put spurs to his horse and rapidly disappeared.

The result of this amusement was another of the same sort, but upon a more enlarged scale. Of course, we had some sporting characters among us; and as the thing was a novelty, it excited considerable interest. I was urged to undertake a second match, against *time*, being assured that I should not want *backers*. I never understood *gambling*, but *backers* I did not require. The question was, who would make bets *against* me? I believe I might have taken odds to an unlimited amount; for that which was proposed they in general considered to be an impracticable thing. My purse being but light and my confidence in myself not overweening, I went no deeper than twenty *Nap[oleon]s* on my own account, though others placed such reliance on my judgement, that heavy bets were taken on both sides. What the match was to be, I shall not state; for after all, it claims no distinction; but it raised the whole country during its performance and shewed the natives an English feat, which none of them however *brave*, could imitate.

My engagement was to walk a certain number of miles, within a given a number of hours. I had my choice of the kingdom for ground; but I could find none level enough and at the same time of extent adequate to my purpose. There was however, adjoining D[esvres], a pasture not quite level, but nearly so, the circuit of which I found to be half an English mile. I did not like this arena and had expressed a wish to wait till the regiment went down to the *bruyere*,[69] where I should find a long and even course of two measured miles. It appeared however, that this could not take place till my limits, as to time should be exceeded; and I was therefore reduced to the necessity of looking about nearer home. Finding nothing practicable but the field aforesaid and finding also that the weather was becoming precarious, I abandoned the design altogether, resolving to pay *half-forfeit*.

The evening previous to the last day upon which the match could be attempted, Joe B [Castley], (my *umpire*) came out of the mess-room

---

69. Note by Smith – The heath, the military and race ground near St Omer.

and informed me that *half-forfeit* would not be taken, the other parties conceiving that no engagement had been made upon that understanding; and that I must either play or pay *the whole*. We both thought the case a hard one; however I said that I would *try it*, sink or swim and advised them all to be upon the *field* by six o'clock next morning: for my own part, I would go home, have a mutton chop, get to bed immediately, eat another in the morning and set them all at defiance. I was absolutely *wroth* and resolved to try the match out of *sheer spite*.

I rose at four; and on calling my umpire, found that he had just gone to bed.[70] I then returned home and read a book, calling again at six: he was more drowsy now than at first. I depended naturally, upon him to see the ground measured and staked; but all this I had to do for myself. The armourer furnished a chain and some carpenters cut the stakes (which in a circle were indispensable). But first, in measuring the ground and then in staking it out, I went twice over it, before the match commenced and had a deal of trouble and vexation, which ought to have been taken off my hands. At length, about half past nine, when all was arranged, my umpire came to his duty. J B [Castley] should have been more alive; for he was a heavy backer so was his reverence [Tunney], who won four or five times the money I did myself; and he afterwards said that he wished me to make another match, for he had such confidence in my judgement and perseverance, that he would go to any amount.

We won the match by two minutes and a half. The day was at first unfavourable and the ground almost dangerous to a pedestrian. I never was so stressed. Soon after the commencement, a tent had been pitched, where all the *beau monde* for leagues around began, *l'apres-midi* to assemble. It was a veritable holiday, though in the middle of harvest. The *authorities* came, the *cure* came and *ladies* came in numbers. As it was understood at what hour the enterprise would terminate, either one way or the other, towards the close there was even a crowd; and all amiable as a French *crowd* is, and delighted upon this occasion, as it was I was fain to carry a stick and sometimes to call upon a bystander to keep the path clear; for there was no time for expostulation, one word and two blows.

---

70. Note by Smith – I dare say he did not believe I was in earnest.

I started at a quarter before ten (instead of four, as had been arranged). When the match commenced, I had taken a single cup of coffee but had eaten *nothing*. When half the distance had been performed, I had gained a quarter of an hour upon the whole time. Chiswick was ready in the tent to wash my feet and change my shoes and stockings; during which process I swallowed some bread and cheese, the first article I had eaten that day and drank a glass or two of claret. But I could not sit *down*. Walking in a circle, so contracted as that of half a mile above thirty times without a halt, made me so giddy, that when I stopped I fell.

The quarter of an hour being expended, I set out again, fresher than at first and S [Robinson] advised me to take a few turns in the reverse direction. I attempted this; but found it would not do, the disposal of the field being against progress. At length I found the ground so heavy, that I threw off my shoes and walked in my stockings, though the shoes had been made expressly for the occasion. The moment of triumph drew nigh. My last round came. The tent was both the starting and the winning post. A few yards from the goal, about a dozen sergeants and sergeants-major laid hold of me, saying, 'Sir, you have done quite enough; the match is *won*; please to sit down here.' I had no idea of this. There was a splendid chair, decorated with laurel, padded with cushions and covered with carpets, into which I was first forced and afterwards upon the shoulders of these fine fellows, carried amid numerous English *hurras* and French *vives* into the tent.

There I found all the rank and fashion of the vicinity eager to congratulate me upon a thing that I really thought of little consequence. There was my friend, who pocketed fifty pounds by the feat; and J B [Castley] my umpire, who gained about half as much. Several other winners were among the company[71] but there was none of the losing *party* visible. The fact was that (as they afterwards good humouredly confessed) popularity was so exclusively on my side, that whether I was to win or lose, those who had wagered against me ran a risk of being pelted out of the field. So they walked off before matters came to a close. The dean (who was also cure of the parish) was there, with several ladies; and they drank a bumper *a la victoire*. But I could not then enjoy the

---

71. Note by Smith – It came to my knowledge afterwards, that the troopers had been betting *their* five-franc pieces, which I was rather grieved to learn; and which prevented me from making another match, that might have *filled* my own purse.

triumph. I was glad to get home, where S [Robinson] and Chiswick had a warm bath prepared for me. That night I was restless; and for several days felt considerable uneasiness. The ground was of the most unfavourable description; the weather was adverse; the commencement inauspicious and almost *everything* against me. I pocketed about fifteen pounds only by this; but it was a bright day in our dull and monotonous existence and shewed the French people what was meant by English *athletics*.

A few days after this exploit (as I was told by a young lady, who happened to be present), a youth of the place having laughed at my performance and declared his ability even to *exceed* it, took a walk in company with some of the fair sex who had been witnesses. He set off in grand style, walked *twice* round and then *fainted*! The circle is bare owing to the tread of my own feet and is called Mr J[ohn]'s promenade to this day. The rent for the occasion was ten francs! The girls told me, that *they* were the cause of my success, for they had been putting up prayers to the Virgin, during the greater part of the time.

A match on a more extended scale was made after this, to be performed upon the *bruyere*; but I thought it unbecoming a medical officer to set himself up as a sporting character, however confident in his physical powers. I had done enough, so I broke it off. We had enjoyed our little *private* amusement and beyond that, I did not think proper to proceed.

In 1817 it devolved upon Murphy [Egan] and myself to go to the annual reviews; and to the neighbourhood of St Omer we proceeded together. Here, upon the commodious plain already spoken of, the cavalry division was assembled for several weeks previous to the start for the banks of the Scheldt. Larry [Patrick] however, went back to the depot at D[esvres] before this took place, on sick leave; so that I found my way alone, as far as professional support was concerned. This however, was but a slight grievance. During the preparatory six weeks, I was in a very curious place of abode. An accomplished and intelligent captain, one of the best read and best scholars among us, shared a village with me; which, being in the centre of several other temporary cantonments, formed a sort of medical headquarters for the troops which surrounded us. My friend B [Castley] and I had the nasty place to ourselves, though our quarters were nearly a mile asunder. Our practice was, after the performance of duty, to pass the day as much together as possible, either in riding about among the antiquities, or fishing, a sport of which B [Castley] was very fond; and there was a fine trout stream in the neighbourhood. This would do only in fine weather however; but upon rainy days we had a domestic resource in chess. This was the slough in which I found most employment for the pole and pattens. Our plan was to dine at each other's house, two days alternately. At the farm where I resided, there was a large dog to whom I had been kind. This animal (rather ferocious) was always let loose at night; and I need hardly observe, that my hours were not quite so early as those of the household. *Baron*, however, made a point every night that I dined with B [Castley] to meet me in the dark (commonly towards midnight), where three or four lanes intersected one another, to show me as it were the way home, if not to protect me. He never passed this spot; and upon the nights that I came from the other end of the village, I never missed him. He neither barked, nor was friskly; but trotted on quietly and steadily before. It appeared to me that *Baron* was not aware by which lane I was to approach; but he certainly had a perfect knowledge of the fact that I *must* pass by this *quatre-bras*; and there he uniformly took up his post. I love anecdotes of animals; and have always been successful in gaining the good will of horses, children, dogs and cats.[72]

From this place we went to the grand review. It is not my intention to give any description of what I there saw; such belongs to the *public* transactions and *official* narratives of the time; but I am surprised that so few spectators (particularly of our nation) came to see us. Forty thousand

---

72. Note by Smith – The commandant of Coimbra had a poodle, of a most extraordinary character. No one could venture to *caress* him, excepting his master and the servant. Being very much an associate of the commandant, I contrived in a short time to get over *Trusty's* scruples and succeeded completely in obtaining the ascendancy. It happened afterwards that his master and I were both in Lisbon; and Trusty accompanied him one day to dine with me. Going away, the poor fellow lost scent as well as sight, but came back to my billet, at the time not a bad one. I took charge of my friend's dog; but knowing his disposition, shut him up in my bedroom when I retired. In the middle of the night the door was opened and an English voice called, 'Doctor!' 'Whoever you are,' I replied, between sleeping and waking, 'take care; for K*'s dog is here.' *Trusty* had already commenced the growl, and Mr * hastily shut the door, keeping it fast till a light could be procured. He then explained the object of his visit, which was to call me to the town-major's, where a gentleman had been taken ill. He was much alarmed at the awful intimation of the canine presence; for K*'s dog was *notorious*. I had a spaniel of my own, which distinguished itself very much as a soldier's dog; and afterwards was much admired even in London. It died in my house, long after I was placed upon half-pay. I had the creature from the litter; and could fill almost a volume with its history. Among other fancies (being a female) it had a liking for the cat and always nursed, sometimes even suckled the kittens.

of the finest troops in Europe (the majority English) will perhaps, never be seen together in warlike trim again. There was all the science and practice of a general action, without any of the mischances. We heard the noise of cannon and of musquetry and we saw the formation and movements of large bodies, both of cavalry and infantry; rivers were crossed by pontoon bridges, skirmishers were thrown out and (with the exception of slaughter) everything was perfect. Panoramas are very well for London; I have seen several; among others that of Waterloo; but the *silence* and the fixed position of all the objects, appeared quite incongruous.

The march down and back to stationary quarters, was a pleasant interruption of the monotony which attached to our mode of life during the rest of the year. French Flanders is a rich country and more particularly interesting on account of its military history. We had there an opportunity of becoming acquainted with the nature of an artificial barrier, formed by a succession or cluster, of regularly fortified towns.

In all, I believe there were four of these reviews, I attended *two* only, the reasons for which would by no means interest the reader. He is already aware that in 1816, I was left with the hospital; in 1817, S [Robinson] staid at D[esvres]; and Murphy [Egan] took himself thither when we started from *Artois* into *Flanders*. In 1818 there were two; I went to the first, but was excused going to the second, got up in honour of the Emperor Alexander, the Grand Duke Constantine[73] and some other *persons* of greater notoriety than myself. J B [Castley] also got off this campaign; so did *Larry* [Patrick]; and we three, as well as the parson, who cared little for military spectacles, gathered into the headquarter village (about a league from St Omer) where we did little but laugh for a week, I mean that J B [James Castley] and I laughed at Larry [Patrick], for his troubles came upon him here thick and three fold; but, as usual, they were all of the ludicrous sort and brought upon him by his own curiosity and absurdity.

I shall relate one or two. The year prior to that of which I am now speaking, the temporary headquarters of the regiment had been in the same neighbourhood, and Murphy [Egan] was lodged *en prime*, in a chateau. He thought it vulgar however, to dine in his billet and was in

---

73. The Grand Duke Konstantin Pavlovich was Tsar Alexander's younger brother and heir presumptive to the childless tsar.

the habit of travelling two or three miles every evening to join a little mess in some other commune. What trouble this gave a servant, or what distress it might inflict upon a horse, were matters for consideration with which the peculiarly constituted mind of Doctor Murphy [Egan] had no acquaintance whatever. For my own part and perhaps Joe [James] will not kill me for saying, that for his also, we preferred a *cotelette* [chop] (remember that *chops* in France are the *operators*, the *patients* being called as I have just named them) with a couple of *muttons*,[74] at our domicile to two courses with four or six *waxes* and a ride of half a dozen miles in the evening. Murphy's [Egan's] notions however, were finer: and I must do him the justice to say, that he was welcome in all regimental directions; in fact, he was worth any money in the estimation of all. But at the period in question, Larry [Patrick] (though high among the officers) was so fallen in the opinion of the plebeians, that the *bat-men* had unanimously voted him to Coventry. Jock had long left him: and after that forbearing fellow gave him up, it was no place for any man to take.

Hereby Murphy [Egan] became like a barrack-yard, which 'fatigue men' are appointed to clean. He was absolutely a duty for the soldiers in turn to perform. Orders were given for a man to go on *fatigue* to Dr Murphy [Egan], to be relieved every three days! The *menage* [members of the household] under this system, may be imagined, but all my powers are inadequate to *describe* it. One evening the doctor had wearied his 'fatigue', by staying out (though by no means to a late hour), till the fellow, a huge lumbering Lancashire man, got into his *master's* bed. In that situation Murphy [Egan] found him (quite dressed, booted and spurred), between *the very sheets*! This was intolerable. 'Get up, you scoundrel! How daur you go into me bed?' 'Humph.' 'Come out o'me bed, you rascal!' 'Humph,' again. 'If you don't git our o'me bed, I'll *putt* you in the gard-house.' 'Who are *you*? What do you want?' 'I want you to rise out o' hat and git out o' me house.' 'I waunt gy out o' no owse to night, so you be dammed whoever you is.' 'I'm your master, Sir.' 'You *lie*; I have no master but the king.' By this time Murphy [Egan] was almost frantic, but *physical* force would have been exercisable in vanity and burlesque upon a brawny tall 'vellow' such as the intruder; so Larry [Patrick] ran for the Adjutant, who happened to have J B [James Castley] with him at the moment and they both, upon hearing Murphy's [Egan's] grievance, repaired to the scene

---

74. Note by Smith – Candles, not *sheep*.

of annoyance, which was but a few yards distant. Turnbull[75] was still enjoying his first sleep among the 'clover,' when the parties walked in; Murphy [Egan] was spokesman.

M [Egan], 'You scounthrel, here's the Adjutant, and Misther Burton [Castley] come, will you get out of me bed now?'

T[urnbull], 'Humph?'

M [Egan], 'I'll *pull* you out by the ligs if you don't move.'

T[urnbull], (*in a very drowsy tone.*) 'What's the matter?'

M [Egan], 'The matter! The matter! Why you are in my bed.'

T[urnbull], 'Well, that need'nt hinder you to come; there's room enough for us both, isn't there? Can't you lie down and keep yourself quiet? What's the use of making a noise?'

This was carrying insolence and insubordination rather too far and the Adjutant very properly marched Turnbull into the guard-house. Thus, one of the finest soldiers of the regiment, through waiting *for*, rather than *upon*, Assistant Surgeon Murphy [Egan], got into a scrape. I believe however that he got out of it next morning.

When J B [James Castley], Larry [Patrick] and myself (the year after the foregoing event) were tripled up, on the occasion more particularly under *review*, Dr Murphy [Egan] had *Slapsus Slingo* in his service. One day, B [Castley] and I had taken a drive to St Omer and upon our return met Larry [Patrick], riding my best horse (which had been accommodated in the stable where his own stood) in the direction we had left. I was not a little surprised; but explanation I could get none, more than that he had been robbed and was in pursuit of the thief. He was too well mounted to be stopped; so we had little help for it but going on. As soon as the gig was put up, we repaired to Murphy's [Egan's] quarters, to ascertain what was the matter. There we heard a doleful story, how Larry [Patrick] had quarrelled over night in the stable with *Slapsus*, how the master had taken to his sword and the groom to a pitchfork, how the doctor had been left in bed till midday, without any one to brush his clothes or clean his boots and how at last, it was discovered that *Slingo* had run away at a very early hour in the morning; and how *Monsieur Morphi* [Egan] had taken my horse (his own being in a sad neglected condition) to pursue the fugitive. In the end he made nothing of the matter and was for a time, again under '*fatigue.*'

---

75. There is no Turnbull listed in the regiment, he has again given a false name.

This draws me towards the termination of our French career. The three and a half years had now expired and arrangements began to be made for the evacuation of the French territory. After the last review we had a change of distribution, by which for my own part, I became a gainer. The last three weeks I spent in France, were passed in the chateau of a *noble* family, where I was treated with the greatest kindness and hospitality. The elder brother had been a wanderer in consequence of his devotedness to the Bourbons and nothing, in the opinion of them all, was good enough for an Englishman. The next had staid in the family mansion and preserved the property, but both were ultras; the Count (an *émigré*) more so in his manner, however, than his brother, who was married and had a family of six beautiful children. Mons De T*** had an air of melancholy resignation about him, which is only to be found in persons of reflection, who have buffeted with adversity. He spoke often to me of his lot, in former days, how little he expected ever more to cross the threshold of his fathers, how much they owed to us, and how much they had to fear from our departure. He was one of those who *avowed* the wish that the British army should not quit the country for at least the full term of five years.[76] Quit it however, even at the time in question we did; and I must now quit an *occupation* which has interested me nearly as much as did the transactions it has been its object to record; the 'reminiscences' have been almost as interesting as were the *realities*.

We embarked at Calais, landed safely in England; and in the course of a march from Ramsgate[77] to Portsmouth, I received sentence of *half-pay*,

---

76. Note by Smith – The original conjecture was, that the Army of Occupation might have to remain in the French territory for five years; though there was a stipulation, that if things wrought well, they should retire at the end of three. At first a hundred and fifty thousand men were retained; but after a short period, the force was reduced to a hundred and twenty thousand; at which it continued till the final evacuation, which took place at the end of the third year and a few months from the date of their entrance. As my regiment was among the first to arrive, so was it among the last to leave. The hotter ultras viewed our departure with concern: but this has been already stated; and the records of the day will fully explain things which can here be matter of incidental allusion only.
77. Note by Smith – Ramsgate was not the destination of our vessel when it left Calais. The scene of embarkation, (by the way) was a singular one and may admit of a brief allusion. We were supplied with numerous conveyances, (none of these however, fit to be longboats to Captain D's magnificent frigate) and as fast as we reached the quay, we were hurried on board the nearest vessel, 'promiscuously.' The trip being a short one, we paid no regard to convenience and huddled together upon deck, the best way we could. My spaniel had never been on the briny element before and had manifested so

being convicted of the crime of *juniority*. It came, however, from *Fredrick*, Duke of York, who never gave pain to the humblest and was always the friend of the poorest.

The work commenced with an *apology* and with an *apology* I feel it necessary to conclude. Offence, I trust, I have given in no quarter and neither real names nor initials have been introduced. Parties acquainted with the details, will readily identify; but to do so will puzzle others. The apology however, is due on the score of the apparently idle and trifling life described in these volumes. 'To kill time', that most precious of all possessions, of which when robbed we cannot regain what we lose and of which every man of reflection and particularly every Christian, ought to know the value, is a common phrase; but it is worthy only of a maniac to spend his thoughts and his exertions in the destruction of that which is of all concerns, the most valuable. But we did not generally speaking, kill *our* time, under the circumstances in which we were placed. We had many disadvantages to contend with and few resources. I have not stated how much we *read*, how much we *wrote*, how much we *conversed* upon useful topics, or how much we *observed*, (a practice always conducive to the formation of a useful character); and if it be taken into account, as far as the author is involved, that not a day passed over his head in which he was not to a certain degree, the minister of relief to suffering humanity, the period of '*Occupation*' ought not to be that of his existence to which he is most reluctant to look back.

## FINIS

---

strong a fancy for a swim, that Chiswick was obliged to hold her *by the cuff*, during the greater part of the passage. We happened to be on board a Ramsgate craftsman, (crafty enough and anxious of course, to get home to his wife and his tea, instead of going to Dover) and the tide not serving for the early part of the evening at Dover, our skipper represented that it would be hazardous to try that capricious harbour, that we should be unable to cross the bar till midnight, that the night looked 'wild and windy' and that if we stood for Dover, he could not answer for consequences. My military companion thereupon, consulted with me as to what should be done: and we reasoned that if there was danger to the horses, we ought to avoid it, not being on our proper element and the skipper being a better judge of these matters than ourselves. The consequence was, that we bore up for Ramsgate; and thus for my own part, I left off where I began. I had now been nearly three years and a half in France and during the greater part of the time, within sight of England; but fate seemed long determined that I should not see either *Dover* or *Calais*, the gates of European intercourse. In Calais I do not suppose we stopped more than twenty minutes on the occasion of embarking; and Dover I did not see until two days after quitting Ramsgate on our march round the coast.

# Bibliography

Bamford, Andrew, *Gallantry and Discipline: The 12th Light Dragoons at War with Wellington* (Barnsley, 2014).
Bamford, Andrew, *With Wellington's Outposts, The Peninsular and Waterloo Letters of John Vandeleur* (Barnsley, 2015).
Cannon, Richard, *Historical Record of the Twelfth, or the Prince of Wales's Royal Regiment of Lancers* (London, 1842).
Dalton, Charles, *The Waterloo Roll Call* (London, 1904).
Hay, Captain William, *Reminiscences 1808-15 Under Wellington* (Cambridge, 1992).
Philippart, John, *The Royal Military Calendar* (London, 1820).
War Office, *Army Lists* (Various).

**Web**
Challis, Lionel S., *Peninsular Roll Call* (The Napoleon Series).

# Index

Abbeville fn 152, fn 153, 185, 186
Andrews, Captain 12 LD 2
Argueil 162, 165, 166

Bacqueville en Caux fn 166, fn 169
Baird, Sergeant William 12 LD fn 86
Barry, Cornet St George 12 LD fn 130
Bavay 111, 112, 113, 114, 132, fn 212
Berry, Charles Ferdinand de Bourbon, Duc de fn 131
Bertie, Lieutenant Lindsey 12 LD fn 54, fn 66, fn 91, 195
Blücher, Field Marshal Prince 48, 69, 112, 119, 126, 143
Boulogne 179, 197, 199, 200, 201, 211, 213, 219, 220, 228, 229, 230, 240, 241
Bridger, Major James 12 LD fn 4, fn 130, 195
Burdett, Sir Francis 3

Caldas, Dr Antonio de Almeida fn 147
Cambrai 150, 203, 213, 216, 217, 218, 237
Carruthers, Regimental Sergeant Major John 12 LD fn 76, 196
Castlereagh, Robert Stewart Viscount 2, 142
Castley, Veterinary Surgeon James 12 LD 16, 17, 23, 49, 121, 129, 142, 157, fn 163, 167, 172, 174, 176, 178, 185, 187, 192, 233, 234, 235, 241, 242, 243, 244, 245, 246, 247, 248, 249
Caulaincourt, General Auguste fn 157
Chabert, General Theodore 30
Clinton, Lieutenant General Sir Henry 128
Cochrane, Lord Thomas 3
Coimbra 109, 145, 146, 147, 148, fn 248
Cole, Captain Honourable William 12 LD fn 4
Combermere, Lieutenant General Stapleton Cotton, Lord 201
Courbevoie 128, 130, 133, 137, 138, 139

Craufurd, Captain Alexander 2nd Ceylon Regiment fn 107
Craufurd, Captain Thomas 3rd Foot Guards fn 107

Decrès, Admiral 125
Delancey, Deputy Quartermaster General Sir William fn 59
Desvres fn 197, 198, 199, 202, fn 203, fn 212, 229, 230, 233, 234, 234, 240, 242, 245, 247
Dieppe fn 165, 166, 170, 174, 175, 176
Dugny 158, 162

Eeklo 28
Egan, Assistant Surgeon Patrick 12 LD 12, 13, 14, 15, 16, fn 49, 51, 64, 130, 135, 136, 137, 138, 145, fn 151, 155, 167, 168, 178, 179, 180, 181, 182, 185, 186, 193, 206, 207, 230, 231, 232, 236–9, 240, 245, 247, 248–9,
Enghien 54, 55
Estinnes au Val 111

Fane, Major General Henry 201
Forges-les-Eaux fn 145, 158, 162, 166, 174, 175, 183
Forrest, Private Jonathan 12 LD fn 153
Fuller, Colonel William, 1 Dragoon Guards fn 98
Fulton, Lieutenant Richard 12 LD 5

Ghent 29, 31, fn 32, 38, 68, 74, 113
Goderich, Lord 2
Goldsmid, Lieutenant Albert 12 LD 4, fn 5
Gordon, George, Marquess of Huntly 9
Goussainville 123, 124
Grant, Inspector of Hospitals Sir James fn 97
Griffiths, Lieutenant John 12 LD fn 16
Grouchy, Marshal Emmanuel 119

Hamilton, Colonel James Scots Greys fn 98
Hay, Lieutenant Colonel James 16 LD fn 75
Hay, Lieutenant William 12 LD fn 5, fn 9, fn 39, fn 54, fn 55, fn 58, fn 61, fn 62, fn 64, fn 68, fn 70, fn 71, fn 119, fn 153, fn 188, fn 195, fn 209
Heydon, Lieutenant William 12 LD fn 9
Horse Guards fn 2
*Howe*, HMS fn 8
Hume, Deputy Inspector of Hospitals Robert 80

Kempt, Major General Sir James 117, fn 142
Kent, Edward Augustus, Duke of 6, fn 114

La Haye Sainte 64, 70, 85, 106
Leech, Lieutenant 12 LD fn 130
Lennox Charles, Duke of Richmond fn 54, fn 136
Ligny, Battle of 55, 130
Lockhart, Cornet John 12 LD 54, fn 66, 68, fn 91, 92, 195, fn 196
Louis XVIII, King 29, 38, 112–13, fn 131, 134, 161, fn 169, 170, 171, 174

Mackay, Captain Robert 79 Foot fn 99
Mickelthwaite, Lieutenant 12 LD fn 130
Mont St Jean 7, 64, 65, 70, 71, 93–107

Neuilly 128, 129, 133,
Nivelles 56, 57, 97, 107, 108, fn 198

Orange, William Prince of 38, 49, fn 100, 142
Ostend 11, 20, 21, 25, 26, fn 65
Otway, Paymaster William 12 LD fn 16, 17–18, 19, 23, 52, 174, fn 175, 183, fn 184,
Oudenaarde 32, 37, 38

Pack, Major General Sir Dennis fn 10, fn 116
Penniston, Corporal John 12 LD fn 171
Pommereuil fn 119
Ponsonby, Lieutenant Colonel The Honourable Frederick 12 LD 3, 13, 14, fn 54, fn 71, 76, 77, 80, fn 81, fn 107, 116, fn 128

Power, Private Edward 12 LD fn 153
Puteaux 129, 130, 131

Quatre Bras 56, 58, 59, 84, fn 99, 110
Quill, Assistant Surgeon Maurice 31 Foot 231

Ramsgate 11, 16, 19, 250, fn 251
Reed, Lieutenant Thomas 12 LD fn 150
Richardson, Private William 12 LD fn 152, fn 153, 185, 186
Ricquebourg 120, 122
Robinson, Surgeon Benjamin 12 LD fn 11, 14, 15, 16, 18, 19, 70, 73, 82, 106, 107, 137, 224, 236, 237, 238, 239, 240, 244, 245, 247
Ronse 32, 33, 36, 38

Sandys, Captain 12 LD fn 2, 92
Santander 145
Schendelbeke 48, 50
Schwarzenberg, Field Marshal Karl Prince von 49
Sidley, Quartermaster Richard 12 LD fn 166, fn 169
St John, Cornet William 12 LD fn 216
St Omer fn 174, 194, fn 242, 245, 247, 249
Stanhope, Honourable Augustus fn 215
Stawell, Captain Samson 12 LD fn 138, fn 141
Steenkirk 56

Talavera, Battle of fn 12, 13, 135
Taylor, Deputy Inspector of Hospitals William fn 107
Tunney, Chaplain Robert fn 108, 118, fn 198, 202, 243

Uxbridge, Henry Paget Lord 39, 48, 68, fn 88, fn 201

Vandeleur, Lieutenant John 12 LD fn 77
Vandeleur, Major General Sir John Ormsby fn 67, 68

Wallace, Captain 12 LD fn 2
Webb, Captain 12 LD fn 2
Wellington, Duke of 37, fn 38, 48, fn 65, 68, 69, fn 70, 78, fn 110, 112, fn 114, 142, 143, 147, fn 181, 203
Wetzig, Surgeon Gottlieb 1st Line KGL fn 114